Blood Vessel Changes in Hypertension: Structure and Function

Volume II

Editor
Robert M. K. W. Lee, Ph.D.
Associate Professor
Department of Anaesthesiology
McMaster University
Hamilton, Ontario
Canada

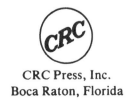

CRC Press, Inc.
Boca Raton, Florida

Library of Congress Cataloging-in-Publication Data

Blood vessel changes in hypertension: structure and function/
  editor. Robert M.K.W. Lee.
      p. cm.
    Includes bibliographies and index.
    ISBN 0-8493-4883-8 (v. 1). ISBN 0-8493-4884-6 (v. 2)
    1. Hypertension—Pathophysiology. 2. Blood -vessels—
Pathophysiology. I. Lee. Robert M. K. W., 1943—
    [DNLM: 1. Blood Vessels—physiopathology. 2. Hypertension—
physiopathology. 3. Vascular Resistance. WG 340 B6647]
RC685.H8B596 1988
616.1'3207—dc19
DNLM/DLC
for Library of Congress
                                                      88-22208
                                                       CIP

Direct all inquiries to CRC Press, Inc., 2000 Corporate Blvd., N.W., Boca Raton, Florida, 33431.

© 1989 by CRC Press, Inc.

International Standard Book Number 0-8493-4883-8 (V.1)
International Standard Book Number 0-8493-4884-6 (V.2)

Library of Congress Card Number 88-22208
Printed in the United States

Dedicated to my

Father   Lee Kyin Yuh   李鏡郁

Mother   Hu Yee Tsu   胡玉翠

Wife   Wong Lin Swen   王寧蓀

ACKNOWLEDGMENTS

I thank Ms. Sheila Seaman for her secretarial assistance. Supported by the Heart and Stroke Foundation of Ontario and the Ontario Ministry of Health

PREFACE

In many forms of hypertension, a thickening of the arterial vessel wall is observed. This is usually due to the increase of smooth muscle mass in the media. The amplifying effects of such structural changes in the regulation of blood pressure, have been elegantly demonstrated by the blood flow measurement and perfusion studies of Professor B. Folkow and his colleagues in humans with essential hypertension, and in various animal models. However, whether such structural changes are primary changes associated with the development of hypertension, or whether they are secondary adaptive changes responsible for the maintenance of hypertension, is still unclear. This is mainly because cardiovascular changes are so intimately associated with blood pressure changes that it is difficult to alter one without affecting the other. Nevertheless, recent studies using various approaches have yielded exciting new findings on the structural and functional alterations of the blood vessels in hypertension. These findings are essential in our understanding of the etiology of hypertension. The specific purpose of this book, is to provide critical review and thoughts on the following topics:

Structural changes in relation to
* Connective tissue
* Cerebral vessel structure and innervation
* Smooth muscle cell hypertrophy and/or hyperplasia
* Rarefactions of microvessels
* The effects of antihypertensive therapy on vessel structure and function

Functional changes in terms of
* Contractile properties of resistance vessels
* Reactivity and sensitivity changes
* Mechanical properties of the arteries
* Endothelial and smooth muscle cell interactions
* Neural and local control of arteries and microcirculation
* Vascular smooth muscle membrane potential

One unique feature is the inclusion of a chapter on vascular changes in pulmonary hypertension. It is evident that there are several common structural changes in the arteries from the systemic and pulmonary circulation which are associated with hypertension.

These chapters are written by established researchers well respected in their areas, providing comprehensive and insightful reviews, and directions for future research. This book should be of major interest to researchers involved in the study of hypertension and the biology of the blood vessels.

Robert M. K. W. Lee

THE EDITOR

Robert M. K. W. Lee, Ph.D. is an Associate Professor in the Department of Anaesthesia, Faculty of Health Sciences, McMaster University, Hamilton, Ontario, Canada. Dr. Lee graduated in 1966 from the University of Mandalay with a B.Sc. (Honors) in Zoology (First Class) and obtained his M.Sc. in Zoology (summa cum laude) in 1969 from the University of Rangoon, Burma. In 1975 he received his Ph.D. in Entomology from the University of Alberta, Edmonton, Alberta, Canada.

Dr. Lee is a member of the American Physiological Society, Canadian Hypertension Society, Canadian Association of Anatomists, European Society for Microcirculation, Microcirculatory Society, International Society for Stereology, Society for Quantitative Morphology, and Microscopical Society of Canada. He has received a Centennial Fellowship from the Medical Research Council of Canada, and a Rose-Levy Rosenstadt Fellowship from the Rose-Levy Rosenstadt Foundation. He is currently a Career Scientist supported by the Ontario Ministry of Health.

Dr. Lee has presented over 40 papers at national and international meetings, and approximately 10 invited lectures at international meetings. He has published over 50 research papers and contributed review chapters in 2 books. His current major research interests include the role of the sympathetic nervous system and structural changes of the blood vessels in the development of hypertension.

CONTRIBUTORS

Volume I

Robert H. Cox, Ph.D.
Professor
Department of Physiology
University of Pennsylvania
Philadelphia, Pennsylvania

Hiroyuki Ito, M.D.
Associate Professor
Department of Pathology
Kinki University School of Medicine
Sayama, Osaka, Japan

J. Michael Kay, M.D.
Professor
Department of Pathology
McMaster University
Hamilton, Ontario, Canada

Michael J. Mulvany, Ph.D.
Lecturer
Biophysics Institute
Aarhus University
Aarhus, Denmark

Gary K. Owens, Ph.D.
Associate Professor
Department of Physiology
University of Virginia
Charlottesville, Virginia

Christopher R. Triggle, Ph.D.
Professor
Department of Basic Medical Sciences
Memorial University of Newfoundland
St. John's, Newfoundland, Canada

CONTRIBUTORS

Volume II

D. W. Cheung, Ph.D.
Associate Professor
Department of Pharmacology
University of Toronto
Toronto, Ontario, Canada

Haruhisa Hashimoto,M.D.
Chief of Cardiology
Department of Internal Medicine
Yoshida General Hospital
Yoshida Ehime, Japan

Robert Maung Kyaw Win Lee, Ph.D.
Associate Professor
Department of Anaesthesia
McMaster University
Hamilton, Ontario, Canada

Tony J.-F. Lee, Ph.D.
Associate Professor
Department of Pharmacology
School of Medicine
Southern Illinois University
Springfield, Illinois

Alex L. Loeb, Ph.D.
Assistant Professor
Department of Anaesthesia
University of Pennsylvania
Philadelphia, Pennsylvania

Julian H. Lombard, Ph.D.
Associate Professor
Department of Physiology
Medical College of Wisconsin
Milwaukee, Wisconsin

M. J. MacKay, Ph.D.
Department of Pharmacology
University of Toronto
Toronto, Ontario, Canada

George Osol, Ph.D.
Assistant Professor
Department of Physiology and Biophysics
   and Obstetrics and Gynecology
College of Medicine
University of Vermont
Burlington, Vermont

Michael J. Peach, Ph.D.
Professor
Department of Pharmacology
University of Virginia School of
   Medicine
Charlottesville, Virginia

Russell L. Prewitt, Ph.D.
Associate Professor
Department of Physiology
Eastern Virginia Medical School
Norfolk, Virginia

D. Lowell Stacy, Ph.D.
Senior Scientist
Glaxo One
Chapel Hill, North Carolina

William J. Stekiel, Ph.D.
Professor
Department of Physiology
Medical College of Wisconsin
Milwaukee, Wisconsin

TABLE OF CONTENTS

Volume I

TABLE OF CONTENTS

Volume II

Chapter 1

ALTERED CEREBRAL VESSEL INNERVATION IN HYPERTENSION

Tony J.-F. Lee

TABLE OF CONTENTS

I. INTRODUCTION

Morphological, physiological, and pharmacological studies have shown that brain blood vessels of several species receive sympathetic vasoconstrictor and nonsympathetic vasodilator nerves.[38,48,64] The distribution of these two types of nerves varies among species and regions.[48,52,56] The functional significance of cerebral vessel sympathetic innervation in controlling normal cerebral blood flow has been shown to be minimal.[4,33] The sympathetic innervation however becomes functionally more important in animals with acute or chronic hypertension.[33,60,63] On the other hand, the functional significance of the nonsympathetic innervation in controlling cerebral circulation during hypertension has been less understood. This has been attributed in part to the unknown nature of vasodilator transmitter and the origin of these nerves.[51] This chapter will focus on the altered nerve-muscle relationship in large cerebral arterial walls in chronic hypertension.

II. GRANULAR AND AGRANULAR VESICLE-CONTAINING NERVES

When fixed in $KMnO_4$, the adrenergic, sympathetic nerve terminals in a variety of preparations are characterized by the presence of many small and a few large dense core granular vesicles.[37,48,55] Accordingly, the nerve terminals containing exclusively agranular vesicles are nonadrenergic, nonsympathetic nerves.[38,48,52,64] In those studies, 6-hydroxydopamine (6OHDA) was given intravenously (i.v.) or intraperitoneally (i.p.) to animals shortly before the experiments. Presumably, 6OHDA is taken up specifically by the adrenergic nerve terminals to improve the granulation of the dense core vesicles.[38,48,52] Based on the vesicle inclusions, the adrenergic nerve or granular vesicle-containing nerve (AVN) terminals can be differentiated (Figure 1). In comparing the innervation pattern in cerebral blood vessels between normotensive and hypertensive animals, 6OHDA was not given to animals by i.v. or i.p. routes since potential differences may exist in the cerebral arterial wall (such as endothelial cells or blood-brain barrier) between hypertensive and normotensive animals which may affect the transport of 6OHDA to the nerve terminals.[55] The isolated brain arteries were therefore incubated with 6OHDA *in vitro* as described by Aprigliano and Hermsmeyer.[2] In cerebral arteries from all species examined, AVN and GVN were found only in the adventitial layer.[48,52,55,69]

III. AVN AND GVN TERMINALS IN CEREBRAL ARTERIES OF NORMOTENSIVE ANIMALS

Following superior cervical ganglionectomy, the GVN completely disappeared while the AVN persisted in pial vessels.[48,52,55,69] This result indicates that the GVN are adrenergic of superior cervical ganglionic origin and the AVN are nonadrenergic and nonsympathetic. The origin of the latter nerves, however, is not positively determined.[38,48,50,52,64]

The relative ratio of AVN and GVN terminals varies among species and among regions even within species (Table 1). The large cerebral arterial walls at the base of the normal adult cat and rat brains have been found to contain more AVN (60%) than GVN (40%) terminals.[48,55] The rabbit basilar arterial wall, on the contrary, contains predominantly GVN (98%) and very few AVN (2%) terminals.[52] In peripheral arteries such as the rabbit ear and saphenous arteries, only GVN are found.[52]

Results from *in vitro* tissue bath studies have indicated that transmural stimulation of the intramural nerves results in vasodilation exclusively in the cat cerebral arteries, predominantly vasoconstriction in the rabbit basilar arteries, and vasoconstriction exclusively in the rabbit ear and saphenous arteries.[49,52,53,57,59] This positive morphopharmacological correlation suggests that GVN (sympathetic) are vasoconstrictor nerves and AVN (nonsympathetic) are dilator nerves.[48,49] This observation also seems to hold true for the rat cerebral artery.[17,36]

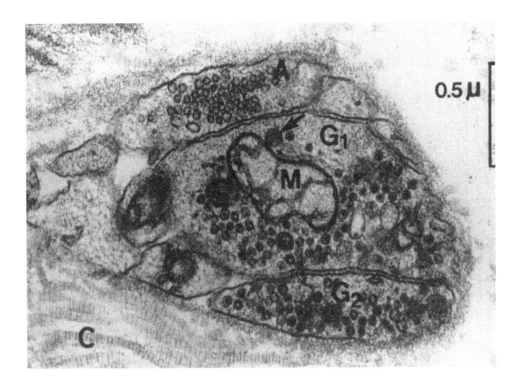

FIGURE 1. Electron micrographs of dual innervation of anterior cerebral arteries of the cat fixed in 2% potassium permanganate. Two types of varicosities can be identified based on the vesicle inclusion. One contains many small dense-core GVN, as indicated by G, and the other contains many small AVN, as indicated by A. Occasionally, large size vesicles (arrow) can be seen. Tissues were preincubated in 6-hydroxydopamine (10^{-4} M) *in vitro* for 15 min before fixation. Collagen (c).

Table 1
PERCENTAGES OF AVN AND GVN TERMINALS IN CEREBRAL ARTERIES

Species	Artery	AVN	GVN	Ref.
Rabbit	Basilar	2	98	52
	Anterior cerebral	40	60	Saito and Lee, unpublished data
Cat	Basilar	63	37	48
	Middle cerebral	54	46	48
	Anterior cerebral	60	40	48
	Pial branch	12	88	48
Rat (WKY)	Basilar	80	20	55
	Middle cerebral	75	25	55
	Anterior cerebral	60	40	55
Rat (SHR)	Basilar	62	40	55
	Middle cerebral	52	48	55
	Anterior cerebral	30	70	55
Rat (RHR)	Basilar	60	40	69
	Middle cerebral	62	38	69
	Anterior cerebral	46	54	69

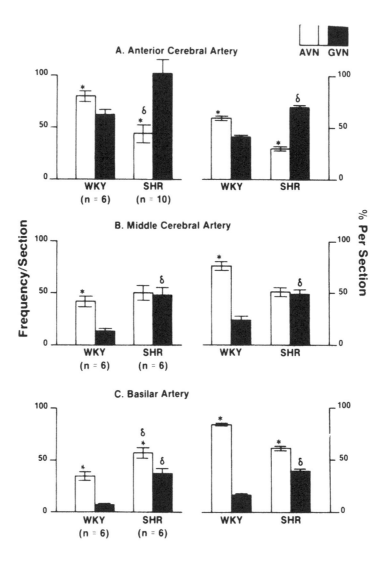

FIGURE 2. GVN and AVN in the adventitial layer of anterior cerebral (panel A), middle cerebral (panel B), and basilar (panel C) arteries in SHR and normotensive WKY. Left panel shows absolute number (mean ± SEM) of nerve terminals observed in each transverse section of the blood vessel wall. Right panel shows the percentage (mean ± SEM) of AVN and GVN of total nerve endings per transverse section. (Panel A) Anterior cerebral artery; there are significantly more AVN (60%) than GVN (40%) in WKY. The number of GVN (70%) is significantly higher than that of AVN (30%) in SHR. (Panel B) Middle cerebral artery; there are significantly more AVN (75%) than GVN (25%) in WKY. In SHR, AVN and GVN become equal in number. (Panel C) Basilar artery; there are significantly more AVN (80%) than GVN (20%) in WKY. In SHR, both AVN and GVN increase. However, the precent difference between AVN (60%) and GVN (40%) becomes smaller than that in WKY. * indicates significantly different (p <0.025) from GVN (paired t-test); d indicates significantly different (p <0.025) from the respective type of nerve endings in WKY (unpaired t-test), n (number of sections).[55]

Similar to that found in the cat, the major cerebral arteries of the normotensive Wistar-Kyoto rat (WKY) receive more AVN terminals than GVN terminals per cross section throughout the adventitial layer (Figure 2). The density of the GVN terminals per cross section varied from region to region and was found highest in the anterior cerebral artery and lowest in the basilar artery. Results from frequency-nerve terminal distribution with varying synaptic cleft distances (Figure 3) further reveal that all WKY cerebral arteries examined contain more AVN than GVN terminals in close synaptic cleft distance. This is similar to that found in the respective regions of the normal cat cerebral arteries.[48] Results from *in vitro* pharmacological studies indicate that cerebral arteries of the cat never constrict, but relax exclusively upon transmural nerve stimulation (TNS).[49,53,59] The relaxation was not affected by blocking the sympathetic transmission,[53] suggesting that the sympathetic nerves play an insignificant role in the TNS-induced responses in normotensive cat. Results from some *in vivo* studies also support that the sympathetic innervation to the cat cerebral arteries was not functional in controlling brain circulation during normotensive or hypotensive experiences.[3,6,34] Although direct measurement of the neurogenic response of the isolated cerebral artery of the rat has not been examined, the similar innervation pattern of WKY cerebral arteries to that of cat cerebral arteries suggests that the vasodilator nerves are predominant in cerebral artery of the normotensive WKY.

IV. AVN AND GVN TERMINALS IN CEREBRAL ARTERIES OF HYPERTENSIVE ANIMALS

A. The Spontaneously Hypertensive Rat (SHR)

The total GVN terminals per cross section in cerebral arteries of the SHR are found to be consistently higher than those in the respective arteries of the WKY (Figure 3). Meanwhile, the AVN terminals per arterial cross section are found to be significantly fewer in some regions such as the anterior cerebral artery. However, they are not different in the middle cerebral artery or the basilar artery in SHR compared to those in WKY (Figure 3). Therefore, in the SHR, the GVN terminals per cross section throughout the adventitial layers absolutely outnumber the AVN terminals in the anterior cerebral artery, and the ratio of total GVN over AVN in middle cerebral and basilar arteries also becomes greater in SHR than in WKY (Figure 4).

B. The Nongenetically Renal Hypertensive Rat (RHR)

Chronic renal hypertension was induced in 7-week-old normotensive male WKY rats by placing a silver clip (internal diameter, 0.25 mm) over the left renal artery through a left lumbar incision and was followed 1 week later by contralateral nephrectomy.[69] RHR were identified with tail arterial systolic pressure higher than 160 mmHg and were sacrificed at 21 to 24 weeks of age. In RHR, both the AVN and GVN terminals were found to be significantly decreased or unchanged in most cerebral arteries examined (Figure 5). This finding contrasts to that found in SHR in that the GVN terminals were significantly increased in all cerebral arteries examined, while the AVN terminals were decreased in some regions.[55]

These results demonstrate that autonomic nerves undergo some changes when animals become hypertensive. Alterations in the pattern of autonomic nerves, however, are different depending on the type of hypertensive model.

V. CATECHOLAMINE FLUORESCENCE IN CEREBRAL ARTERIES OF THE HYPERTENSIVE RAT

A. The SHR

The catecholamine fluorescence observed in cerebral arteries of WKY seems to parallel the density of the GVN per cross section in the respective arteries. The anterior cerebral arteries receive the densest and the basilar arteries receive the sparsest catecholamine fluorescence. These results are somewhat similar to that found in rat cerebral arteries reported by others.[44] In WKY, the proximal end of basilar arteries is found to receive extremely sparse or no sympathetic innervation and the small branches of pial arteries receive no sympathetic innervation. These two arteries in SHR, however, receive significantly denser sympathetic innervation (Figure 6).

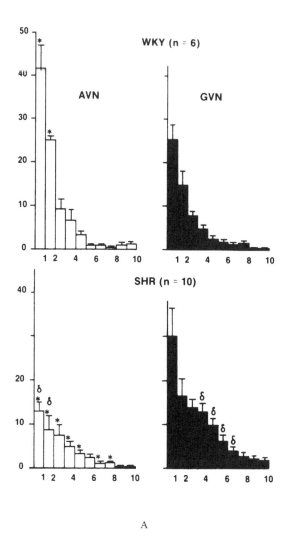

A

FIGURE 3. Distribution of GVN and AVN terminals with various synaptic cleft distances in (A) anterior cerebral artery, (B)
middle cerebral artery, and (C) basilar artery of WKY and SHR.
The ordinate indicates frequency of nerve terminals per transverse section (mean ± SEM), and the abscissa represents synaptic
or neuromuscular distances in mm. * indicates significantly
different (p <0.025, paired t-test) from the GVN terminals within
the same synaptic cleft range. d indicates significantly different
(p <0.025, unpaired t-test) from their respective type of nerve
terminals within the same synaptic cleft range in WKY, n
(number of sections). (From Lee, T. J. -F. and Saito, A., *Circ.
Res.*, 55, 392, 1984. With permission.)

These results together with the general elevation of GVN in all arteries examined suggest that
the vascular sympathetic innervation is denser in most of the brain regions in SHR than in WKY.

B. The Nongenetically RHR

Our preliminary results indicate that the catecholamine fluorescence in cerebral arteries from
a 21-week-old RHR (one-kidney, one-clip; 1K-1C) was not appreciably different from that of
age-matched WKY.[69] Since GVN or sympathetic nerve terminals decrease in these arteries, it
is possible that this type of hypertension is characterized by a defect primarily in autonomic
nerve terminals.

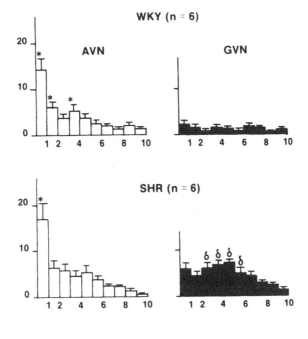

FIGURE 3B.

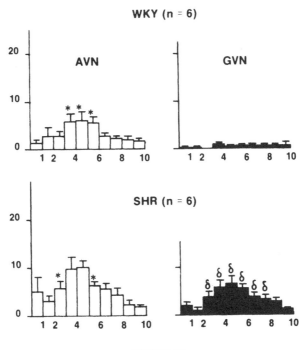

FIGURE 3C.

VI. ENDOGENOUS NOREPINEPHRINE (NE) CONTENTS IN CEREBRAL ARTERIES OF CHRONIC HYPERTENSION

A. The SHR

The endogenous NE content of cerebral arteries is also found to be greater in SHR than in WKY. For example, the NE content was about 2.5 times higher in basilar arteries of SHR than

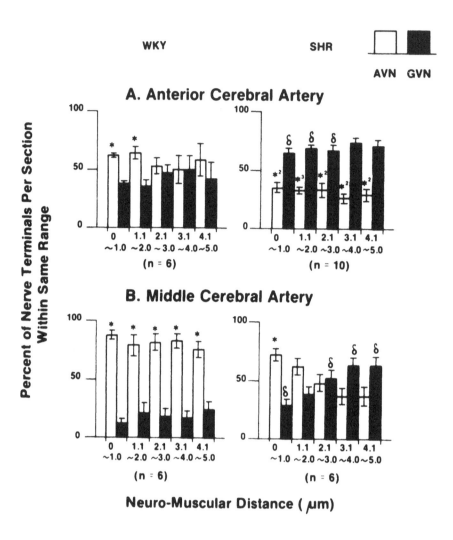

FIGURE 4. Percentage (mean ± SEM) of AVN and GVN terminals within the same synaptic cleft or neuromuscular distance in anterior cerebral arteries (panel A) and middle cerebral arteries (panel B) of WKY and SHR. * indicates significantly different (*p* <0.025, paired *t*-test) from GVN terminals within the same range. d indicates significantly different (*p* <0.025, unpaired *t*-test) from their respective type of nerve terminals within the same synaptic cleft or neuromuscular distance in WKY, n (number of sections). (From Lee, T. J.-F. and Saito, A., *Circ. Res.*, 55, 392, 1984. With permission.)

in those of WKY based on content per tissue wet weight.[55] However, the wet weight per unit length of the basilar artery is also 1.5 times heavier in SHR than in WKY. The dry weight of cerebral arterial preparation was also heavier in SHR than WKY. These results are consistent with an increase in muscle mass in SHR arteries,[55] although a potential increase in vascular water content cannot be ruled out. Therefore, true total content of NE per unit length of the basilar artery should be 1.5 times higher than the estimated concentration based on content per wet weight. Thus, the corrected NE content per unit length will be 3.75 times (2.5 × 1.5) higher in SHR than in WKY. This corrected value parallels the difference found for the GVN terminals between cerebral arteries of SHR and WKY.[55] These results suggest that the elevated NE content in cerebral arteries of SHR is most likely due to an elevated number of GVN or sympathetic nerve terminals, although several other factors such as an accelerated biosynthesis, increased reuptake of NE, or the presence of more storage vesicles per varicosity[8,27] cannot be ruled out.

Elevated NE content in several peripheral blood vessels of SHR has been reported by some,[24,31,32] but not by others who do not verify this change.[78] Nevertheless, neuronal NE uptake in these vascular preparations has consistently been shown to increase in SHR.[61,65,78,80,84] Since the weight per unit length of both cerebral arteries[55] and several peripheral arteries[24,28] is greater in SHR than in WKY, expression of NE concentration by microgram content per tissue wet weight[78] may underestimate the NE content of the arterial preparations from hypertensive animals.

B. The Nongenetically RHR

The NE content in RHR cerebral arteries has not been examined. However, it is possible that the NE content will decrease in cerebral arteries of the RHR compared to those of WKY. This is based on the observation that sympathetic nerve terminals or GVN terminals decrease in these arteries.[69] Interestingly, the concentrations of NE have been reported to decrease in mesenteric artery and heart in renal hypertensive animals.[25,26]

VII. SYNAPTIC CLEFT DISTANCE

The synaptic cleft distance of varicosity from the smooth muscle cells is another determinant for functional significance of a given innervation.[7,48,52,74] Presumably, the more intimate the synaptic cleft, the higher the concentration of the transmitter at the postsynaptic receptors would be, and therefore, the larger the response for a given amount of transmitter release. The synaptic concentration of the transmitter would be expected to recede with the cube of the distance from nerve terminals.[7] However, based on the frequency-synaptic cleft distance distribution relationship (Figures 3 and 5), the relative number of AVN and GVN terminals in each respective synaptic cleft distance can be compared.

A. The SHR

In the anterior cerebral arteries, the GVN terminals at close synaptic distance ($<3\,\mu$m) are not different between SHR and WKY, but they significantly elevate at synaptic cleft distance between 3 and 7 μm in SHR (Figure 3). In the same artery, the AVN terminals with close synaptic cleft distance ($<2\,\mu$m), however, are significantly less in SHR than in WKY. The GVN terminals in middle cerebral and basilar arteries are also consistently higher (between 2 and 8 μm from the smooth muscle cells) in SHR than in WKY, while the AVN terminals at any synaptic range in these two arteries are not significantly different between SHR and WKY. The increase in GVN terminals in these SHR arteries results in a greater ratio of GVN over AVN terminals within each synaptic range (Figure 4). These results further suggest that the sympathetic adrenergic vasoconstriction may become more prominent in cerebral arteries of SHR than of WKY.

B. The Nongenetically RHR

In the anterior cerebral artery, both AVN terminals with neuromuscular distances less than 7 μm and GVN terminals with neuromuscular distances less than 2 μm were significantly fewer in RHR than NR ($p < 0.05$). Both AVN terminals with neuromuscular distances less than 4 μm and GVN terminals with neuromuscular distances less than 1 μm decreased in the basilar artery of RHR (Figure 5). The reduction of AVN and GVN with close neuromuscular distances in cerebral arteries of RHR suggests that the functional innervation in cerebral blood vessels in these animals may be weakened or impaired. This finding corresponds to the reported impaired function of sympathetic nerves in peripheral tissues of the renal hypertensive animal.[21,83]

VIII. ORIGINS OF SYMPATHETIC AND NONSYMPATHETIC NERVES IN CEREBRAL PIAL VESSELS OF HYPERTENSIVE ANIMALS

The origin of the elevated sympathetic adrenergic nerves or GVN in cerebral pial arteries

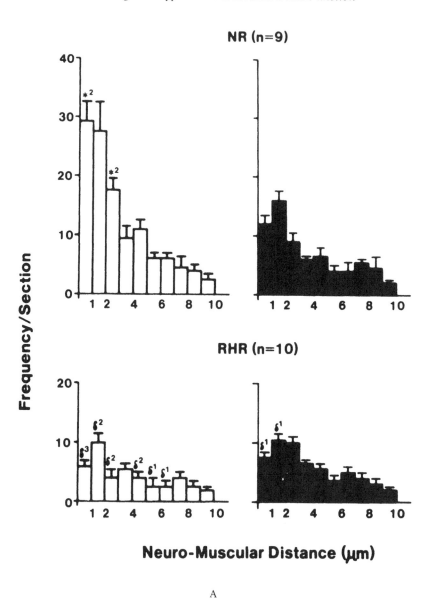

FIGURE 5. Distribution of synaptic distances between nerve endings and the membrane of the nearest smooth muscle cells in anterior cerebral (A), middle cerebral (B), and basilar arteries (C) of NR and RHR. The left and right panels show histograms of AVN and GVN, respectively. There were more AVN than GVN in the anterior cerebral artery, with a synaptic cleft of less than 3.0 mm in NR. There were significantly fewer AVN, with neuromuscular distances less than 7.0 mm, and GVN, with neuromuscular distances less than 2.0 mm, in RHR than in NR. In the middle cerebral artery, there was no difference in the distribution of AVN and GVN between NR and RHR. In the basilar artery, there were significantly fewer AVN and GVN in RHR than in NR in close neuromuscular distances. * = significantly different from GVN with same synaptic cleft range (paired *t*-test): *[1] = $p < 0.05$, *[2] = $p < 0.01$, *[3] = $p < 0.001$; d = significantly different from the respective type of nerve in NR with the same cleft range; d[1] = $p < 0.05$, d[2] = $p < 0.01$, d[3] = $p < 0.001$. (from Saito, A. and Lee, T. J. -F., *Hypertension,* 4, 514, 1985. With permission.)

(except the vertebral artery) of the SHR is believed to be entirely from the superior cervical ganglia, since removal of these ganglia results in a complete disappearance of GVN and the catecholamine fluorescence. This is consistent to that found in the SHR stroke-prone rat.[66] By contrast, the origin of the cerebral vasodilator nerves has not been positively determined. It has

NR (n=9)

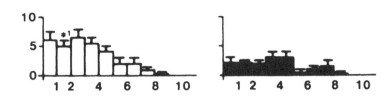

RHR (n=9)

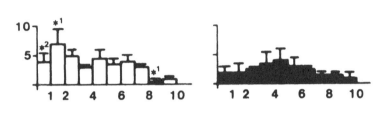

Neuro-Muscular Distance (μm)

FIGURE 5B.

NR (n=9)

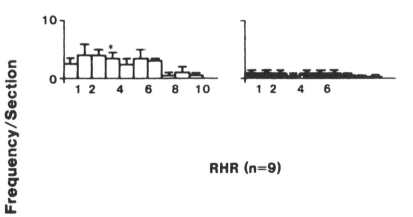

RHR (n=9)

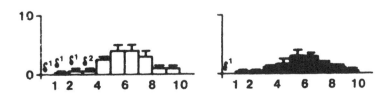

Neuro-Muscular Distance (μm)

FIGURE 5C.

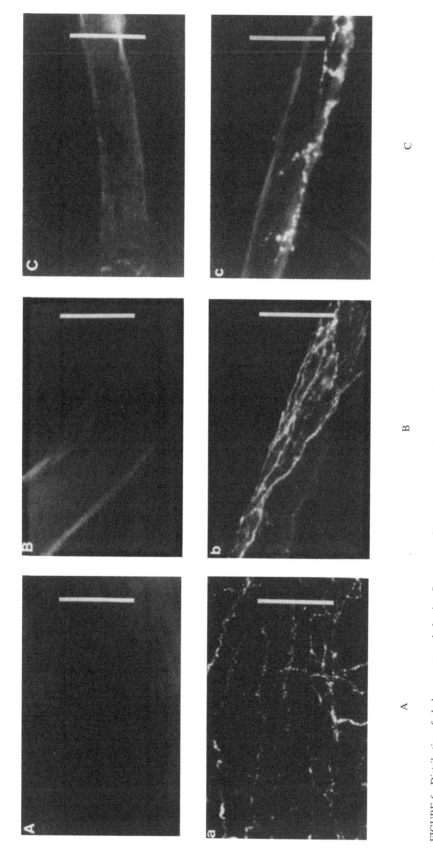

FIGURE 6.   Distribution of whole-mount catecholamine-fluorescence fibers in cerebral arteries of WKY (panels A to C) and SHR (panels a to c). In WKY no fluorescence is found in the vertebral artery (panel A) and the small branch of middle cerebral artery (panels B and C). On the other hand, the vertebral artery (panel a) and small branches of middle cerebral arteries (pane b and c) of SHR receive significant amounts of catecholamine fluorescence. Vertebral arteries (panels A, a) were cut open before fixation for inducing catecholamine fluorescence. Bars represent 100 mm. (From Lee, T. J.-F., and Saito, A., *Circ. Res.*, *55*, 392, 1984. With permission.)

been suggested that the cerebral vasodilator nerves are carried via the superficial petrosal nerves which originate from the geniculate ganglion.[11,77] However, results from some *in vivo* studies failed to show a change in cerebral blood flow during electrical stimulation of the petrosal nerves.[9,70] Furthermore, it has been suggested that the cerebral blood vessels of the dog may be innervated by multiple dilator pathways.[42] It has been reported that the total AVN terminals per cross section decrease in the anterior cerebral artery remain unchanged in the middle cerebral artery and the basilar artery in SHR and decrease in both the anterior cerebral and basilar arteries in RHR (Figures 3 and 5). These results suggest that the rat cerebral blood vessels may receive AVN from more than one source and that their activities may vary with different types of hypertension.[50]

IX. IS ALTERED CEREBRAL VESSEL INNERVATION IN CHRONIC HYPERTENSION A RESULT OF HIGH BLOOD PRESSURE?

It is intriguing that the decrease of AVN terminals in the anterior cerebral artery only occurs in close synaptic cleft distance (<2 μm), while the elevated GVN terminals occur primarily in wider synaptic cleft distance (between 3 and 8 μm) in SHR cerebral arteries (Figure 3). It has been suggested that high blood pressure may extrude nerves from the arterial wall in the sheep carotid artery.[43] However, high blood pressure is unlikely to be the primary factor in the reduction of nerve endings with close synaptic cleft distance in cerebral arteries, since there was no appreciable difference in the distribution of AVN terminals in both middle cerebral and basilar arteries between WKY and SHR. The increase in GVN terminals in SHR cerebral arteries is probably not due to high blood pressure either. In RHR, both the AVN and GVN terminals per cross section decrease in the anterior cerebral and basilar arteries.[69] These results suggest that alteration of AVN and GVN in hypertensive animals may be due to factors other than the high blood pressure itself.

X. FUNCTIONAL SIGNIFICANCE OF CEREBRAL VESSEL INNERVATION IN CHRONIC HYPERTENSION

It is generally accepted that the response of the vascular smooth muscle cells during electrical nerve stimulation is determined by the synaptic concentration of transmitter released from the nerve endings and the sensitity of postsynaptic effector cells.[7,76,79] The release of NE transmitter upon nerve stimulation or K^+ solution in several peripheral vascular preparations has been shown to increase in SHR.[19,24] This is not suprising if these arteries, such as mesenteric arteries and caudal of the rat,[10,58] also contain more adrenergic nerve terminals. The vascular smooth muscles have also been shown to be more sensitive to exogenously applied NE in SHR than in WKY.[12,19,35,61,78,80] These results favor that sympathetic vasoconstriction in some vascular beds in SHR would be expected to be enhanced.

The exact pattern of transmitter release in the SHR cerebral artery has not been determined, although release of NE and acetylcholine from cerebral arteries of other species upon TNS has been demonstrated.[13,15,16] Since the increased GVN terminals in SHR cerebral arteries occur primarily in the wide synaptic distance, it is questionable whether the neurogenic vasoconstriction is enhanced in SHR cerebral arteries. However, cerebral blood vessels, which differ from most peripheral blood vessels, receive dual vasoconstrictor and dilator nerves. With few exceptions,[54] cerebral vasoconstrictor nerves are sympathetic nerves (GVN) and vasodilator nerves are nonsympathetic nerves (AVN).[48,49,52,65] Acetylcholine (ACH)-, substance P (SP)-, vasoactive intestinal polypeptide (VIP)-, peptide H1 (pH1)-, and calcitonin gene-related peptide (CGRP)-like substances have been shown to be associated wityh nonsympathetic nerves in cerebral arteries.[13,18,51,56,68a] Following chronic sympathectomy, AVN is still present while GVN completely disappeared,[48,52] suggesting that ACh-, SP-,VIP-, pH1-, and CGRP-like substances are associated with AVN. However, recent studies have suggested that a VIP-like substance is a vasodilator and ACh and SP are potential vasonconstrictors.[47,49,56] Cholinergic nerves may be preganglionic and/or ACh may coexist with a dilator transmitter,[51] and SP-containing fibers may be sensory in nature.[14] The suggestion that AVN are vasodilator nerves and GVN are vasoconstrictor nerves[48,49,52] is still acceptable.

It has been demonstrated that AVN and GVN terminals are frequently found in close apposition in cerebral arteries.[38,48,64] This close relationship between GVN and AVN terminals suggests a possible functional axo-axonal interaction. Release of NE from sympathetic nerve terminals in cerebral arteries has been shown to be inhibited by a potential transmitter such as acetylcholine.[15,16] This result implies that release of transmitters from sympathetic nerve terminals may be inhibited by substance(s) released from the neighboring AVN terminals. Thus, any change in ratio of AVN/GVN terminals in cerebral arteries between WKY and SHR should alter the interaction between AVN and GVN terminals. It has been shown that the ratio of AVN/GVN terminals, especially those with close synaptic distances, decreased in most SHR cerebral arteries. This result may suggest a decreased presynaptic inhibition of transmitter release from GVN in the SHR cerebral artery which facilitates release of transmitter from sympathetic nerve terminals and results in a greater synaptic transmitter concentration. Together with the findings that the SHR cerebral arteries contain elevated muscle layers[55,62] and may become more sensitive to a vasoactive agent,[81] it is possible that the cerebral neurogenic vasoconstriction is enhanced in SHR.

Results from several *in vivo* physiological studies have also demonstrated that sympathetic nerves become more functional in controlling brain circulation during acute or chronic hypertensions.[6,30,33,60,63,67] The sympathetic nerves of superior cervical ganglionic orgin have been shown to become more active[60] and may release a "trophic" factor. This may be the cause of hypertrophy of the vascular smooth muscle and, therefore, serve an important protective role against stroke during chronic hypertension.[6,30,33,60,67]

Furthermore, it has been shown that in chronic arterial hypertension, both the lower and upper limits of cerebral blood flow (CBF) autoregulation are reset to higher blood pressures. Such hypertensive adaptation of the lower limit has been found in man,[72] baboon,[40] and rat.[5,22,68] Hypertensive adaptation of the upper limit of autoregulation has been found in baboon.[71] It is therefore interesting to note that GVN were increased in all cerebral arteries of SHR compared to WKY. On the other hand, both GVN and AVN terminals were decreased in cerebral arteries of RHR (Figure 5). These results suggest that the active neurogenic vasodilation for increasing cerebral blood flow may be impaired in both RHR and SHR and that the vasoconstriction may be improved in SHR and weakened in RHR. Indeed both RHR and SHR have been shown to be more susceptible to ischemic brain damage than normotensive WKY following acute hypotension.[5] RHR, but not NR or SHR, suffer brain ischemia and edema following a sudden increase in blood pressure, presumably due to rupture of the blood-brain barrier induced by high blood pressure.[23,39] Taken together, it is possible that GVN and AVN are important factors involved in setting the respective upper and lower limits of the autoregulatory maintenance of cerebral blood flow. Since significant variations in regional cerebral vessel innervation exist, it is possible that the upper and lower limits of the autoregulatory plateau differ from region to region and from species to species. This hypothesis is in line with the recent reports by Sadoshima and Heistad[68] that the lower limit of the autoregulatory pleateau differs in various regions of the brain in stroke-prone SHR.

XI. CONCLUDING REMARKS

Both pial and intraparenchymal vessels are important in controlling brain circulation. CBF in SHR has been shown to be relatively normal compared to that of WKY.[20,75] Thus, cerebral vasculature must adapt to preserve and regulate blood flow at elevated arterial pressure. Since cerebral arteries contribute significantly to cerebral autoregulation[45] and 40 to 50% of the total cerebral blood resistance occurs in large arterial vessels,[29,73] examination of changes in the large cerebral arteries will provide some insight into the adaptation process which occurs during hypertension.

Results from morphological studies indicate that cerebral vasodilator and constrictor nerves undergo changes during chronic hypertension. Although the catecholamine fluorescence fibers (or axonal fibers) in cerebral arteries are altered in SHR but not appreciably in RHR, sympathetic and nonsympathetic nerve terminals significantly change in both genetic and nongenetic hypertension. These results suggest that defects in autonomic nerve terminals may be related to hypertension. The alteration in nerve terminals however varies among types of hypertension. The increased sympathetic adrenergic activity in peripheral vascular beds has been postulated to cause and maintain hypertension.[1,82] In early hypertension, there are signs of a net increase of adrenergic influence of the heart,[41] but at least in established hypertension this seems due more to a withdrawal of parasympathetic.[46] The increased sympathetic activity in adult SHR brain arteries[60,67] is accompanied by an increase of sympathetic vasoconstrictor nerves in most, and a greater decrease of nonsympathetic vasodilator nerves in some brain regions (Figure 3). The increased sympathetic activity and therefore hypertrophy of the smooth muscle layer in cerebral arteries of SHR is thought to have a beneficial protective effect against brain lesions such as stroke.[6,30,60,67] On the other hand, a decrease in both vasodilator and constrictor nerve terminals in RHR cerebral arteries (Figure 5) suggests that the RHR-type hypertension is prone to ischemic damage.

The observation that an increase in sympathetic activity in SHR cerebral arteries and a decrease in sympathetic function in RHR cerebral arteries may have important clinical implication. Treatments of these two types of hypertension should therefore be varied. Drugs that block sympathetic transmission should be given with caution to patients with essential hypertension of the RHR type. Blocking sympathetic transmission may further decrease the already weakened sympathetic activity in this type of hypertension. It may precipitate brain lesions such as a stroke upon a sudden surge in systemic blood pressure.

The lower and upper limits of cerebral blood flow autoregulation are shown to reset to high blood pressures. Based on morphological data that sympathetic nerves in cerebral arteries decrease in RHR, the upper limit in RHR may not necessarily reset to a higher blood pressure. The clear difference in innervation pattern in brain blood vessels between different types of hypertension strongly indicates that a generalization on CBF autoregulation cannot be made until the individual model of hypertension has been examined.

ACKNOWLEDGMENTS

This work was supported by a grant from the National Institutes of Health (HL 27763), a Grant-in-Aid from the American Heart Association (83-1040), with funds contributed in part from the American Heart Association/Illinois Affiliate, and funds from Southern Illinois University School of Medicine. The author thanks Ms. Salie Fluckiger for preparation of the manuscript.

REFERENCES

1. **Abboud, F. M.,** The sympathetic system in hypertension. State-of-the-art review, *Hypertension,* 4 (Suppl. II), 208, 1982.
2. **Aprigliano, O. and Hermsmeyer, K.,** *In vitro* denervation of the portal vein and caudal artery of the rat, *J. Pharmacol. Exp. Ther.*, 190, 568, 1976.

3. **Alm, A. and Bill, A.,** The effect of stimulation of the cervical sympathetic claim on retinal oxygen tension and on uveal, retinal and cerebral blood flow in cats, *Acta Physiol. Scand.,* 88, 83, 1973.

4. **Araki, H., Su, C., and Lee, T. J.-F.,** Effect of superior cervical ganglioectomy on the sensitivity of rabbit ear artery and cerebral arteries of rabbit and cat to vasoactive agents, *J. Pharmacol. Exp. Ther.,* 220, 49, 1982.

5. **Barry, D. I., Standgaard, S., Graham, D. I., Braendstrup, O., Svendsen, U. G., Vorstrup, S., Hemmingsten, R., and Bolwig, T. G.,** Cerebral blood flow in rats with renal and spontaneous hypertension: resetting of the lower limit of autoregulation, *J. Cerebral Blood Flow Metab.,* 2, 347, 1982.

6. **Beausang-Linder, M. and Bill, A.,** Cerebral circulation in acute arterial hypertension — protective effects of sympathetic nervous activity, *Acta Physiol. Scand.,* 111, 193, 1981.

7. **Bevan, J. A. and Su, C.,** Variations of intra- and perisynaptic adrenergic transmitter concentrations with width of synaptic cleft in vascular tissues, *J. Pharmacol. Exp. Ther.,* 190, 30, 1974.

8. **Burnstock, G., Gannon, B., and Iwayama, T.,** Sympathetic innervation of vascular smooth muscle in normal and hypertensive animals, *Circ. Res.,* 27 (Suppl. II), 5, 1970.

9. **Busija, D. W. and Heistad, D. D.,** Effects of cholinergic nerves on cerebral blood flow in cats, *Circ. Res.,* 48, 62, 1981.

10. **Cassis, L. A., Stitzel, R. E., and Head, R. J.,** Hypernoradrenergic innervation of the caudal artery of the spontaneously hypertensive rat: an influence upon neuroeffector mechanism, *J. Pharmacol. Exp. Ther.,* 234, 792, 1985.

11. **Chorobski, J. and Penfield, W.,** Cerebral vasodilator nerves and their pathway from the medulla oblongata, *Arch. Neurol. Psychiatry,* 28, 1257, 1932.

12. **Collis, M. G. and Vanhoutte, P. M. ,** Vascular reactivity of isolated perfused kidneys from male and female spontaneously hypertensive rats, *Circ. Res.,* 41, 759, 1977.

13. **Duckles, S. P.,** Evidence for a functional cholinergic innervation of cerebral arteries, *J. Pharmacol. Exp. Ther.,* 217, 544, 1981.

14. **Duckles, S. P. and Buck, S. H.,** Substance P in cerebral vasculature: depletion by capsaicin suggests a sensory role, *Brain Res.,* 245, 171, 1982.

15. **Duckles, S. P. and Kennedy, C. D.,** Cerebral blood vessels: effects of exogenous acetylcholine and field stimulation on norepinephrine release, *J. Pharmacol. Exp. Ther.,* 222, 562, 1982.

16. **Edvinsson, L., Falck, B., and Owman, C.,** Possibility for a cholinergic action on smooth muscalature and on sympathetic axons in brain vessels medicated by muscarinic and nicotinic receptors, *J. Pharmacol. Exp. Ther.,* 200, 117, 1977.

17. **Edvinsson, L.,** Sympathetic control of cerebral circulation, *TIPS,* 5, 425, 1982.

18. **Edvinsson, L., McCulloh, J., and Uddman, R.,** Substance P: immunohistochemical localization and effect upon cat pial arteries *in vitro* and *in vivo, J. Physiol.,* 318, 251, 1981.

19. **Ekas, R. D. and Lokhandwala, M. F.,** Sympathetic nerve function and vascular reactivity in spontaneously hypertensive rats, *Am. J. Physiol.,* 241, R379, 1981.

20. **Ferrone, R. A., Walsh, G. M., Tsuchiya, M., and Frohlich, E. D.,** Comparison of hemodynamics in conscious spontaneously and renal hypertensive rats, *Am. J. Physiol.,* 236, H403, 1979.

21. **Fink, G. D. and Brody, M. J.,** Impaired neurogenic control of renal vasculature in renal hypertensive rats, *Am. J. Physiol.,* 238, H770, 1980.

22. **Fujishima, M. and Omae, T.,** Lower limit of cerebral autoregulation in normotensive and spontaneously hypertensive rats, *Experientia,* 32, 1019, 1976.

23. **Fujishima, M., Onomiya, K., Oniki, H., Ogata, J., and Omae, T.,** Effects of acute hypertension on brain metabolism in normotensive, renaovascular hypertensive and spontaneously hypertensive rats, *Stroke,* 9, 349, 1978.

24. **Galloway, M. P. and Westfall, T. C.,** The release of endogenous norepinephrine from the coccygeal artery of spontaneously hypertensive and Wistar-Kyoto rats, *Circ. Res.,* 51, 225, 1982.

25. **Garrett, J., Castro-Travares, J., and Branco, D.,** Uptake and metabolism of norepinephrine by blood vessels of perinephritic hypertensive dogs, *Blood Vessels,* 18, 100, 1981.

26. **Goldstein, B. M., Lai, F. M., Herzlinger, H., and Cervoni, P.,** Disposition of catecholamines in cardiovascular tissues of aorta coarcted hypertensive rats, *Life Sci.,* 31; 1633, 1982.

27. **Graham, J. D. P., Lever, J. D., and Sprigg, T. L. B.,** Adrenergic innervation of the small vessels in the pancreas of the rat and changes observed during early renal hypertension, *Circ. Res.,* 26 (Suppl. II), 25, 1970; 27 (Suppl. II), 32, 1970.

28. **Greenberg, S. and Wilborn, W.,** Functional and structural changes in veins in spontaneous hypertension, *Arch. Int. Pharmacodyn. Ther.,* 258, 208, 1982.

29. **Harper, S. L., Bohlen, H. G., and Rubin, M. J.,** Arterial and microvascular contributions to cerebral cortical autoregulation in rats, *Am. J. Physiol.,* 246, H17, 1984.

30. **Hart, M. N., Heistad, D. D., and Brody, M. J.,** Effect of chronic hypertension and sympathetic denervation on wall/lumen ratio of cerebral vessels, *Hypertension,* 2, 419, 1980.

31. **Head, R. J. and Berkowitz, B. A.,** Vascular and circulating catecholamines in diabetes and hypertension, in *Catecholamines: Basic and Clinical Frontiers,* Usdin, E., Kopin, I. J., and Barchas, I., Eds., Pergamon Press, Elmsford, NY, 1979, 1518.

32. **Head, R. J., Cassis, L. A., Robinsson, R. L., Westfall, D. P., and Stitzel, R. E.,** Altered catecholamine contents in vascular and nonvascular tissues in genetically hypertensive rats, *Blood Vessels,* 22, 196, 1985.

33. **Heistad, D. D.,** Effects of nerves on cerebral vessels in stroke, cerebral edema, hypertension, *J. Lab. Clin. Med.,* 99, 139, 1982.

34. **Heistad, D. D., Marcus, M. L., and Gross, P. M.,** Effects of sympathetic nerves on cerebral vessels in dog, cat and monkey, *Am. J. Physiol.,* 235, 4544, 1978.

35. **Hermsmeyer, K.,** Cellular basis for increased sensitivity of vascular smooth muscle in spontaneously hypertensive rats, *Circ. Res.,* 38 (Suppl. II), 53, 1967.

36. **Hirst, G. D. S., Neild, T. O., and Silverberg, G. D.,** Norepinephrine receptors on the rat basilar arteries, *J. Physiol. (London),* 328, 351, 1982.

37. **Hökfelt, T. and Jonsson, G.,** Studies on reaction and binding of monoamines after fixation and process for electron microscopy with special reference to fixation with potassium permanganate, *Histochemie,* 16, 45, 1968.

38. **Iwayama, T., Furness, J. B., and Burnstock, G.,** Dual adrenergic and cholinergic innervation of the cerebral arteries of the cat, *Circ. Res.,* 26, 35, 1970.

39. **Johnasson, B. B. and Linder, L. -E.,** Hypertension and brain edema: an experimental study on acute and chronic hypertension in the rat, *J. Neurol. Neurosurg. Psychiatry,* 44, 402, 1981.

40. **Jones, J. V., Fitch, W., MacKenzie, E. T., Strandgaard, S., and Harper, A. M.,** Lower limit of cerebral blood flow autoregulation in experimental renovascular hypertension in the baboon, *Circ. Res.,* 39, 555, 1976.

41. **Julius, S., Pascual, A. V., and London, R.,** Role of parasympathetic inhibition in the hyperkinetic type of borderline hypertension, *Circulation,* 44, 413, 1971.

42. **Kameyama, S., Ishii, R., and Kobayashi, K.,** Cholinergic innervation of the cerebral blood vessels in the dog and effect of electrical stimulation of ciliary ganglion, in *Cerebral Blood Flow: Effects of Nerves and Neurotransmitters,* Vol. 14, Heistad, D. D. and Marcus, M. L., Eds., Elsevier, Amsterdam, 1982, 447.

43. **Keatinge, W. R. and Torrie, C.,** Action of sympathetic nerves on inner and outer muscle of sheep carotid artery and effect of pressure on nerve distribution, *J. Physiol.,* 257, 699, 1976.

44. **Kobayashi, S., Tsukahara, S., Sugita, K., and Nagata, T.,** Adrenergic and cholinergic innervation of rat cerebral arteries, *Histochemistry,* 70, 129, 1981.

45. **Kontos, H. A., Wei, E. P., Navari, R. M., Levasseur, J. E., Rosenblum, W. I., and Patterson, J. L.,** Responses of cerebral arteries and arterials to acute hypotension and hypertension, *Am. J. Physiol.,* 234, H371, 1978.

46. **Korner, P. I., Shaw, J., Uther, J. B., West, M. J., McRitchie, R. J., and Richards, J. G.,** Autonomic and nonautonomic circulatory components in essential hypertension in man, *Circulation,* 48, 107, 1973.

47. **Larsson, L. I., Edvinsson, L., Fahrenkrug, J., Hakanson, J., Owman, C., Schaff-Alitzke de Muckadell, O., and Sundler, F.,** Immunohistochemical localization of a vasodilator polypeptide (VIP) in cerebrovascular nerves, *Brain Res.,* 113, 400, 1976.

48. **Lee, T. J. -F.,** Ultrastructural distribution of vasodilator and constrictor nerves in cat cerebral arteries, *Circ. Res.,* 49, 971, 1981.

49. **Lee, T. J. -F.,** Morphopharmacological study of cerebral vasodilator and constrictor nerves, in *Neurogenic Control of Brain Circulation,* Heistad, D. D. and Marcus, M. L., Eds., Elsevier, Amsterdam, 1982, 431.

50. **Lee, T. J. -F.,** Cholinergic mechanisms in cerebral circulation, in *Trends in Autonomic Pharmacology,* Vol. 3, Kalsner, S., Ed., Urban & Schwarzenberg, Baltimore, MD, 1985, 187.

51. **Lee, T. J. -F.,** Sympathetic and nonsympathetic transmitter mechanisms in cerebral vasodilation and constriction, in *Neural Regulation of Brain Circulation,* Owman, C. and Hardebo, J. E., Eds., Elsevier, Amsterdam, 1986, 285.

52. **Lee, T. J. -F., Chiueh, C. C., and Adams, M.,** Synaptic transmission of vasoconstrictor nerves in rabbit basilar artery, *Eur. J. Pharmacol.,* 61, 55, 1980.

53. **Lee, T. J. -F., Hume, W. R., Su, C., and Bevan, J. A.,** Neurogenic vasodilation of cat cerebral arteries, *Circ. Res.,* 42, 535, 1978.

54. **Lee, T. J. -F., Kinkead, L. R., and Sarwinski, S.,** Norepinephrine and acetycholine transmitter mechanisms in large arteries of the pig, *J. Cereb. Blood Flow Metab.,* 2, 439, 1982.

55. **Lee, T. J. -F. and Saito, A.,** Altered cerebral vessel innervation in the spontaneously hypertensive rat, *Circ. Res.,* 55, 392, 1984.

56. **Lee, T. J. -F., Saito, A., and Berezin, I.,** Vasoactive intestinal polypeptide-like substance: the potential transmitter for cerebral vasodilation, *Science,* 224, 898, 1984.

57. **Lee, T. J. -F., Su, C., and Bevan, J. A.,** Neurogenic sympathetic vasoconstriction of rabbit basilar artery, *Circ. Res.,* 39, 120, 1976.

58. **Lee, R. M. K. W., Forrest, J. B., and Daniel, E. E.,** Ultrastructural changes in mesenteric arteries from spontaneously hypertensive rats, *Blood Vessels,* 20, 72, 1983.

59. **Medgett, I. C. and Langer, S. Z.,** Characterization of smooth muscle α-adrenoceptors and of responses to electrical stimulation in the cat isolated perfused middle cerebral arteries, *Naunyn Schmiedebergs Arch. Pharmacol.,* 323, 24, 1983.

60. **Mueller, S. M. and Ertel, B. S.,** Association between sympathetic nerve activity and cerebrovascular protection in young spontaneously hypertensive rats, *Stroke,* 14, 88, 1983.
61. **Mulvany, M. J., Aalkjaer, C., and Christensen, J.,** Changes in noradrenaline sensitivity and morphology of arterial resistance vessels during development of high blood pressure in spontaneously hypertensive rats, *Hypertension,* 2, 664, 1980.
62. **Nordberg, C., Fredrikssen, K., and Johansson, B. B. C.,** The morphometry of consecutive segments in cerebral arteries of normotensive and hypertensive rats, *Stroke,* 16, 313, 1985.
63. **Nordborg, C. and Johansson, B. B.,** The ratio between media thickness and radius in cerebral arteries and arterioles of SHR and NR, *Jpn. Heart J.,* 20 (Suppl. I), 290, 1979.
64. **Owman, C., Edvinsson, L., and Nielsen, K. C.,** Autonomic neuroreceptor mechanisms in brain vessels, *Blood Vessels,* 11, 2, 1974.
65. **Rho, J. H., Newman, B., and Alexander, N.,** Altered *in vitro* uptake of norepinephrine by cardovascular tissues of spontaneously hypertensive rats. I. Meseneteric artery, *Hypertension,* 3, 704, 1981.
66. **Sadoshima, S., Busija, D. W., Brody, M. J., and Heistad, D. D.,** Sympathetic nerve protect against stroke in stroke-prone hypertensive rats. A preliminary study, *Hypertension,* 3 (Suppl. I), 1, 1981.
67. **Sadoshima, S. and Heistad, D. D.,** Sympathetic nerves protect the blood-brain barrier in stroke-prone spontaneously hypertensive rats, *Hypertension,* 4, 904, 1982.
68. **Sadoshima, S., and Heistad, D. D.,** Regional cerebral blood during hypotension in normotensive and stroke-prone spontaneously hypertensive rats: effect of sympathetic denervation, *Stroke,* 14, 575, 1983.
68a. **Saito, A., Kimura, S., Uchiyama, Y., Shoji, T., Lee, T. J. -F., and Goto, K.,** Calcitonin gene-related peptide (CGRP) and blood vessel function, in *Vascular Neuroeffector Mechanisms,* Bevan, J. A., Majewski, H., Maxwell, R. A., and Story, D. F., Eds., TCSU PRESS, in press, 1987.
69. **Saito, A. and Lee, T. J. -F.,** Autonomic innervation of the brain arteries decreases in renal hypertensive rats, *Hypertension,* 4, 514, 1985.
70. **Scremin, O. U., Sonnenschein, R. R., and Rubinstein, E. H.,** Cholinergic cerebral vasodilation: lack of involvement of cranial parasympathetic nerves, *J. Cereb. Blood Flow Metab.,* 3, 362, 1983.
71. **Strandgaard, S., MacKenzie, E. T., Sengupta, D., Rowan, J. O., Lassen, N. A., and Harper, A. M.,** Upper limit of autoregulation of cerebral blood flow in the baboon, *Circ. Res.,* 34, 435, 1974.
72. **Strandgaard, S., Olesen, J., Skinhoj, E., and Lassen, N. A.,** Autoregulation of brain circulation in severe arterial hypertension, *Br. Med. J.,* 1, 507, 1973.
73. **Stromberg, D. D. and Fox, J. R.,** Pressure in the pial arterial microcirculation of the cat during changes in systemic arterial pressure, *Cir. Res.,* 32, 229, 1972.
74. **Su, C. and Lee, T. J. -F.,** Regional variation of adrenergic and nonadrenergic nerves in blood vessels, in *Vascular Neuroeffector Mechanisms,* Bevan, J. A., Burnstock, G., Johansson, B., Maxwell, R. A., and Nedergaard, O. A., Eds., S. Karger, Basel, 1975, 35.
75. **Tobia, A. J., Lee, J. Y., and Walsh, G. M.,** Regional blood flow and vascular resistance in the spontaneously hypertensive rat, *Cardiovasc. Res.,* 8, 758, 1974.
76. **Vanhoutte, P. M.,** Adrenergic neuroeffector interaction in the blood vessel wall, *Fed. Proc.,* 37, 181, 1978.
77. **Vasquez, J. and Purves, M. J.,** Studies on the dilator pathway to cerebral blood vessels, in *Neurogenic Control of the Brain Circulation,* Owman, C. and Edvinsson, L., Eds., Plenum Press, Oxford, 1977, 59.
78. **Webb, R. C., Vanhoutte, P. M., and Bohr, D. F.,** Adrenergic neurotransmission in vascular smooth muscle from spontaneously hypertensive rats, *Hypertension,* 3, 93, 1981.
79. **Westfall, T. C.,** Local regulation of adrenergic neurotransmission, *Physiol. Rev.,* 57, 659, 1977.
80. **Whall, C. W., Myers, M. M., and Halpern, W.,** Norepinephrine sensitivity, tension development and neuronal uptake in resistance arteries from spontaneously hypertensive and normotensive rats, *Blood Vessels,* 17, 1, 1980.
81. **Winquist, R. J. and Bohr, D. F.,** Structural and functional changes in cerebral arteries from spontaneously hypertensive rats, *Hypertension,* 5, 292, 1983.
82. **Zimmerman, B. G.,** Peripheral neurogenic factors in acute and chronic alteration of arterial pressure, *Circ. Res.,* 53, 121, 1983.
83. **Zimmerman, B. G., Friedman, P. L., and Wong, P. C.,** Depressed adrenergic nerve function in tibial arteries of two-kidney, one-clip Goldblatt hypertensive dogs, *Blood Vessels,* 19, 311, 1982.
84. **Zsoter, T. T., Sirko, S., Wolchinsky, C., Kadar, D., and Endrenyi, L.,** Adrenergic activity in arteries of spontaneously hypertensive rats, *Can. J. Physiol. Pharmacol.,* 59, 1104, 1981.

Chapter 2

THE CEREBRAL VASCULATURE IN CHRONIC AND ACUTE HYPERTENSION

George Osol

TABLE OF CONTENTS

I. INTRODUCTION

Cerebrovascular disease takes a severe toll on our society. In the U.S., stroke is the third leading cause of death, and is the most life-threatening neurological disease of adult life.[1,2] The likelihood of stroke increases with the severity of hypertension and even mild elevations in blood pressure are associated with increased risk.[3] It is significant that, although hypertension is the major risk factor for vascular brain disease, the mechanisms through which damage to the vasculature occurs are still a subject of debate. This chapter attempts to provide an overview of our current knowledge about the effects of chronic and acute hypertension on the cerebral vasculature.

The end point of cerebrovascular disease is damage to the parenchyma of the brain. Unlike many other organs in the body, the brain depends exclusively on glucose as an energy source to fuel metabolism. Because its storage capacity is practically nonexistent, even short-term interruptions in the supply of glucose or oxygen can have catastrophic effects and produce irreversible and often tragic neurologic deficits.

The human brain is avaricious in its metabolic demands and, stated most simply, the task of the cerebral circulation is to ensure a continuous supply of blood to every area of the brain. Comprising only 2% of the adult body weight, the human brain receives an estimated 15 to 20% of the cardiac output[3] (but only about 3% in the dog, cat, rabbit and rat[4]), and maintains its blood flow at relatively stable levels despite occasionally large fluctuations in blood pressure.[5-7] This process, termed autoregulation, is effected through a variety of mechanisms.[8,9] The complex interplay between neural, myogenic, and metabolic influences determines both the efficiency of autoregulation and the pressure range over which it occurs.

Each of these mechanisms is affected by chronic hypertension. It is not surprising, then, that although the clinical symptoms of hypertension-related cerebrovascular disease are sometimes abrupt (e.g., aneurysmal hemorrhage), in many cases the underlying pathogenesis is gradual and progressive.[10] Thus, many cerebrovascular accidents may be viewed as an acute culmination of much more gradual pathogenic mechanisms which lead to a local or general disordering of normal blood flow.

For some types of cerebrovascular accidents, the pathologic basis is congenital (in saccular or "berry" aneurysms, for example). Sometimes, its origin is extracranial. A prominent example of the latter is embolic stroke, which is usually a manifestation of heart disease.[11] Emboli originating from the heart or carotid bifurcations are carried into the brain, only to lodge in one of the major cerebral arteries. Depending on the location, thrombolytic activity, and the degree of collateral circulation, the extent of injury may be minor and completely reversible (a transient ischemic episode), permanent, or even lethal.

Regarding the cerebral circulation specifically, it has been suggested that at least two distinct pathological processes are at play in hypertension-induced cerebrovascular damage, and that they can best be separated on the basis of vessel size and type.[12] The evidence supporting this hypothesis is histologic, since in the larger intracranial and extracranial arteries of hypertensive patients, complex atherosclerotic lesions are the dominant finding. These are common at bifurcations and include plaques, ulcerations, subintimal hemorrhages, and formation of intraluminal thrombi. In smaller vessels, hyalin necrosis, the formation of micoraneurysms, and lipid degeneration of the arterial wall are more commonly observed.[3,10] Hypertension-induced rupture of diseased large and small arteries may occur, possibly as a result of localized cellular degeneration within the arterial wall.[13]

II. CLINICAL OBSERVATIONS

Four major cerebrovascular illnesses are strongly associated with hypertension: cerebral infarction, lacunar infarction, hypertensive encephalopathy, and hypertensive brain hemorrhage. The vessel size and location, and type of lesions which are observed varies with the disease.[3,10,12]

Cerebral infarctions are most often associated with focal areas of damage in the major cerebral arteries.

Lacunar infarctions are more commonly observed in the smaller penetrating vessels, and may occur through a variety of mechanisms such as intravascular coagulation, fibrinoid necrosis, embolism, inflammation, and severe sclerosis.

In hypertensive encephalopathy, which can occur at any age, the pathologic findings include fibrinoid necrosis of arterioles, thrombosis of small arterioles and capillaries, petechial hemorrhages and perivascular exudates.[10]

There may also be a predilection for damage to specific regions of the brain.[3,10] For example, hypertensive hemorrhage occurs predominantly (about 80%) in the cerebral hemispheres, whereas lipohyaline degeneration of perforating vessels leads to aneurysmal rupture, frequently along the lenticulostriate and thalamostriate vessels. Lacunar infarctions are situated most often in the putamen, globus pallius, cerebral white matter, or brain stem. The vascular damage in hypertensive encephalopathy is usually attributed to a sudden and excessive elevation of blood pressure,[14,15] and pathologic findings consist primarily of fibrinoid necrosis or rupture of smaller arterioles and capillaries.[3,10] Arterial lesions in hypertensive encephalopathy occur predominantly in the brain stem and basal ganglia and to a lesser extent, in the cerebral hemispheres.[3]

As mentioned above, autoregulatory mechanisms are altered in chronic hypertension. That some of these changes are compensatory and beneficial becomes apparent when one considers that normotensive patients are more susceptible to hypertensive encephalopathy from sudden pressure elevation than chronic hypertensives. The cerebral vasculature of a chronic hypertensive can withstand pressures up to 250/150 mmHg because the upper limit of autoregulation has been shifted through structural and functional adaptation.[14] Since the lower limit of autoregulation is also shifted to higher pressures, the same patient may be more vulnerable to ischemia from a level of hypotension which is normally well tolerated.[17] Chronic antihypertensive therapy may restore autoregulatory limits to normal values.[16]

Although hypertension is associated with the development of atherosclerotic lesions, its primary effect may be to accelerate rather than initiate this process. For example, the frequency of large cerebral infarcts was found to be similar in normo- and hypertensives.[17] Carotid occlusion was found more commonly in normotensives (25 vs. 9% in NT vs. HT).[18] Conversely, large and small intracerebral hemorrhages and small infarcts were found almost exclusively in hypertensives. These observations suggest that factors other than hypertension are primary determinants of atherothrombotic infarction due to carotid disease. Once initiated, hypertension may hasten the atherosclerotic process and appears to be a major factor in the development of disease in medium and small cerebral arteries.

Hypertension-induced damage to the cerebral vasculature may be associated with at least one form of dementia, defined here as an irreversible and usually progressive loss of cognitive and intellectual functions. In one study, the intellectual function of newly diagnosed untreated hypertensive men having diastolic blood pressures in excess of 105 mmHg was compared with that of normotensive controls.[19] A significant impairment of attention span and vigilance was reported in the hypertensive group. Previously, Wilkie and Eisdorfer[20] also reported significantly greater intellectual loss, measured over a 10-year period, in hypertensive patients when compared with matched normotensive controls. Finally, Ladurner et al. compared stroke patients with and without evidence of intellectual deficits and found hypertension to be the only risk factor which was significantly associated with dementia.[21] Although the results of these studies are intriguing, further investigation of underlying mechanisms is required before any definitive conclusions can be reached. Certainly, there are other mechanisms which may lead to dementia. This syndrome is difficult to study with clinical precision and, for obvious reasons, the usefulness of animal models is limited. Pending the development of more specific diagnostic tools, the relative importance of hypertension-induced vascular disease as a cause for dementia remains to be determined.

In summary, chronic hypertension is clearly damaging to the cerebral vasculature and has been termed the "preeminent precursor of stroke".[2] Approximately two thirds of diagnosed stroke cases are due to ischemia and infarction secondary to occlusive disease of the small- and medium-sized cerebral arteries. Subarachnoid and intraparenchymatous hemorrhages are observed in about 14% of stroke cases. Subarachnoid hemorrhage,which is twice as common as intracerebral hemorrhage, is usually associated with rupture of saccular aneurysms in the Circle of Willis, or in proximal segments of large cerebral arteries. Cerebral embolism, which accounts for most of the remaining patients with stroke, is associated most often with cardiac disease.

III. ANIMAL MODELS OF CHRONIC HYPERTENSION

Laboratory experiments using animal models of chronic and acute hypertension have provided a wealth of information about the nature, location, and extent of structural and functional changes within the cerebral vasculature over time. Since its introduction by Okamoto and Aoki in 1963,[22] the spontaneously hypertensive rat (SHR) has become the most widely studied animal model of chronic hypertension. A substrain which develops a high incidence of strokes, the spontaneously hypertensive stroke-prone (SHRSP) rat was introduced more recently[23] and its use is becoming widespread as well.

An in-depth evaluation of the relevance of these rat models to human essential hypertension is beyond the scope of this chapter, but the interested reader is referred to two review articles which make a case for[24] and against[25] the suitability of the spontaneously hypertensive rat as a model of human essential hypertension. Suffice it to say that Alexander Pope may have been correct in writing that "The proper study of mankind is man", and the saying that essential hypertension, the human disease, may yet prove to be a good model for understanding the disease in the rat is not without merit.

On the other hand, there are a number of similarities between the SHR and the essentially hypertensive human; i.e., the pattern of development (gradual) and absolute levels of hypertension, changes in vascular structure and reactivity, occurrence of vascular pathology, and responsiveness to antihypertensive treatment.

Caution is most warranted in evaluating the types of effects which are clearly influenced by environmental factors superimposed on a long aging process, and by absolute differences in arterial size. The latter dictate that the magnitude of physical forces acting on the vascular wall (wall tension and shear stress) may be substantially different in larger animals and man. Hence, the location, incidence, and rate of development of lesions may be qualitatively different as well. Large variations in diet, patterns of stress, etc. in man vs. laboratory mammals are also potentially significant factors. This is particularly evident with respect to models which relate hypertension to the development of atherosclerosis or dementia.

The remainder of this chapter deals with information obtained through experiments with animal models of hypertension. In addition to the SHR and SHRSP, other valuable genetic rat models of hypertension have been developed. The list, by no means exhaustive, includes: the Dahl rat, in which salt-sensitive and salt-resistant strains have been developed;[26,27] the New Zealand strain of Smirk and Hall;[28] and the Milan strain.[29] Two relatively recent models are the Lyon strain, developed in France[30] and the Sabra strain[31] originated in Israel.

A useful large animal model is the deoxycorticosterone acetate (DOCA)-hypertensive pig, studied by Bohr and his co-workers.[32]

For studies of acute hypertension, rats, cats, rabbits, and baboons have all been used (see below).

IV. CEREBRAL BLOOD FLOW AUTOREGULATION IN NORMOTENSIVES

The first direct observations of cerebral autoregulation were made more than 50 years ago.[33,34] Using a cranial window technique, in which the pial circulation is made visible, Fog and his associates varied the arterial pressure in cats and observed that pial arteries constricted when blood pressure increased and dilated when it was decreased. From these early studies, and from many subsequent investigations, the concept has emerged that cerebral blood flow (CBF) is relatively constant over a wide range of arterial pressures.

Before reviewing the effects of hypertension on CBF, several considerations are in order:

1. In discussing autoregulation of CBF, the term relatively should be emphasized, since CBF is not invariant, changing approximately 0.4 to 0.6%/mmHg change in arterial pressure.[35-39] This amount is not insignificant since, for a 100-mmHg increase in pressure, CBF increases approximately 50%.

2. Although CBF autoregulation occurs over a wide range of arterial pressures, there is a "lower limit" of autoregulation,[5] so that further decreases in arterial pressure result in decreases in CBF and may lead to underperfusion and ischemia. Notably, the results of Haggendahl and Johansson[40] and MacKenzie and et al.[41] demonstrate that dilation at the lower pressure limit of autoregulation is not maximal, i.e., vasodilating stimuli such as hypercapnea produce further increases in pial artery diameter and cerebral blood flow.

3. An "upper limit" of autoregulation also exists,[42] above which further increases in pressure induce a "breakthrough" in which arteries are no longer able to withstand the distending pressure and are forced to dilate. When this occurs, CBF increases rapidly, and pathologic consequences such as cerebral edema and arteriolar rupture may ensue.[43,44]

4. Autoregulation of CBF should be considered from both a global and regional standpoint. Global, or hemispheric autoregulation may be preserved in spite of regional disruptions which may induce local damage, yet have a negligible effect on total CBF.[14]

5. The anatomy of the vasculature is such that some regions of the brain are inherently more vulnerable to damage from sudden reductions in blood flow. Most often, these are the "boundary zones" — areas of the brain which are supplied by the terminal branches of two major cerebral arteries, with few collaterals. During hypertension these areas are most likely to be affected.[45] Furthermore, autoregulation may be better preserved in some areas of the brain (brain stem) than in others (cerebrum), due to differences in segmental resistance.[46]

6. CBF is regulated through a variety of mechanisms.[8,9,39] For the most part, the contribution of each mechanism is determined by anatomical location and physiologic state of the animal. Hence, it is believed that the control of blood flow through larger, proximal cerebral arteries is qualitatively different from that of smaller, downstream vessels. Likewise, the importance of a particular mechanism may depend on the level of arterial pressure.[39] This becomes evident when one considers CBF autoregulation in chronic hypertension.

7. Unlike some other vascular beds, a significant portion (39 to 51% of total cerebrovascular resistance, or 60 to 70% of precapillary cerebral vascular resistance[47,48]) of cerebrovascular resistance can be attributed to large arteries. Therefore, all cerebral arteries — large and small — potentially contribute to CBF autoregulation.

Several investigators measured changes in the diameter of cerebral arteries as a function of systemic arterial presssure. In cats, Kontos et al.[49] and MacKenzie et al.[50,51] found that larger arteries were more responsive than smaller arterioles at normal and increased arterial pressures. At systemic pressures below 90 mmHg, arterioles with resting diameters of less than 50 μm dilated proportionately more to decreases in arterial pressure. Harper et al. measured cerebral arterial and microvascular pressures and blood flow in rats and found that 20 to 70 μm arterioles responded by proportionately equal changes in diameter, and that microvascular pressures were a linear function of arterial pressure.[52] Based on these findings, CBF autoregulation in several species appears to involve both large and small arteries. Furthermore, there may be a hierarchy of responsiveness such that the contribution of larger arteries is greater at higher systemic pressures, thereby protecting smaller downstream vessels from excessive pressure elevation.

V. CBF AUTOREGULATION IN CHRONIC HYPERTENSION

In hypertensive humans, and in laboratory animal models of chronic hypertension, the absolute values of CBF are approximately equal to those measured in normotensives, usually about 50 ml/100 g/min.[5,53] Since capillary pressures are comparable,[54] and systemic arterial pressures are significantly elevated, for flow to remain within normal values in hypertension, cerebrovascular resistance must be increased. As described below, in Sections X and XI, this increase appears to have both structural and functional components.

The limits of the autoregulatory pressure range can be determined by acutely changing systemic blood pressure with stimuli which do not directly affect the cerebral vasculature.[9] Due to the presence of a blood-brain barrier, which restricts the passage of most substances into the vascular wall,[55] intravenous infusions of angiotensin II or norepinephrine increase systemic arterial pressure in a dose-dependent manner without directly constricting cerebral arteries. Hypotension can be induced in a variety of ways such as infusion of trimetaphan (in humans[56]) or adenosine triphosphate (ATP), electrical stimulation of the right vagus nerve, decreasing venous return by placing a snare around the inferior vena cava, or arterial bleeding.[49]

By simultaneously measuring blood pressure and CBF, or by observing the cerebral vasculature directly through a cranial window, the autoregulatory pressure range can be approximated. The shape of the pressure-flow curve in an autoregulatory bed such as the brain is sigmoidal, having a relatively flat central plateau which delineates the range of arterial pressures (abscissa) over which flow (ordinate) is relatively constant. The lower pressure limit is defined as the pressure at which a significant decrease in CBF is first noted, or at which arterial dilation to a reduction in pressure is no longer observed. The upper pressure limit corresponds to the point at which CBF begins to increase sharply following an increase in pressure. If cerebral arteries are observed directly, dilation occurs above the upper pressure limit, instead of autoregulatory constriction. This phenomenon of autoregulatory "breakthrough"[15] has been implicated in the pathogenesis of acute hypertensive encephalopathy and is antagonistic to the earlier concept of hypertensive cerebral vasospasm.[57-60]

A number of studies have shown that the autoregulatory pressure range in normotensives is approximately between 50 and 175 mmHg of arterial pressure.[39] In chronically hypertensive humans,[61] rats,[62,63] and baboons,[64] the lower limit of autoregulation is shifted toward higher pressures. For example, in one clinical study,[61] the lower limit in normotensives was reached at a mean systemic pressure of 50 to 70 mmHg, and the lowest blood pressure which could be tolerated without the patient experiencing mild symptoms of brain hypoperfusion was 35 to 40 mmHg. In hypertensives, the corresponding values were 85 to 150 and 50 to 85 mmHg, respectively. Subjective symptoms of hypoperfusion (dizziness) were experienced when global CBF was reduced to about 70% of normal resting level.[9] Studies of renal and spontaneously hypertensive rats[62,63] and of baboons with renovascular hypertension[64] have yielded similar results.

Sadoshima et al.[65] measured the upper limit of cerebral autoregulation in spontaneously hypertensive rats and found that the elevation towards higher pressures was gradual, with average values increasing from 118 mmHg at 4 weeks to 180 mmHg at 3 months and 208 mmHg at 6 months. They concluded that the upward shift of CBF autoregulation was closely related to an elevation in basal blood pressure, which was also correlated with an increased thickness of the vessel wall.

Having defined the pressure limits of the autoregulatory range, a question may be raised as to whether the efficiency of the regulatory mechanisms is altered, i.e., does the slope of the pressure-flow relationship change in chronic hypertension? Because the slope varies with the level of absolute pressure, to be valid, comparisons should be made for the same change in pressure or flow. To my knowledge, this question has not been addressed quantitatively *in vivo*. It is difficult to answer by examining the published data since there is considerable variability, and most studies have attempted to characterize either the lower or upper pressure limits of autoregulation and not the entire range. Unfortunately, this limitation precludes an evaluation of the slope within the central portion of the autoregulatory range.

We attempted to answer this question *in vitro* by using excised segments of posterior cerebral arteries from adult (16- to 30-week-old) normotensive (WKY) and hypertensive (SHR) rats.[66] Cylindrical arterial segments (100 to 200 µm I.D.) were mounted on microcannulae and subjected to random changes in transmural pressure. Lumen diameter was measured and, in addition to the pressure range over which constriction occurred in response to pressure increases, and dilation to pressure decreases, a gain index was calculated to provide a quantitative measure of the efficiency. This gain index is predictive of the change in flow which would have occurred through a cylinder at the initial and final pressure and diameter. Flow was assumed to be dependent on the fourth power of the diameter, according to Poiseuille's Law. Since the *in vitro* system virtually eliminates metabolic or neural influences normally present *in vivo,* the diameter responses appear be of purely myogenic origin, although endothelial influences cannot be eliminated. The myogenic pressure ranges averaged 49 to 145 mmHg in the WKY and 64 to 181 mmHg in SHR. In addition to this shift in pressure range, the myogenic gain of diameter responses to pressure change in SHR was weaker than in WKY rats; the former maintained essentially a constant diameter over the myogenic pressure range, whereas arteries from the normotensives decreased in diameter with increasing pressure. When hypertension was prevented in SHRSP rats by treatment with MK-421 (a converting enzyme inhibitor) from the time of weaning, myogenic responses (range and gain) were comparable to those of normotensive (WKY) controls. This finding implicates blood pressure history as a major determinant of myogenic responsiveness.

One limitation of this study was that only one segment of the cerebral vasculature was examined. If the pattern holds true for smaller and larger arteries, and unless compensatory neural influences develop, these data suggest that hypertension induces a decrease in arterial contractility, suggesting that the efficiency of autoregulatory mechanisms may be attenuated.

As a result of the 30 to 50 mmHg upwards shift in the lower pressure limit of autoregulation in chronic hypertensives,[61-64,67] a legitimate concern might be the possibility of inducing cerebral ischemia by overly vigorous antihypertensive therapy.[68,69] This unfortunate situation has occurred in several instances in man during acute treatment of malignant hypertension.[70-72] In chronically hypertensive rats with renal or spontaneous hypertension, Barry et al.[73] administered dihydralazine intravenously and measured blood flow using the [133]Xenon injection technique modified for studies on rats.[74] Animals were sacrificed by perfusion with a fixative at the time when the lowest mean arterial pressure (about 50 mmHg) was reached, and the brain subsequently examined. Ischemic lesions were found in two out of six renal hypertensive, and two out of five spontaneously hypertensive rats. These results are somewhat complicated by a more recent discovery[75] that dihydralazine can, paradoxically, dilate or induce repeated vasospasm in rat pial arteries. Therefore, the ischemia maybe due to a direct effect of the drug on the cerebral vasculature and not simply to the reduction in arterial pressure. However, the same investigators obtained similar results (ischemia in 5 out of 12 hypertensive rats) using diazoxide, which is used clinically in the management of acute hypertensive crises and which may not directly affect cerebral arteries.[76] More recently, in a study of spontaneously hypertensive rats, it was found that captopril, an angiotensin-converting enzyme inhibitor, produced an immediate shift in the autoregulatory range, decreasing the upper and lower pressure limits by about 25 and 55 mmHg, respectively.[77] The authors speculated that this potentially beneficial action was attributed to an inhibitory effect on the luminal membrane of larger inflow-tract cerebral arteries. By inhibiting the action of angiotensin converting enzyme and attenuating angiotensin-II induced vasoconstrictory tone, resistance in the proximal vasculature was reduced, and normal blood flow could be maintained at lower levels of perfusion pressure.

In practice, treatment of chronic hypertensives does not usually result in cerebral ischemia for several reasons:[61] (1) The brain is able to compensate for decreases in blood flow to some extent by increasing the efficiency of oxygen extraction. (2) The lower limit of autoregulation is sufficiently low to allow considerable room for therapeutic adjustments in pressure. (3) During prolonged treatment, there is often a readaptation of the vasculature so as to reset the autoregulatory pressure range to lower pressures. This was demonstrated by Vorstrup et al. in a study with renal hypertensive rats.[78] They found that after 2 months of antihypertensive treatment (with reserpine, dihydralazine, and hydrochlorothiazide) the lower limit of autoregulation had decreased from 90 to 109 mmHg to 50 to 69 mmHg, values which were identical with those of normotensive controls. It was inferred that this phenomenon reflected a reversal of hypertension-induced cerebrovascular hypertrophy or hyperplasia.

In summary, it appears that the risk of provoking cerebral ischemia with antihypertensive treatment can be restricted to four clinical settings:

1. During initial treatment of patients with accelerated malignant hypertension[68,69]
2. In elderly hypertensives which have a diminished capacity for adaptive changes[79]
3. In patients with atheromatous stenosis of the large extra- or intracranial arteries or variations in the vascular anatomy of the circle of Willis[80]
4. In acute stroke patients with transient hypertension[81]

A more detailed description of pharmacological considerations may be found in the review by Strandgaard and Paulson.[6]

VI. EFFECTS OF ACUTE HYPERTENSION ON CEREBRAL ARTERY DIAMETER AND BLOOD FLOW

This review is mainly concerned with the effects of chronic hypertension on the cerebral vasculature. Nevertheless, it is worthwhile to examine the effects of sudden elevations in blood pressure on cerebrovascular behavior. Acute responses, which are easily induced in a laboratory setting, afford a glimpse into the physical limits and possible mechanisms of hypertensive damage to the cerebral vasculature.

Although acute hypertension is usually induced experimentally, it is worth noting that blood pressure in man is quite variable, and the "normal" pattern is that of some average pressure upon which considerable fluctuations are imposed by emotional or physical stimuli. For example, transient hypotension may be induced by sudden postural change, and transient hypertension is well documented during periods of emotional or physical stress. The size of the elevations can be significant; in weightlifters, for example, systolic pressures in excess of 300 mmHg have been recorded.

Experimental studies have shown that when the systemic pressure is suddenly elevated above the upper limit of CBF autoregulation, the distending forces acting on the vascular wall may be overcome, leading to forced dilatation[49,50,83,84] of the arteries and disruption of the blood brain barrier.[8,15,45,49,86-88] As might be expected from the previous discussion of autoregulatory pressure limits, in terms of absolute pressure, smaller increases are required to produce vascular damage in normotensives than in hypertensives.

There is also evidence for regional heterogeneity in cerebral autoregulatory mechanisms. Baumbach and Heistad[89] induced acute hypertension in cats by aortic obstruction and intravenous infusion of norepinephrine or angiotensin. Regional cerebral blood flow was measured using isotope-labeled microspheres, and the permeability of the blood-brain barrier was examined by infusing ^{125}I-albumin or Evans blue dye. Severe hypertension (mean arterial pressure was elevated to about 187 mmHg) increased blood flow 159% in the cerebrum, 106% in the cerebellum, and 58% in the brain stem. The authors speculated that regional heterogeneity in autoregulatory responses to sudden pressure elevation may be attributed to differences in the fraction of systemic arterial pressure which is transmitted to smaller arteries. In support of this hypothesis, they cited a study in which pressure gradients in the human brain were predicted from measurements of arterial length and radius obtained from acrylic casts of the human cerebral vasculature.[90] Based on differences in the ratio of radius to length in arteries in the cerebral cortex and basal ganglia, a steeper pressure gradient was predicted in the latter, suggesting that structural patterns may underlie the observed differences. Blood-brain barrier dysfunction during acute hypertension also occurred preferentially in the cerebrum in cats[41,89] but not rats,[91] a finding which is another reminder of species differences in the architecture and physiology of the cerebral circulation.

During an episode of acute hypertension, cerebral arteries often develop areas of uneven constriction, a phenomenon which has been called the "sausage-" or "bead-string" phenomenon.[49,50,83,84,89,92] Originally thought to represent areas of excesssive constriction, or "hypertensive vasospasm",[57-60] more recent studies suggest that the narrowed portions possess autoregulatory tone and that the wider segments have undergone forced dilatation and loss of reactivity to changes in transmural pressure.[49,50,84] Some potentially harmful hemodynamic consequences of forced dilatation are

1.   A decrease in flow resistance and the subsequent exposure of smaller, downstream vessels to excessive transmural pressures may lead to blood-brain barrier damage and edema, or rupture. For this reason, sudden forced dilatation may be a crucial event in hypertensive encephalopathy or in hemorrhagic stroke.
2.   Segmental differences in lumen diameter may lead to increased flow turbulence, shear, and endothelial damage, initiating a positive feedback cycle through which further vascular damage would occur.
3.   An increase in flow to one territory of a major artery could produce an intracerebral steal phenomenon, decreasing blood flow to areas in which perfusion is already marginal, such as the watershed or boundary zones between two major arteries in which ischemic lesions tend to cluster.[93,94]

In an impresssive series of studies, Kontos et al. have defined an underlying mechanism through which vascular damage leading to forced dilatation may occur. Working with anesthetized cats, they found that acute severe elevations of arterial pressure (systolic pressures >170 mmHg) induced by angiotensin II or norepinephrine infusion produced forced dilations of the pial arteries.[49] The responses were size-dependent, with smaller (<100 µm) arteries dilating while larger vessels (>200 µm) remained constricted. With further elevations in pressure (>200 mmHg), dilations were observed in large arteries as well. This dilation was frequently irreversible and was accompanied by a loss of responsiveness to hypercapnea, a powerful vasoconstrictor stimulus, and by passive responses to changes in blood pressure. Scanning and transmission electron microscopy revealed discrete areas of destructive endothelial lesions, but no evidence of platelet aggregation.[84] Lesions were also seen within vascular smooth muscle cells of every artery studied, although the percentage of affected cells was small (5%). The oxygen consumption of pial arterioles which underwent forced dilation was significantly reduced.

Pretreatment with cyclooxygenase inhibitors (indomethacin or AHR-5850) or topical application of scavengers of free oxygen radicals (mannitol or superoxide dismutase) prevented both the dilation and the structural damage associated with sudden hypertension. More recent studies, summarized by Kontos[95] have substantiated these initial observations, and have produced results which are consistent with the view that acute hypertension stimulates the release of some autacoid, possibly bradykinin, which stimulates arachidonate release from membrane phospholipids, possibly through activation of phospholipase C. Increased arachidonate concentrations initiate cyclooxygenase-mediated prostaglandin synthesis within the vascular wall. During the subsequent action of prostaglandin hydroperoxidase, there is production and release of a superoxide anion radical which enters the cerebral extracellular space via an anion channel and, by dismutation, gives rise to hydrogen peroxide. The combination leads to the generation of hydroxyl radicals, which damage the endothelium and vascular smooth muscle and render the artery unreactive to normally present vasoactive stimuli. More recently, it was shown that topical application of arachidonate on the brain surface increased permeability to I-labeled albumin or horseradish peroxidase.[96] These changes were primarily observed in penetrating and intraparenchymal arterioles, although larger arteries and veins occasionally displayed focal endothelial lesions as well.

VII. ACUTE HYPERTENSION AND THE BLOOD-BRAIN BARRIER

Damage to the blood-brain barrier in acute hypertension is also well documented and the "breakthrough" phenomenon has been described in several animal species, and in humans.[9] The rate and amplitude of pressure change appear to be important determinants of subsequent damage. Haggendal and Johansson, working with cats, observed extravasation of Evans blue into the brain when blood pressure was increased suddenly. Stepwise increases to the same level did not produce similar damage.[97]

The systemic pressure at which autoregulatory breakthrough occurs in the cerebral circulation may be surprisingly well-defined. Skinhoj and Strandgaard[98] measured cerebral blood flow as a function of systemic blood pressure in two patients using the ^{133}Xe intracarotid injection method. In the first patient, CBF was almost constant between 110 to 145 mmHg. When blood pressure reached 155 mmHg, CBF increased by approximately 75% almost uniformly throughout the hemisphere. In the second, cerebral autoregulation was normal in the range of 110 to 162 mmHg; at 164 mmHg, CBF suddenly doubled. Subjectively, this patient felt somewhat dizzy and developed a slight headache.

There is a high degree of consistency in the pattern of vascular events which have been observed during experimentally induced hypertension. As pressure exceeds the upper limit of autoregulation, pial constriction is overcome by dilation of small (<100 μm) arteries which is initially focal (the "sausage string" phenomenon) and then becomes widespread. CBF increases markedly, and there is often a disruption of the blood-brain barrier as evidenced by extravasation of protein-bound dye into the brain tissue. The precise segment of the cerebral vasculature in which disruption first occurs has been more difficult to identify.

Using histological methods, i.e., electron microscopy for horseradish peroxidase localization, BBB disruption was reported in arterioles and capillaries.[99-103] In contrast, others found veins to be the primary site of involvement.[101,102] Recently, Mayhan and Heistad[104] were able to provide additional evidence for the latter. Their objectives were to determine where BBB disruption first occurred, and whether molecular size was a factor. The study was also designed to explore the effect of rate of blood pressure elevation on BBB damage, a variable which was not controlled in earlier studies. Sprague-Dawley rats were studied using intravital fluorescent microscopy of pial vessels during perfusion with fluorescein-labeled (FITC) dextrans ranging in molecular weight from 4,000 to 70,000 Da. When mean arterial pressure was increased gradually (92 to 172 mmHg in 2.9 min) by intravenous infusion of phenylephrine, all leaky sites were found to be venular. More rapid elevation of systemic pressure (89 to 167 mmHg in 1.7 min) produced venular disruption as well, although in 8 out of 18 experiments there was diffuse extravasation of FITC-dextran from arterioles (40 to 60 μm) in 5 to 10 min.

Another observation related an effect of rate of pressure elevation on the type of damage incurred. Specifically, leakage of small molecular weight dextran (4 K) was greater than that of heavier molecules (20 and 70 K) following a gradual increase in arterial pressure; with a more rapid change permeability was increased to a similar extent irrespective of molecular weight.[104] The rationale for this experiment was based on the proposed mechanisms for endothelial transport and BBB damage. Two mechanisms of BBB disruption are currently thought to exist.

One (size-independent) is vesicular, and several studies have provided evidence for an increased number and turnover rate of pinocytotic vesicles within endothelial cells during acute hypertension.[99-101,105,106] There is also one report of pinocytotic vesicles fusing to form transendothelial channels.[106]

The other system involves physical separation of endothelial cell-to-cell junctions, and this formation of intercellular pores would predict some dependency on molecular size.[107] This pattern of increased permeability is characteristic of hyperosmotic BBB disruption, in which a shrinking of endothelial cells might take place. In an electron microscopic study with rabbits, Hansson et al. found that following acute hypertension, horseradish peroxidase could penetrate cerebral arterioles through vesicular and, occasionally, pore (tight-junction rupture) mechanisms.[108] In another study of metaraminol-induced hypertension in rats, exclusively vesicular transport of HRP was observed.[109]

In conclusion, the data predominantly favor an augmentation of endothelial vesicular transport mechanisms in acutely induced hypertension, although more subtle damage (such as produced by gradual pressure elevation) may involve separation of tight junctions as well. Differences between the venous and arterial endothelium may also exist; clearly, a greater understanding of the mechanisms is required prior to reaching any firm conclusion.

A third mechanism by which BBB damage could occur is through excessive constriction, or vasospasm. Excessive constriction has been shown to produce damage to the vascular wall.[110,111] Considering the available evidence, however, it is difficult to sustain a belief in the older, "hypertensive vasospasm" hypothesis which gained acceptance in the 1950s and 1960s.[57-60] This hypothesis postulated prolonged vasospasm and ischemia to be the cause of BBB damage and cerebral edema in hypertensive encephalopathy. The evidence presented above, obtained from direct observation of pial vessels and the reported resistance of BBB to ischemia (it remains preserved for up to 12 h after death[112]), argue against its veracity.

Although species differences may exist, an attractive reconciliation of both hypotheses is that, following transient hypertension, forced dilatation may produce an intracerebral "steal" phenomenon, shunting blood away from areas of already marginal perfusion. In one study, rebound cerebral hypoperfusion was reported in New Zealand white rabbits following acute, transient hypertension induced by angiotensin infusion.[45] During pressure elevation, CBF increased about 44%; when pressure was returned to normal, CBF decreased 22% below normal within 5 min and then gradually increased during the next hour. Focal areas of severely decreased cortical flow (at least 2 standard deviations from the mean, or about 40 ml/100 g/min) were observed. These were localized predominantly in the cortex, clustering in arterial boundary zones, and were well circumscribed, having the shape of a truncated cone with its base at the cortical surface and the apex at the transition zone between gray and white matter.

In gerbils, Ito et al. studied the effects of a combination of transient ischemia (30 min to 6 h), produced by occluding the left carotid artery, followed by 30 min of reperfusion at normotensive or hypertensive levels.[113] Even relatively mild hypertension (MAP 157 mmHg) significantly increased the number of HRP-labeled endothelial vesicles. In summary, acute elevations of arterial pressure above the upper autoregulatory limit induce forced dilatation, loss of arterial autoregulatory responsiveness, and large increases in CBF. Damage to the vascular smooth muscle and endothelium has been observed and may be induced by a sudden release of oxygen-free radicals which occurs as a by-product of prostaglandin synthesis within the vascular wall. BBB damage, manifested by increased transendothelial vesicular transport as well as interendothelial gap formation, occurs. The rate of pressure change may determine the location and type of endothelial damage. For gradual changes in pressure, the initial site of BBB breakdown appears to be in venules and small veins. Forced dilatation may produce an intracerebral steal and shunt blood away from cortical areas, such as the boundary zones between two major arteries, resulting in focal ischemia, or expose smaller, downstream vessels to excessive distending presures and rupture. Severe endothelial damage may also lead to a breakdown of anticoagulant mechanisms and initiate focal arterial thrombosis and ischemia.

VIII. CHRONIC HYPERTENSION AND THE BLOOD-BRAIN BARRIER

Byrom reported focal BBB damage in renal hypertensive rats, made visible by trypan blue extravasation in 1954.[57] More recently, Giacomelli et al. observed damage to endothelial tight junctions shown with horseradish peroxidase.[114] This was mainly apparent in dilated segments of cortical arterioles. An increase in the number of endothelial pinocytic vesicles but intact tight junctions has also been reported.[115,116]

In another study, there was no ultrastructural evidence for increased transendothelial permeability in the SHR.[117] Only the trunk of the middle cerebral artery was examined, however, so that damage in other areas of the cerebral vasculature would not have been detected. Using a freeze-fracture technique, Majack and Bhalla found that interendothelial junctions in SHR were characterized by a twofold increase over controls in the number of tight-junctional strands and in average apical-basal depth.[118] They interpreted this observation, made in 12- to 16-month-old rats, as evidence for adaptive endothelial changes in chronic hypertension, which increase the adhesive forces between neighboring endothelial cells and prevent increases in paracellular permeability. The junctional morphology of cerebral arteries from 3-week-old SHR and WKY rats was identical, suggesting that this adaptation was induced during the development of high blood pressure.

The specific model of chronic hypertension, and the nature of the intervention used to disrupt the barrier, are also important variables in asessing the state of the BBB. In chronically hypertensive rats (SHR), the BBB appears to be less resistant to damage from acute pressure elevation than that of normotensive WKY.[119] This effect may be due to a combination of vascular hypertrophy and of reflex sympathetic mechanisms which induce vasoconstriction of larger arteries and decrease wall stress. When hyperosmotic stimuli which stress the BBB without invoking sympathetic constrictor reflexes are used, the BBB in the SHRSP appears to be more susceptible to disruption.[120]

Focal disruptions of the BBB were also found in SHRSP rats which manifested signs of neurological dysfunction, and occasionally in age-matched control animals which appeared normal.[121] Within the experimental group, a gradation of damage was observed, ranging from focal areas of mild edema to ischemic infarction or hemorrhage. Regional CBF was decreased only when the edema was severe or in areas of hemorrhage or ischemia. This observation of edema preceding a reduction in regional CBF argues for disruption of the BBB, and not vasospasm, as the initiating event in hypertensive encephalopathy.

Ischemic infarctions were associated with blood flow reductions in the homologous region of the contralateral hemisphere, a phenomenon termed "diaschisis".[122] The degree of diaschisis was correlated with the severity of ischemia.[121]

Results from studies on rats with renovascular hypertension have shown increased susceptibility to disruption under basal conditions, and during acute increases in arterial pressure.[56,123,124]

IX. THE ROLE OF THE SYMPATHETIC NERVOUS SYSTEM IN THE CEREBRAL CIRCULATION IN NORMOTENSION AND HYPERTENSION

Several lines of experimental evidence suggest that the sympathetic system exerts a protective influence on the cerebral vasculature in both acute and chronic hypertension.

When processed for catecholamine fluorescence, considerable variation in the density of cerebral adrenergic innervation has been reported, with greatest amounts present in the anterior and middle cerebral arteries, and little or no fluorescence in vertebral or basilar arteries.[125] In the SHR, however, there is evidence of an increased density of innervation, higher endogenous norepinephrine content, and a significantly elevated incidence of granular vesicle-containing nerves, which are characteristic of sympathetic nerve terminals.[126] The cerebral circulation may also possess dilator nerves containing agranular vesicles; the number of which was found to decrease or stay unchanged in the SHR.[126] Assuming similar sensitivity of vascular smooth muscle to norepinephrine, these results suggest that sympathetic influences on the cerebral circulation are augmented in this model of chronic hypertension.

In normotensive animals, the effects of sympathetic stimulation on CBF vary with species, but are generally relatively minor. In cats or dogs, flow is unchanged; in monkeys and rabbits, CBF decreases by about 25%.[127] Likewise, sympathetic denervation does not increase CBF in normotensives,[128,129] suggesting that the contribution of the sympathetic nervous system to vascular tone in the cerebral circulation is usually minimal. It should be remembered, however, that the control of flow autoregulation is complex, and other autoregulatory mechanisms (myogenic, metabolic) may compensate for changes in sympathetic influence. Thus, sympathetic stimulation constricts large pial arteries by 7 to 12% in cats, but autoregulatory dilation of downstream vessels maintains CBF at relatively normal levels.[130,131]

During an episode of acute hypertension, electrical stimulation of sympathetic nerves attenuates disruption of the BBB and the increase in CBF in cats.[132,133] This appears to be due to a vasoconstrictor effect on large cerebral arteries which increases proximal resistance, thereby decreasing pressure in small pial arteries.[134]

In rats with chronic hypertension (SHRSP), surgical interruption of the sympathetic nerves in one cerebral hemisphere at a young age (1 month) was correlated with a large increase in eventual BBB disruption on the denervated side (in 12 out of 12 rats). By comparison, the contralateral innervated hemisphere in which BBB disruption was observed occurred in only 3 out of 12 rats.[135] In a later study, it was found that unilateral ganglionectomy increased the incidence of stroke by 62.5%, relative to a sham-operated group with similar systolic arterial pressures. Cerebral hemorrhage and infarction almost always (79% of the time) developed in the denervated hemisphere. The age at which ganglionectomy is performed is important, since the incidence of stroke did not increase in the denervated hemisphere when surgery was postponed until the animals were 3 months old.

One mechanism through which the sympathetic nervous system may exert a protective effect on the cerebral circulation may be by inducing structural changes in the arterial wall. In normotensives, Bevan et al. demonstrated a trophic influence of the sympathetic nerves on cerebral artery mass in normotensives. In their study with rabbits, unilateral ganglionectomy resulted in 20 and 12% reductions in the mass of middle and posterior cerebral arteries, respectively, 8 to 10 weeks after denervation.[137]

In SHRSP rats, sympathetic denervation significantly attenuated the development of vascular hypertrophy in parenchymal but not pial cerebral arteries.[138] This trophic effect may be the primary mechanism by which the sympathetic system exerts a protective effect on the cerebral circulation in chronic hypertension, although a functional component (decrease in vasoconstrictor influence) may be present in chronic hypertensives as well, especially during sudden elevations in pressure.[127]

Werber and Heistad unilaterally denervated 1-month-old SHRSP and WKY rats.[88] One year later, they cut the superior cervical sympathetic nerve contralateral to the chronic ganglionectomy to eliminate immediate sympathetic vasoconstrictor effects. By measuring both intravascular pressures and CBF, large and small artery resistances were calculated. Under control conditions, large cerebral artery resistance was increased twofold in SHRSP, as compared with WKY, rats. This effect was more prominent (threefold increase in large-artery resistance) under maximally dilated conditions. Chronic denervation did not affect large or small artery resistance under control conditions; during maximal dilation, the resistance of chronically denervated large cerebral arteries in SHRSP was 29% lower ($p < 0.05$) than that of innervated arteries. These results suggest that the arterial caliber under activated conditions is not affected by denervation, but that the loss of a trophic sympathetic influence on larger arteries becomes unmasked when dilation is induced.

A protective effect of the sympathetic system on the cerebral circulation through hypertrophy of the arterial wall, and increased basal tone is an appealing concept. The need for caution in extrapolating SHR or SHRSP data to humans, or even to other rat models of hypertension is evident, however, when one considers the complexity of genetic, environmental, and nutritional interactions. For example, Dahl salt-sensitive rats were unilaterally ganglionectomized in the same laboratory and at the same age (1 month) as the above-mentioned SHRSPs.[139] These animals eventually developed strokes in the dorsal neocortex with hemorrhage, edema, and infarction, as well as fibrinoid necrosis of the cerebral arteries. The incidence and location of strokes, however, was similar in the innervated and denervated hemispheres. Furthermore, the type of diet ingested was found to be of critical importance to survival. After 4 months, all 37 of the rats on Japanese chow had died, whereas more than 50% of the animals on American chow were still alive. The active dietary ingredient has not been identified. Although Tobian et al.[140] reported a dramatic decrease in mortality in SHRSP rats fed the Japanese diet supplemented with potassium, in the previous study,[139] potassium levels were higher in the Japanese formulation, indicating that other components are involved.

In summary, an increase in the density of cerebral adrenergic innervation and perivascular norepinephrine content has been described. A sympathetic trophic influence on the growth of cerebral arteries has been documented; in hypertension, it may promote hypertrophy of the vascular wall and increase the wall to lumen ratio. In addition, vasoconstriction of larger cerebral arteries may further diminish the level of wall stress and increase vascular resistance. In acute hypertension, reflex sympathetic vasoconstriction of proximal cerebral arteries increases large artery resistance and protects smaller, downstream arteries from exposure to excessive distending pressures. Through these trophic and tonic neural mechanisms, the incidence of forced dilatation and subsequent BBB damage may be minimized in some, but not all, models of chronic hypertension.

X. STRUCTURAL AND BIOCHEMICAL CHANGES IN CEREBRAL ARTERIES IN CHRONIC HYPERTENSION

The most common structural change in cerebral arteries from chronically hypertensive rats is a hypertrophy of the vascular wall and an increase in the wall to lumen ratio. The extent of wall hypertrophy and the size of artery in which it is greatest may depend on age and animal model used, and on methods of tissue preparation for morphometric analysis. Body weight may be another important factor since, compared with WKY controls, the body weight of SHR and SHRSP rats is often reduced.

Structural changes within the aorta of genetically hypertensive rats may begin early in life, possibly before birth.[141] Nordborg and Johansson[142,143] measured significantly greater media to lumen ratios in larger (>80 μm) cerebral arteries of 15-day-old spontaneously hypertensive rats when compared with Wistar-Kyoto controls. When 200-day-old animals were examined, statistically significant increases in wall to lumen ratios were seen in small but not large cerebral arteries.[144] Genetic influences were also evident; significant differences in media to radius ratios were seen in 20- to 80-μm pial arteries of SHR vs. local Wistar controls; when a different normotensive control (Wistar-Kyoto) was used, significant differences were detected only in pial arteries with a lumen diameter of 20 μm or less. In a more recent study, media to radius ratios were found to be consistently higher in 7- and 12-month-old SHR and SHRSP rats in some but not all cerebral arteries examined, and over a wide (5 to 400 μm) range of arterial sizes.[145,146]

For hemodynamic significance, it is important to determine whether a hypertrophied vascular wall is also indicative of decreased lumen caliber. Hypertrophic adaptation could occur from smooth muscle cell proliferation at the medio-adventitial border and result in a thicker vascular wall without any change in internal radius. Nevertheless, during activation, when the thickness of the vascular wall increases, encroachment upon the lumen may occur. This principle was developed by Folkow[147] and is termed "structural autoregulation". Hypertrophy and vasoconstriction both favor a reduction in wall stress which, by definition, is the product of transmural pressure and radius (wall tension), divided by the thickness of the vascular wall.

The results of several studies suggest that arterial caliber is, in fact, reduced in the cerebral circulation of SHR and SHRSP rats. Brayden et al.[148] examined posterior cerebral arteries from 25-week-old WKY and SHR rats and measured a significant reduction in the inside radius of arteries from the hypertensive strain over the entire range of transmural pressures from 0 to 100 mmHg. Similar results were obtained with arteries from SHR but not SHRSP rats of the same age, although the SHRSP vessels did have a significantly higher wall to radius ratio. Wall hypertrophy was absent in age-matched SHRSP in which systolic blood pressures were kept at normotensive levels, suggesting that the effect is directly attributable to elevation of blood pressure and not genetic factors.[149]

Johansson et al.[150] monitored pial artery lumen diameter *in vivo* in 6-month-old SHR and WKY rats using a closed cranial window under normocapnic and hypercapnic conditions. Arteries in the parasagittal parietal region were observed using an intravital microscope attached to a video camera. Under both resting conditions and during maximal dilation, the diameter of SHR arteries was significantly smaller than WKY. However, presumably due to the thicker wall, the percent increase in diameter from resting levels was greater in the SHR (~55% vs. 37%).

Other mechanical and biochemical differences have been reported in cerebral arteries from hypertensive animals. The DNA content of SHR posterior cerebral arteries was elevated by 26% when compared with normotensive controls, presumably due to a comparable (28%) thickening of the medial layer.[148] The relative percentage of smooth muscle cells in the media (about 72%) was unchanged, and connective tissue (collagen and elastin) concentrations were similar. Hence, although passive distension ratios were less for the SHR, the stress-elastic modulus relationship was similar. When activated with high concentrations of KCl, arteries from hypertensives developed a similar amount of active wall tension. However, the normalized active smooth muscle cell stress was significantly (20%) decreased. This observation was supplemented with measurements of actin and myosin. When normalized to DNA content, the actin and myosin contents of SHR cerebral arteries were decreased 25 and 49%, respectively.

In summary, cerebral arteries from chronically hypertensive rats generally exhibit a hypertrophy of the vascular wall. Structural changes may be observed early in life, and become more pronounced with age and severity of hypertension. Media to lumen ratios are often increased, and some evidence exists for lumen narrowing. These changes may counteract the expected increase in wall stress and contribute to structural autoregulation. The amount of biochemical evidence is limited, but suggests the possibility of decreased contractility based on reductions in vascular smooth muscle cell actin and myosin content. Passive distensibility is decreased *in vitro*, but some preliminary *in vivo* evidence suggests that under normal, partially activated conditions, cerebral arteries in the SHRSP are more distensible than in the WKY rat.[151]

In addition to these changes, chronic hypertension produces structural changes which are more localized and characteristic of pathologic rather than purely adaptive processes. These were discussed in Sections I and II and are acceleration of atheroma formation in large arteries and fibrinoid necrosis, lipohyalin degeneration, and endothelial and smooth muscle vacuolization in the smaller arteries of the brain.[3,10,12,146]

Since length is another determinant of resistance, the geometric pattern of the vasculature or arterial rarefaction may also play a role in the development of hypertension. In this connection, it was discovered that young (1 month) normotensive WKY rats do not develop lesions from rapid occlusion of the middle cerebral artery.[152] Other animals, such as adult cats[153,154] or monkeys[155-157] develop irreversible brain lesions.

Coyle and Jokelainen subsequently found that age-matched SHRSP developed gross cortical lesions ipsilateral to the ligation whereas WKY rats did not.[158] The apparent reason is the existence of a well-developed dorsal collateral arterial supply from the anterior and posterior cerebral arteries in the young WKY. This system is poorly developed in the SHRSP.

An increase in vascular resistance due to arterial rarefaction in SHR was suggested by Hutchins and Darnell.[159] In the cerebral vasculature, rarefaction was noted in rats with renal and deoxycorticosterone-saline hypertension.[160] Conversely, in SHR rats ranging in age from 3 to 27 months, Knox[161] and Harper and Bohlen[54] did not observe a decrease in capillary or arterial density. Based on these findings, it appears likely that differences in the architecture of the vascular bed exist in various animal models of chronic hypertension. The extent of these differences may vary, and their hemodynamic importance is not well understood at this time.

XI. VASCULAR TONE AND REACTIVITY IN CHRONIC HYPERTENSION

Local and general changes in CBF autoregulation in hypertension, and structural (hypertrophy) and functional evidence (influence of the sympathetic nervous system) for increased resistance within the cerebral vasculature have already been reviewed. In this final section, hypertension-induced alterations in the dynamic properties of cerebral arteries will be considered.

Most cerebral arteries studied *in vivo*[49,50,150] or *in vitro*[66,149,162,168] possess a substantial amount of intrinsic tone. This is to say that, under *in situ* conditions, cerebral arteries may be induced to dilate anywhere from 25 to 50% above their resting diameter if vasodilating stimuli such as hypercapnea or papaverine are administered. Due to the presence of a BBB, intravenous infusions of many vasoactive agents such as ATP, norepinephrine, and angiotensin have little or no direct effect on cerebrovascular resistance and arterial diameter. When applied topically to the adventitial surface, these same interventions elicit potent constrictor or dilator effects.

The importance of endothelial thromboresistant and barrier functions in the brain has been recognized for some time. Since Furchgott and Zawadski discovered that acetylcholine induced the release of endothelial-derived relaxing factor (EDRF),[163] our perception of this tissue must be expanded to include the potential for active endothelial modulation of vascular smooth muscle cell tone and reactivity. In addition to possibly several types of EDRF, the vascular endothelium also produces prostacyclin,[164] a potent vasodilating agent and an inhibitor of platelet aggregation. Unfortunately, compared with the level of knowledge about large arteries such as the aorta, the amount of available information specific to endothelial regulatory function in cerebral arteries is extremely small, and virtually nothing is known of how this influence is affected by chronic hypertension.

In other arteries such as the aorta, significant changes in endothelial function have been observed in chronic hypertensives. For example, the normal vasodilating response to ACh is altered in favor of contraction in the aorta of SHR rats.[166] If similar changes occur in resistance-sized arteries, clearly, the potential for increasing vascular resistance by active modulation of tone and reactivity is significant. Any current review article would be incomplete without mention of this fact, and pertinent literature on endothelial regulation of cerebral artery diameter will doubtless be forthcoming. As described above, acute hypertension is known to induce structural changes in the endothelium, which may alter permeability. In one report,[167] associated changes in endothelial surface charge were also described, with loss or marked reduction of anionic groups in the cerebral arteriolar endothelium. Changes in surface charge or permeablity may indirectly alter vascular reactivity by permitting normally excluded vasoactive substances (histamine, serotonin) to come into contact with smooth muscle cell membranes.

As mentioned above, pial arteries *in vivo* operate in a partially constricted state. Studies on isolated, pressurized cerebral arteries from calves[162] and rats[66,149,168] have shown that a similar degree of intrinsic tone is present in an artery which is removed from *in vivo* neurogenic and metabolic influences. Therefore, activation appears to result from mechanisms intrinsic to the vascular wall. Active responses to stretch[169] or changes in transmural pressure which favor autoregulation of blood flow have been observed in large and small cerebral arteries from several species.[66,149,162,168] When activated with high concentrations of serotonin or potassium, rat cerebral arteries are capable of 70 to 75% reductions in lumen diameter.[66,149] According to Poiseiulle's Law, this range of constriction can theoretically produce a 256-fold change in flow.

Arteries from SHR or SHRSP rats are capable of a similar degree of maximal constriction and, in terms of percent reduction in diameter due to intrinsic tone (measured *in vitro* at a transmural pressure of 100 mmHg), develop approximately the same level of myogenic tone; lumen diameters are reduced by approximately 35%.[66,149] Although the myogenic pressure range is shifted toward higher pressures, the hypertensive vessels have a diminished capacity to constrict to changes in transmural pressure. These observations correlate with the findings of a study[148] in which smooth muscle cell actin and myosin concentrations were decreased in posterior cerebral arteries from SHR vs. WKY rats. The effect appears to be directly related to the elevation in blood pressure since treatment of SHRSP rats with an antihypertensive agent (MK 421, a converting enzyme inhibitor) from the time of weaning lowered the upper myogenic pressure limit and increased the strength of myogenic diameter responses to levels which were comparable to those previously found in normotensive WKY rats.[149]

In *in vitro*, as in *in vivo*, sudden increases in transmural pressure beyond the upper limit of the myogenic pressure range induce spontaneous dilations, forced dilation, and diminished reactivity to subsequent changes in pressure or pharmacologic stimulation.[66] In a study of arterial mechanics using excised pressurized cerebral vessels taken from normotensive rats, Halpern et al. found that, when arteries were activated with a 125-mM potassium depolarizing solution and then subjected to increasing pressure, the transmural pressure and internal radius at which forced dilatation occurred was closely correlated with the zero media tension point, calculated by using the general tension equation which is applicable to thick-walled cylinders. Zero tension was attained in depolarizing solution only when transmural pressures were on the order of 200 to 250 mmHg.[170] The implication is that, in the physiological pressure range, the vessel media is normally in a state of compression (negative wall tension). Although there are no available data on hypertensives, this observation deserves mention as it may afford a glimpse into the sometimes not-so-obvious mechanical forces which operate within the vascular wall, and which may be related to the mechanism of forced dilatation. The importance of using the general tension equation, which takes media thickness into account (and not the LaPlace formulation, which is designed for thin-walled cylinders) in the study of small-artery mechanics, becomes obvious. In arteries from hypertensives, in which the media is hypertrophied, this argument assumes even greater importance.

Pressure-dependent membrane depolarization and action potential generation have been demonstrated in cat and rat cerebral arteries.[171,172] Resting membrane potentials (E_m) were similar in SHR and WKY arteries at a transmural pressure of 0 mmHg. As pressure was elevated, there were significant reductions in Em arterial muscle from both strains. The slope of the relationship between Em and transmural pressure was significantly greater in SHR cerebral arterial muscle, suggesting that myogenic depolarization was exaggerated in chronic hypertension.

SHR and SHRSP cerebral arteries also display rhythmic oscillations in diameter which are absent in most preparations from WKY rats.[66,173,175] These oscillations have been reported in other arteries from hypertensive rats during exogenous activation with norepinephrine[174] and, in cerebral arteries, can be correlated with cyclic depolarizations in membrane potential.[173]

The underlying mechanism may be due to calcium-induced potassium efflux, as the rhythmic vasomotion can be abolished by calcium blockade with MnCl or diltiazem, by Na/K pump inhibition with ouabain, or by incubation in potassium-free physiological saline. Furthermore, rhythmic contractions can be induced in cerebral arteries from normotensives by exposure to tetraethylammonium (TEA), a potassium channel blocker.[175]

Spontaneous tone in cerebral arteries is sensitive to calcium entry blockade with diltiazem. When the sensitivity of cerebral arteries from age-matched SHRSP and WKY rats was compared, no differences could be detected.[176] Calculated IC_{50} values were 7.7×10^{-7} M (SHRSP) and 8.9×10^{-7} M (WKY), a difference which was not statistically significant. In another case, when a single dose (10^{-5} M) of verapamil was applied, the percent change in external diameter was significantly greater in SHR compared with WKY arteries pressurized to 40, 100, or 140 mmHg.[172] This finding was interpreted as evidence for an increased calcium conductance in cerebral artery smooth muscle from hypertensive rats. As our understanding of the mechanisms of action of various calcium entry blockers is improved, a more unified concept of how chronic hypertension affects vascular smooth muscle calcium dynamics may emerge.

Many studies have demonstrated functional changes in isolated blood vessels from hypertensive animals. There are considerable quantitative and qualitative differences among vascular beds. In the cerebral vasculature, Winquist and Bohr[177] studied the reactivity of ring segments of basilar arteries from normotensive WKY and hypertensive SHR rats. Animals were 3 to 5 months old at the time of sacrifice and were selected for similar body weights. Cerebral arteries from hypertensives required less stretch to achieve a given level of passive force. At a particular level of passive force, however, the levels of active force generated by a potassium depolarizing solution was significantly decreased in SHR basilar arteries. Eight out of 14 SHR vessels developed phasic activity superimposed on tonic contraction, and this activity was dependent on the presence of extracellular calcium.

Although calcium was necessary for contraction, WKY arteries were more sensitive to the constrictor effects of exogenous Ca^{++} and the maximum contractile response to a readdition of calcium to potassium depolarizing solution was significantly greater. Conversely, arteries from SHR were more sensitive to serotonin, and developed a level of tension which constituted a greater percentage of that developed in potassium depolarizing solution.

Relaxation to isoproterenol was similar in SHR and WKY arteries, but the maximal amount of relaxation was greater in WKY (51 vs. 30% in the SHR). Elevating extracellular calcium concentrations from 1.6 mM to 20 mM, an intervention which is known to have a relaxing effect on vascular smooth muscle,[178] produced greater maximal relaxation in WKY (91 vs. 76%), although this difference was significant only at a 90% level of confidence ($p < 0.1$). The concentration of calcium required to inhibit 40 mM KCl contraction by 50% was significantly less (IC_{50} for WKY = 8.3×10^{-3} M; for SHR = 12×10^{-3} M) in arteries from the normotensive strain. These observations are compatible with hypothesis of a decrease in the number of membrane-stabilizing calcium binding sites in vascular smooth muscle from the SHR.[179]

In summary, functional differences in cerebrovascular responsiveness have been measured in chronic hypertension, and their divergence exemplifies the complexity of mechanisms governing arterial function. The level of intrinsic tone may or may not be different in chronic hypertension, and there is some evidence for alterations in the effectiveness of arterial diameter adjustments to rapid changes in transmural pressure. Changes in sensitivity to some, but not other pharmacologic interventions have been reported. Differences in membrane function have been observed, although at present there is no unifying hypothesis to explain divergent findings. As new information on calcium channels in cerebral vascular smooth muscle, and on the cellular processes which link receptor- or stretch-activation and calcium entry is obtained, more complete understanding of the impact of hypertension on these mechanisms will emerge.

"We dance round in a ring and suppose,
But the Secret sits in the middle and knows."

Robert Frost

REFERENCES

1. **Packard, B.,** *Heart and Vascular Diseases*, NIH Publ. No. 84-2357, Vol. 2., 10th Rep. of the Dir., Natl. Heart, Lung, and Blood Institute, Public Health Service, National Institutes of Health, Bethesda, MD, 1982, 27.
2. **Wolf, P. A., Kannel, W. B., and Verter, J.,** Epidemiologic appraisal of hypertension and stroke risk, in *Hypertension and the Brain*, Guthrie, G. P., Jr. and Kotchen, T. A., Eds., Futura Publ., Mount Kisco, NY, 1984, chap. 11.
3. **Conomy, J. P.,** Impact of arterial hypertension on the brain. Brain in hypertension, *Postgrad. Med.,* 68, 86, 1980.
4. **Winn, H. R., Haley, E. C., and Berne, R. M.,** Cerebral blood flow regulation in normotension and hypertension, in *Hypertension and the Brain,* Guthrie, G. P., Jr. and Kotchen, T. A., Eds., Futura Publ., Mount Kisco, NY, 1984, chap. 8.
5. **Lassen, N. A.,** Cerebral blood flow and oxygen consumption in man, *Physiol. Rev.* , 39, 183, 1959.
6. **Strandgaard, S. and Paulson, O. B.,** Cerebral autoregulation, *Stroke,* 15, 413, 1984.
7. **Lassen, N. A.,** Control of cerebral circulation in health and disease, *Circ. Res.,* 34, 749, 1974.
8. **Mchedlishvili, G.,** Physiological mechanisms controlling cerebral blood flow, *Stroke,* 11, 240, 1980.
9. **Strandgaard, S.,** Autoregulation of Cerebral Circulation in Hypertension, FADL's forlag Kobenhavn, 1978.
10. **Dinsdale, H.,** Consequences of elevated arterial pressure in brain, in *Hypertension and the Brain,* Guthrie, G. P. and Kotchen, T. A., Eds., Futura Publ., Mount Kisco, NY, 1984, chap. 10.
11. **Fisher, C. M., Mohr, J. P., and Adams, R. D.,** Cerebrovascular diseases, in Harrison's *Principles of Internal Medicine,* Wintrombe, M. W., Thorn, G. W., Adams, R. D., Braunwald, E., Isselbacher, K. J., and Petersdorf, R. G., Eds., 7th ed., McGraw-Hill , New York, 1974, chap. 326.
12. **Doyle, A. E.,** Vascular complications of hypertension, in *Handbook of Hypertension,* Vol. 1, Robertson, J. I. S., Ed., Elsevier, Amsterdam, 1983, chap. 17.
13. **Takebayashi, S. and Kaneko, M.,** Electron microscopic studies of ruptured arteries in hypertensive intracerebral hemorrhage, *Stroke,* 14, 28, 1983.
14. **Dinsdale, H.B.,** Hypertensive encephalopathy, *Stroke,* 13, 717, 1982.
15. **Johansson, B., Strandgaard, S., and Lassen, N. A.,** On the pathogenesis of hypertensive encephalopathy, *Circ. Res.,* 34-35 (Suppl. 1), 167, 1974.
16. **Strandgaard, S.,** Autoregulation of cerebral blood flow in hypertensive patients, *Circulation,* 53, 720, 1976.
17. **Cole, F. M. and Yates, P. O.,** Comparative incidence of cerebrovascular lesions in normotensive and hypertensive patients, *Neurology (Minneapolis),* 18, 255, 1968.
18. **Harrison, M. J .G. and Marshall, J.,** The results of carotid angiography and cerebral infarction in normotensive and hypertensive subjects, *J. Neurol. Sci.,* 24, 243, 1975
19. **Boller, V., Vrtunski, B., Mack, J. L., and Kim, Y.,** Neuropsychologic correlates of hypertension, *Arch. Neurol.,* 34, 701, 1977.
20. **Wilkie, F. and Eisdorfer, C.,** Intelligence and blood pressure in the aged, *Science,* 172, 959, 1971.
21. **Ladurner, G., Iliff, L. D., and Lechner, G.,** Clinical factors associated with dementia in stroke, *J. Neurol. Psychiatry,* 45, 97, 1982.
22. **Okamoto, K. and Aoki, K.,** Development of a strain of spontaneously hypertensive rats, *Jpn. Circ. J.,* 27, 282, 1963.
23. **Okamoto, K., Yamori, Y., and Nagaoka, A.,** Establishment of the stroke-prone spontaneously hypertensive rats (SHR), *Circ. Res.,* 34-35 (Suppl. 1), 143, 1974.
24. **Trippodo, N. C. and Frohlich, E. D.,** Similarities of genetic (spontaneous) hypertension, man and rat, *Circ. Res.,* 48, 309, 1981.
25. **McGiff, J. C. and Quilley, C. P.,** The rat with spontaneous genetic hypertension is not a suitable model of human essential hypertension, *Circ. Res.,* 48, 455, 1981.
26. **Dahl, L. K., Heine, M., and Tassinari, L.,** Role of genetic factors in susceptibility to experimental hypertension due to chronic excess salt ingestion, *Nature (London),* 194, 480, 1962.
27. **Dahl, L. K., Heine, M., and Tassinari, L.,** Effects of chronic salt ingestion. Evidence that genetic factors play an important role in susceptibility to experimental hypertension, *J. Exp. Med.,* 115, 1173, 1962.
28. **Smirk, F. H. and Hall, W. H.,** Inherited hypertension in rats, *Nature (London),* 182, 727, 1958.
29. **Bianchi, G., Fox, U., and Imbasciati, E.,** The development of a new strain of spontaneously hypertensive rats, *Life Sci.,* 14, 339, 1974.
30. **Renaud, B., Fourniere, S., Denoroy, L., Vincent, M., Pujol, J. F., and Sassard, J.,** Early increase in phenylethanolamine-N-methyltransferase activity in a new strain of spontaneously hypertensive rats, *Brain Res.,* 159, 149, 1978.
31. **Zamir, N., Gutman, Y., and Ben-Ishay, D.,** Hypertension and brain catcholeamine distribution in the Hebrew University Sabra, H and N rats, *Clin. Sci. Mol. Med.,* 55 (Suppl. 4), 105s, 1978.
32. **Terris, J. M., Bereck, K. H., Cohen, E. L., Stanley, J. C., Whitehouse, W. M., Jr., and Bohr, D. F.,** Deoxycorticosterone hypertension in the pig, *Clin. Sci. Mol. Med.,* 51, 303, 1976.

33. **Fog, M.,** Cerebral circulation. The reaction of the pial arteries to a fall in blood pressure. *Arch. Neurol. Psychiatry,* 37, 351, 1937.

34. **Fog, M.,** Cerebral circulation II: reaction of pial arteries to an increase in blood pressure, *Arch. Neurol. Psychiatry,* 41, 260, 1939.

35. **Finnerty, F. A., Witkin, L., and Fazekas, J. F.,** Cerebral hemodynamics during cerebral ischemia induced by acute hypotension, *J. Clin. Invest.,* 33, 1227, 1954.

36. **Moyer, J. H., Miller, S. I., Tanshnek, A. B., Snyder, H., and Bowman, R. O.,** Malignant hypertension and hypertensive encephalopathy, *Am. J. Med.,* 14, 175, 1953.

37. **Moyer, J. H. and Morris, G.,** Cerebral hemodynamics during controlled hypotension induced by the continuous infusion of ganglionic blocking agents (hexamethonium, pendiomide and arfonad), *J. Clin. Invest.,* 33, 1081, 1954.

38. **Moyer, J. H., Morris, G., and Snyder, H.,** A comparison of the cerebral hemodynamic response to aramine and norepinephrine in the normotensive and the hypotensive subject, *Circulation,* 10, 265, 1954.

39. **Heistad, D. D. and Kontos, H. A.,** Cerebral circulation, in *Handbook of Physiology — the Cardiovascular System III,* American Physiological Society, Bethesda, MD, 1983, chap. 5.

40. **Haggendal, E. and Johansson, B.,** Effects of arterial carbon dioxide tension and oxygen saturation on cerebral bloodflow autoregulation in dogs, *Acta Physiol. Scand.,* 66 (Suppl. 258), 27, 1965.

41. **MacKenzie, E. T., Farrar, J. K., Fitch, W., Graham, D. I., Gregory, P. C., and Harper, A. M.,** Effects of hemorrhagic hypotension on the cerebral circulation. I. Cerebral blood flow and pial arteriolar caliber, *Stroke,* 10, 711, 1979.

42. **Symon, L., Held, K., and Dorsch, N. W. C.,** A study of regional autoregulation in the cerebral circulation to increased perfusion pressure in normocapnia and hypercapnia, *Stroke,* 4, 139, 1973.

43. **Lassen, N.A. and Agnoli, A.,** The upper limit of autoregulation of cerebral blood flow, On the pathogenesis of hypertensive encephalopathy, *Scand. J. Clin. Lab. Invest.,* 30, 113, 1972.

44. **Strandgaard, S., Jones, J. V., Mackenzie, E. T., and Harper, A. M.,** Upper-limit of cerebral blood flow autoregulationin experimental renovascular hypertension in the baboon, *Circ. Res.,* 37, 164, 1975.

45. **Dinsdale, H. B., Robertson, D. M., and Haas, R. A.,** Cerebral blood flow in acute hypertension, *Arch. Neurol.,* 31, 80, 1974.

46. **Baumbach, G. L. and Heistad, D. D.,** Heterogeneity of brain blood flow and permeability during acute hypertension, *Am. J.Physiol.,* 249, H629, 1986.

47. **Shapiro, H. M., Stromberg, D. D., Lee, D. R., and Wiederhielm, C. A.,** Dynamic pressures in the pial arterial microcirculation, *Am. J. Physiol.,* 221, 279, 1971.

48. **Tomita, M. F., Gotoh, F., Sato, T., Amano, T., Tanahashi, N., and Tanaka, K.,** Variations in resistance of larger and smaller parts of cerebral arteries with CO_2 inhalation, exsanguination, and vasodilator administration, *Acta Neurol. Scand. Suppl.,* 64, 302, 1977.

49. **Kontos, H. A., Wei, E. P., Navari, R. M., Levasseur, J. E., Rosenblum, W. I., and Patterson, J. L.,** Responses of cerebral arteries and arterioles to acute hypotension and hypertension, *Am. J. Physiol.,* 234, H371, 1978.

50. **MacKenzie, E. T., Strandgaard, S., Graham, D. I., Jones, J. V., Harper, A. M., and Farrar, J. K.,** Effects of acutely induced hypertension in cats on pial arteriolar caliber, local cerebral blood flow, and the blood-brain barrier, *Circ. Res.,* 39, 33, 1976.

51. **MacKenzie, E. T., Farrar, J .K., Fitch, W., Graham, D. I., Gregory, P. C., and Harper, A. M.,** Effects of hemorrhagic hypotension on the cerebral circulation. I. Cerebral bloodflow and pial arteriolar caliber, *Stroke,* 10, 711, 1979.

52. **Harper, S. L., Bohlen, H. G., and Rubin, M. J.,** Arterial and microvascular contributions to cerebral cortical autoregulation in rats, *Am. J. Physiol.,* 246, H17, 1984.

53. **Kety, S. S., Hafkenschiel, J. H., Jeffers, W. A., Leopold, I. H., and Shenkin, H. A.,** The blood flow, vascular resistance and oxygen consumption of the brain in essential hypertension, *J. Clin. Invest.* 27, 511, 1948.

54. **Harper, S. L. and Bohlen, G.,** Mircrovascular adaptation in the cerebral cortex of adult spontaneously hypertensive rats, *Hypertension,* 6, 408, 1984.

55. **Bradbury, M. W. B.,** The blood-brain barrier, *Circ. Res.,* 57, 213, 1985.

56. **Olesen, J.,** Quantitative evaluation of normal and pathological cerebral blood flow regulation to perfusion pressure changes in man, *Arch. Neurol. (Chicago),* 28, 978, 1973.

57. **Byrom, F. B.,** The pathogenesis of hypertensive encephalopathy and its relation to the malignant phase of hypertension, *Lancet,* 2, 201, 1954.

58. **Rodda, R. and Denny-Brown, D.,** The cerebral arterioles in experimental hypertension. I. The nature of arteriolar constriction and its effects on the collateral circulation, *Exp. Hypertension,* 49, 53, 1966.

59. **Meyer, J. S., Waltz, A. G., and Gotoh, F.,** Pathogenesis of cerebral vasospasm in hypertensive encephalopathy. I. Effects of acute increases in intraluminal blood pressure on pial bloodflow, *Neurology (Minneapolis),* 10, 735, 1960.

60. **Meyer, J. S., Waltz, A. G., and Gotoh, F.,** Pathogenesis of cerebral vasospasm in hypertensive encephalopathy. II. The nature of increased irritability of smooth muscle of pial arterioles in renal hypertension, *Neurology (Minneapolis),* 10, 859, 1960.

61. **Strandgaard, S.,** Autoregulation of cerebral blood flow in hypertensive patient. The modifying influence of prolonged antihypertensive treatment on the tolerance to acute, drug-induced hypotension, *Circulation,* 53, 720, 1976.

62. **Barry, D. I., Strandgaard, S., Graham, D. I., Braedenstrup, O., Svendsen, U. G., Vorstrup, S., Hemmingsen, R., and Bolwig, T. G.** Cerebral blood flow in rats with renal and spontaneous hypertension: resetting of the lower limit of autoregulation, *J. Cereb. Blood Flow Metab.,* 2, 347, 1982.

63. **Jones, J. V., Fitch, W., MacKenzie, E. T., Strandgaard, S., and Harper, A. M.,** Lower limit of cerebral blood flow autoregulation in the baboon, *Circ. Res.,* 39, 555, 1976.

64. **Fujishima, M. and Omae, T.,** Lower limit of cerebral autoregulation in normotensive and spontaneously hypertensive rats, *Experientia,* 32, 1019, 1976.

65. **Sadoshima, S., Yoshida, F., Ibayashi, S., Shiokawa, O., and Fujishima, M.,** Upper limit of cerebral autoregulation during the development of hypertension in spontaneously hypertensive rats — effect of sympathetic denervation, *Stroke,* 16, 477, 1985.

66. **Osol, G. and Halpern, W.,** Myogenic properties of cerebral blood vessels from normotensive and hypertensive rats, *Am. J. Physiol.,* 249, H914, 1985.

67. **Strandgaard, S., Olesen, J., Skinhoj, E., and Lassen, N. A.,** Autoregulation of brain circulation in severe arterial hypertension, *Br. Med. J.,* I, 507, 1973.

68. Editorial: Thought for autoregulation in the hypertensive patient, *Lancet,* 2, 510, 1979.

69. Editorial: Dangerous antihypertensive treatment, *Br. Med. J.,* I, 228, 1979.

70. **Ledingham, J. G. G. and Rajagopalan, B.,** Cerebral complications in the treatment of accelerated hypertension, *Q. Med. J.,* 48, 25, 1979.

71. **Graham, D. I.,** Ischaemic brain damage of cerebral perfusion failure type after treatment of severe hypertension, *Br. Med. J.,* 4, 739, 1975.

72. **Cove, D. H., Seddon, M., Fletcher, R. F., and Dakes, D. C.,** Blindness after treatment for malignant hypertension, *Br. Med. J.,* 1, 245, 1979.

73. **Barry, D. I., Strandgaard, S., Graham, D. I., Svendsen, U. G, Braendstrup, O., and Paulson, O.,** Cerebral blood flow during dihydralazine-induced hypotension in hypertensive rats, *Stroke,* 15, 102, 1984.

74. **Hertz, M. M., Hemmingsen, R., and Bolwig, T. B.,** Rapid and repetitive measurements of blood flow and oxygen consumption in the rat brain using intraarterial Xenon injection, *Acta Physiol. Scand.,* 101, 501, 1977.

75. **Auer, L. M., Sayama, I., and Johansson, B. B.,** Cerebrovascular effects of dihydralazine in hypertensive and normotensive rats, *Acta Med. Scand. Suppl.,* 678, 73, 1983.

76. **Barry, D. I., Strandgaard, S., Graham, D. I., Braendstrup, O., Svendsen, U. G., and Bolwig, T. G.,** Effect of diazoxide-induced hypotension on cerebral blood flow in hypertensive rats, *Eur. J. Clin. Invest.,* 13, 201, 1983.

77. **Barry, D. I., Paulson, O. B., Jarden, J. O., Juhler, M., Graham, D. I., and Strandgaard, S.,** Effects of captopril on cerebral blood flow in normotensive and hypertensive rats, *Am. J. Med.,* 76, 79, 1984.

78. **Vorstrup, S., Barry, D. I., Jarden, J. O., Svendsen, U. G., Braendstrup, O., Graham, D. I., and Strandgaard, S.,** Chronic antihypertensive treatment in the rat reverses hypertension-induced changes in cerebral blood flow autoregulation, *Stroke,* 15, 312, 1984.

79. **Jackson, G., Pierscianowski, T. A., Mahon, W., and Condon, J.,** Inappropriate hypertensive therapy in the elderly, *Lancet,* 2, 1317, 1976.

80. **Ruff, R. L., Talman, W. T., and Petito, F.,** Transient ischemic attacks associated with hypotension in hypertensive patients with carotid artery stenosis, *Stroke,* 12, 353, 1981.

81. **Britton, M., DeFaire, U., and Helmers, C.,** Hazards of therapy for excessive hypertension in acute stroke, *Acta Med. Scand.,* 207, 253, 1980.

82. **Lee, R. M. K. W., Ed.,** *Blood Vessels Changes in Hypertension: Structure and Function,* Vols. 1 and 2, CRC Press, Boca Raton, FL, 1989.

83. **Auer, L.,** The pathogenesis of hypertensive encephalopathy, *Acta Neurochir. Suppl.,* 29, 1, 1978.

84. **Kontos, H. A., Wei, E. P., Dietrich, W. D., Navari, R. M., Povlishock, J. T., Ghatak, N. R., Ellis, E. F., and Patterson, J. L., Jr.,** Mechanism of cerebral arteriolar abnormalities after acute hypertension, *Am. J. Physiol.,* 240, H511, 1981.

85. **Heistad, D. D., Marcus, M. L., and Gross, P. M.,** Effects of sympathetic nerves on cerebral vessels in dog, cat, and monkey, *Am. J. Physiol.,* 235, H544, 1978.

86. **Heistad, D. D. and Marcus, M. L.,** Effect of sympathetic stimulation on permeability of the blood-brain barrier to albumin during acute hypertension in cats, *Circ. Res.,* 45, 331, 1979.

87. **Johansson, B., Li, C.-H., Olsson, Y., and Klatzo, I.,** The effect of acute arterial hypertension on the blood-brain barrier to protein tracers, *Acta Neuropathol. (Berlin),* 16, 117, 1970.

88. **Werber, A. H. and Heistad, D. D.,** Effects of chronic hypertension and sympathetic nerves on the cerebral microvasculature of stroke-prone spontaneously hypertensive rats, *Circ. Res.,* 55, 286, 1984.

89. **Baumbach, G. L. and Heistad, D. D.,** Heterogeneity of brain blood flow and permeability in hypertension, *Am. J. Physiol.,* 249, H629, 1985.

90. **Fukasawa, H.,** Hemodynamical studies of cerebral arteries by means of mathematical analysis of vascular casts, *Tohoku J. Exp. Med.,* 99, 255, 1969.

91. **Johansson, B. B.,** Effect of an acute increase of the intravascular pressure on the blood-brain barrier, *Stroke,* 9, 588, 1978.

92. **Farrar, J. K., Jones, J. V., Graham, D. I., Strandgaard, S. ,and MacKenzie, E. T.,** Evidence against cerebral vasospasm during acutely induced hypertension, *Brain Res.,* 104, 176, 1976.

93. **Yamori, Y., Horie, R., Handa, H., Sato, M., and Fukase, M.,** Pathogenetic similarity of strokes in stroke-prone spontaneously hypertensive rats and humans, *Stroke,* 7, 46, 1976.

94. **Robertson, D. M., Dinsdale, H. B., Hayashi, T., and Tu, J.,** Cerebral lesions in adrenal regeneration hypertension, *Am. J. Pathol.,* 59, 115, 1970.

95. **Kontos, H. A.,** Oxygen radicals in cerebral vascular injury, *Circ. Res.,* 57, 508, 1985.

96. **Wei, E. P., Ellison, M. D., Kontos, H. A., and Povlishock, J. T.,** O_2 radicals in arachidonate-induced increased blood-brain barrier permeability to proteins, *Am. J. Physiol.,* 251, H693, 1986.

97. **Haggendal, E. and Johansson, B.,** Pathophysiological aspects of the blood-brain barrier change in acute arterial hypertension, *Eur. Neurol.,* 6, 24, 1972.

98. **Skinhoj, E. and Strandgaard, S.,** Pathogenesis of hypertensive encephalopathy, *Lancet,* 1, 461, 1973.

99. **Baumbach, G. L., Mayhan, W. G., and Heistad, D. D.,** Protection of the blood-brain barrier by hypercapnia during acute hypertension, *Am. J. Physiol.,* 251, H282, 1986.

100. **Hansson, H., Johansson, B. B., and Blomstrand, C.,** Ultrastructural studies on cerebrovascular permeability in acute hypertension, *Acta Neuropathol.,* 32, 187, 1975.

101. **Nag, S., Robertson, D. M., and Dinsdale, H. B.,** Cerebral cortical changes in acute experimental hypertension. An ultrastructural study, *Lab. Invest.,* 36, 150, 1977.

102. **Nag, S., Robertson, D. M., and Dinsdale, H. B.,** Quantitative estimate of pinocytosis in experimental acute hypertension, *Acta Neuropathol.,* 46, 107, 1979.

103. **Povlishock, J. T., Kontos, H. A., Rosenblum, W. I., Becker, D. P., Jenkins, W., and DeWitt, D. S.,** A scanning electron-microscopic analysis of the intraparenchymal brain vasculature following experimental hypertension, *Acta Neuropathol.,* 51, 203, 1980.

104. **Mayhan, W. G. and Heistad, D. D.,** Permeability of blood-brain barrier to various sized molecules, *Am. J. Physiol.,* 248, H712, 1985.

105. **Westergaard, E.,** The blood-brain barrier to horseradish peroxidase under normal and experimental conditions, *Acta Neuropathol.,* 39, 181, 1977.

106. **Farrell, C. L. and Shrivers, R. R.,** Capillary junctions of the rat are not affected by osmotic opening of the blood-brain barrier, *Acta Neuropathol.,* 63, 179, 1984.

107. **Ziylan, Y. A., Robinson, P. J., and Rapoport, S. I.,** Differential blood-brain barrier permeabilities to macromolecules of different sizes after osmotic opening, *J. Cereb. Blood Flow Metab.,* 3, 423, 1983.

108. **Hansson, H. A., Johansson, B., and Blomstrand, C.,** Ultrastructural studies on cerebrovascular permeability in acute hypertension, *Acta Neuropathol.,* 32, 187, 1975.

109. **Bronsted, H. E. and Westergaard, E.,** Vesicular transport of proteins from blood to brain during acute hypertension, *Acta Physiol. Scand.,* 95, 67A, 1975.

110. **Lee, R. M. K .W., Garfield, R. E., Forrest, J. B., and Daniel, E. E.,** Smooth muscle cell herniation in the contracted arterial wall of spontaneously hypertensive and normotensive rats, *Acta Anat.,* 119, 65, 1984.

111. **Joris, I. and Majno, G.,** Endothelial changes induced by arterial spasm, *Am. J. Pathol.,* 102, 346, 1981.

112. **Rappoport, S.I.,** Pathological alterations of the blood-brain barrier, in *Blood-Brain Barrier in Physiology and Medicine,* Raven Press, New York, 1976, 131.

113. **Ito, U., Ohno, K., Yamaguchi, T., Takei, H., Tomita, H., and Inaba, Y.,** Effect of hypertension on blood-brain barrier change after restoration of blood flow in post-ischemic gerbil brains, *Stroke,* 11, 606, 1980.

114. **Giacomelli, F., Wiener, J., and Spiro, D.,** The cellular pathology of experimental hypertension. V. Increased permeability of cerebral arterial vessels, *Am. J. Pathol.,* 59, 133, 1970.

115. **Eto, T., Omae, T., and Yakamoto, T.,** An electron microscope study of hypertensive encephalopathy in the rat with renal hypertension, *Arch. Histol. Jpn.,* 33, 133, 1971.

116. **Hazama, F., Amano, S., Haebara, H., Yamori, Y., and Okamoto, K.,** Pathology and pathogenesis of cerebrovascular lesions in spontaneously hypertensive rats, in *The Cerebral Vessel Wall,* Cervos-Navarro, J., Betz, E., Matakas, F., and Wullenweber, R., Eds., Raven Press, New York, 1976, 245.

117. **Giacomelli, F., Rooney, J., and Wiener, J.,** Cerebrovascular ultrastructure and permeability after carotid artery constriction in experimental hypertension, *Exp. Mol. Pathol.,* 28, 309, 1978.

118. **Majack, R. A. and Bhalla, R. C.,** Ultrastructural characteristics of endothelial permeability pathways in chronic hypertension, *Hypertension,* 3, 586, 1981.

119. **Mueller, S. M. and Heistad, D. D.,** Effect of chronic hypertension on the blood-brain barrier, *Hypertension,* 2, 809, 1980.

120. **Tamaki, K., Sadoshima, S., and Heistad, D. D.,** Increased susceptibility to osmotic disruption of the blood-brain barrier in chronic hypertension, *Hypertension,* 6, 633, 1984.

121. **Tamaki, K., Sadoshima, S., Baumbach, G. L., Iadecola, C., Reis, D. J., and Heistad, D. D.,** Evidence that disruption of the blood-brain barrier precedes reduction in cerebral blood flow in hypertensive encephalopathy, *Hypertension,* 6 (Suppl. 1), 75, 1984.

122. **Slater, R., Reivich, M., Goldberg, H., Banka, R., and Greenberg, J.,** Diaschisis with cerebral infarction, *Stroke,* 8, 684, 1977.

123. **Johansson, B. B. and Linder, L. E.,** The blood-brain barrier in renal hypertensive rats, *Clin. Exp. Hypertension,* 2, 983, 1980.

124. **Mueller, M. and Luft, F.C.,** The blood-brain barrier in renovascular hypertension, *Stroke,* 13, 229, 1982.

125. **Lee, T. J. -F.,** Ultrastructural distribution of vasodilator and constrictor nerves in cat cerebral arteries, *Circ. Res.,* 49, 971, 1981.

126. **Lee, T. J. -F. and Saito, A.,** Altered cerebral vessel innervation in the spontaneously hypertensive rat, *Circ. Res.,* 55, 392, 1984.

127. **Heistad, D. D.,** Effects of nerves on cerebral vessels in stroke, cerebral edema, and hypertension, *J. Lab. Clin. Med.,* 99, 139, 1982.

128. **Sadoshima, S., Thammes, M., and Heistad, D.,** Cerebral blood flow during elevation of intracranial pressure: effects of sympathetic nerves, *Am. J. Physiol.,* 10, H78, 1981.

129. **Mueller, S. M., Heistad, D. D., and Marcus, M. L.,** Total and regional cerebral blood flow during hypotension, hypertension, and hypocapnia: effect of sympathetic denervation in dogs, *Circ. Res.,* 41, 350, 1977.

130. **Kuschinsky, W. and Wahl, J.,** Alpha-receptor stimulation by endogenous and exogenous norepinephrine and blockade by phentolamine in pial arteries of cats, *Circ. Res.,* 37, 168, 1975.

131. **Wei, E. P., Raper, A. J., Kontos, H. A., and Patterson, J. L., Jr.,** Determinants of response of pial arteries to norepinephrine and sympathetic nerve stimulation, *Stroke,* 6, 654, 1975.

132. **Bill, A. and Linder, J.,** Sympathetic control of cerebral blood flow in acute arterial hypertension, *Acta Physiol. Scand.,* 96, 114, 1976.

133. **Beausang-Linder, M. and Bill, A.,** Cerebral circulation in acute arterial hypertension — protective effects of sympathetic nervous activity, *Acta Physiol. Scand., 1*11, 193, 1981.

134. **Heistad, D. D., Marcus, M. L., and Abboud, F. M.,** Role of large arteries in regulation of cerebral blood flow in dogs, *J. Clin. Invest.,* 62, 761, 1978.

135. **Sadoshima, S. and Heistad, D. D.,** Sympathetic nerves protect the blood-brain barrier in stroke-prone spontaneously hypertensive rats, *Hypertension,* 4, 904, 1982.

136. **Sadoshima, S., Busija, D. W., and Heistad, D. D.,** Mechanisms of protection against stroke in stroke-prone spontaneously hypertensive rats, *Am. J. Physiol.,* 244, H406, 1983.

137. **Bevan, R. D., Tsuru, H., and Bevan, J. A.,** Cerebral artery mass in the rabbit is reduced by chronic sympathetic denervation, *Stroke,* 14, 393, 1983.

138. **Hart, M. N., Heistad, D. D., and Brody, M. J.,** Effect of chronic hypertension and sympathetic denervation on wall/lumen ratio of cerebral vessels, *Hypertension,* 2, 419, 1980.

139. **Werber, A. H., Baumbach, G. L., Wagner, D. V., Mark, A. L., and Heistad, D. D.,** Factors that influence stroke in Dahl salt-sensitive rats, *Hypertension,* 7, 59, 1985.

140. **Tobian, L., Lange, F., Ulm, K., Wold, L., and Iwai, J.,** Potassium reduces cerebral hemorrhage and death rate in hypertensive rats, even when blood pressure is not lowered, *Hypertension,* 7 (Suppl. 1), 110, 1985.

141. **Gray, S. D.,** Anatomical and physiological aspects of cardiovascular function in Wistar-Kyoto and spontaneously hypertensive rats at birth, *Clin. Sci.,* 63 (Suppl. 8), 383, 1982.

142. **Nordborg, C. and Johansson, B. B.,** The ratio between thickness of media and internal radius in cerebral, mesenteric, and renal arterial vessels in spontaneously hypertensive rats, *Clin. Sci.,* 57 (Suppl 5), 27, 1979.

143. **Nordborg, C. and Johansson, B. B.,** Morphometric study on cerebral vessels in spontaneously hypertensive rats, *Stroke,* 11, 266, 1980.

144. **Nordborg, C. and Johansson, B. B.,** Cerebral vessels in spontaneously hypertensive rats, *Acta Neuropathol. Suppl.,* 7, 369, 1981.

145. **Nordborg, C., Fredricksson, and Johansson, B. B.,** The morphometry of consecutive segments in cerebral arteries of normotensive and spontaneously hypertensive rats, *Stroke,* 16, 313, 1985.

146. **Johansson, B. B.,** Cerebral vascular bed in hypertension and consequences for the brain, *Hypertension,* 6 (Suppl. 3), 81, 1984.

147. **Folkow, B.,** Structural autoregulation — the local adaptation of vascular beds to chronic changes in pressure, in *Development of the Vascular System,* Ciba Foundation Symposium 100, O' Connor, Ed., Pitman, London, 1983, 56.

148. **Brayden, J. E., Halpern, W., and Brann, L. R.,** Biochemical and mechanical properties of resistance arteries from normotensive and hypertensive rats, *Hypertension,* 5, 17, 1983.

149. **Osol, G. and Halpern, W.,** Effect of antihypertensive treatment on myogenic properties of brain arteries from the stroke-prone rat, *J. Hypertension,* 4 (Suppl. 3), 5517, 1986.

150. **Johansson, B. B., Auer, L. M., and Sayama, I.,** Reaction of pial arteries and veins to hypercapnia in hypertensive and normotensive rats, *Stroke,* 16, 320, 1985.

151. **Baumbach, G. L., Dobrin, P. B., Hart, M. N., and Heistad, D. D.,** Cerebral vascular mechanics in hypertension, *Circulation,* 72 (Suppl. III), 255, 1985.

152. **Coyle, P.,** Middle cerebral artery occlusion in the young rat, *Stroke,* 13, 855, 1982.

153. **Sundt, T. M., Jr. and Waltz, A. G.,** Experimental cerebral infarction: retroorbital, extradural approach for occluding the middle cerebral artery, *Mayo Clin. Proc.,* 41, 159, 1966.

154. **O' Brien, M. D. and Waltz, A. G.,** Transorbital approach for occluding the middle cerebral artery without craniectomy, *Stroke,* 4, 201, 1973.

155. **Waltz, A. G. and Sundt, T. M.,** The microvasculature and microcirculation of the cerebral cortex after arterial occlusion, *Brain,* 90, 681, 1967.

156. **Hudgins, W. R. and Garcia, J. H.,** Transorbital approach to the middle cerebral artery of the squirrel monkey: a technique for experimental cerebral infarction applicable to ultrastructural studies, *Stroke,* 1, 1107, 1970.

157. **Garcia, J. H. and Kamijyo, S.,** Cerebral infarction. Evolution of histopathological changes after occlusion of the middle cerebral artery in primates, *J. Neuropathol. Exp. Neurol.,* 33, 408, 1974.

158. **Coyle, P. and Jokelainen, P. T.,** Differential outcome to middle cerebral artery occlusion in spontaneously hypertensive stroke-prone rats (SHRSP) and Wistar Kyoto (WKY) rats, *Stroke,* 14, 605, 1983.

159. **Hutchins, P. M. and Darnell, A. E.,** Observation of a decreased number of small arterioles in spontaneously hypertensive rats, *Circ. Res.,* 34 (Suppl. I), 161, 1974.

160. **Sokolova, I. A., Radionov, I. M., and Blinkov, S. M.,** Rarefaction of capillary network in the brain of rats with induced DOCA-saline and renal hypertension, *Microvasc. Res.,* 22, 125, 1981.

161. **Knox, C. A.,** Effects of aging and chronic arterial hypertension on the cell populations in the neocortex and archicortex of the rat, *Acta Neuropathol.,* 56, 139, 1982.

162. **Vinall, P. E. and Simeone, F. A.,** Cerebral autoregulation: an in vitro study, *Stroke,* 12, 640, 1981.

163. **Furchgott, R. F. and Zawadski, J. V.,** The obligatory role of endothelial cells in the relaxation of arterial smooth muscle by acetylcholine, *Nature (London),* 288, 373, 1980.

164. **Moncada, S., Herman, A. G., Higgs, E. A., and Vane, J. R.,** Differential formation of prostacyclin (PGX or PGI) by layers of the arterial wall. An explanation for the antithrombotic properties of vascular endothelium, *Thromb. Res.,* 11, 323, 1977.

165. **Bunting, S., Moncada, S., and Vane, J.,** The prostacyclin-thromboxane A2 balance: pathophysiological and therapeutic implications, *Br. Med. Bull.,* 39, 271, 1983.

166. **Luscher, T. F. and Vanhoutte, P. M.,** Endothelium-dependent contractions to acetylcholine in the aorta of the spontaneously hypertensive rat, *Hypertension,* 8, 244, 1986.

167. **Nag, S.,** Cerebral endothelial surface charge in hypertension, *Acta Neuropathol.,* 63, 276, 1984.

168. **Dacey, R. G., Jr. and Duling, B. R.,** A study of rat intracerebral arterioles: methods, morphology and reactivity, *Am. J. Physiol.,* 243, H598, 1982.

169. **Toda, N., Hatano, Y., and Hayashi, S.,** Modification by stretches of the mechanical response of isolated cerebral and extracerebral arteries to vasoactive agents, *Pfluegers Arch.,* 374, 73, 1978.

170. **Halpern, W., Mongeon, S. A., and Root, D. T.,** Stress, tension, and myogenic aspects of small isolated extraparenchymal rat arteries, in *Smooth Muscle Contraction,* Stephens, N. L., Ed., Marcel Dekker, New York, 1984, 427.

171. **Harder, D. R.,** Pressure-dependent membrane depolarization in cat middle cerebral artery, *Circ. Res.,* 55, 197, 1984.

172. **Harder, D. R., Smeda, J., and Lombard, J.,** Ehnanced myogenic depolarization in hypertensive cerebral arterial muscle, *Circ. Res.,* 57, 319, 1985.

173. **Harder, D. R., Brann, L., and Halpern, W.,** Altered membrane electrical properties of smooth muscle cells from small cerebral arteries of hypertensive rats, *Blood Vessels,* 20, 154, 1983.

174. **Lamb, F. S., Myers, H., Hamlin, M. N., and Webb, R.,** Oscillatory contractions in tail arteries from genetically hypertensive rats, *Hypertension,* 7 (Suppl. 1), 25, 1985.

175. **Osol, G. and Halpern, W.,** Spontaneous vasomotion in pressurized cerebral arteries from genetically hypertensive rats, *Am. J. Physiol.,* 254, H28, 1988.

176. **Osol, G., Osol, R., and Halpern, W.,** Effects of diltiazem on myogenic tone in pressurized brain resistance arteries from normotensive and hypertensive rats, in *Proc. Int. Symp. Mech. Trt. Ess. Hypert.,* Aoki, K., Ed., Academic Press, Orlando, FL, 1986, in press.

177. **Winquist, R. J. and Bohr, D. F.,** Structural and functional changes in cerebral arteries from spontaneously hypertensive rats, *Hypertension,* 5, 292, 1983.

178. **Bohr, D. F.,** Vascular smooth muscle: dual effect of calcium, *Science,* 139, 597, 1963.

179. **Holloway, E. T. and Bohr, D. F.,** Reactivity of vascular smooth muscle in hypertensive rats, *Circ. Res.,* 33, 678, 1973.

Chapter 3

ENDOTHELIUM AND SMOOTH MUSCLE INTERACTIONS IN HYPERTENSION

Alex L. Loeb and Michael J. Peach

TABLE OF CONTENTS

I. INTRODUCTION

A. Importance of Endothelium as the Surface of the Vessel

The endothelial cell stands at the interface between the blood and the rest of the body. Although not the load bearing cell in the vessel wall, it is in a prime position to modulate the activity of the load bearing smooth muscle cells. Being located at the vessel lumen, one of the most obvious functions of the endothelium is to act as a barrier to blood-borne elements. In fact, for a long time, the barrier function, which extends to capillary endothelium as well, was thought to be the primary role of the endothelium. These cells were thought to selectively regulate the passage of varied substances between the blood and tissues. Among the first active functions of the endothelium to be determined was the ability to take up, modify, and transport blood-borne agents. The endothelium also can act as an endocrine organ in response to stimuli to release prostaglandins, growth factors, relaxing factors, and constricting substances, all of which have the potential to modulate growth or reactivity of the underlying smooth muscle. In addition, smooth muscle cells and nerve terminals have the ability to synthesize and release substances which can modulate endothelial cell function.

B. Potential Changes in Smooth Muscle-Endothelium Interactions in Hypertension

An increase in blood pressure has the potential to alter many of the normal smooth muscle-endothelium interactions. As will be discussed in detail below, hypertension has been associated with an increase in endothelial permeability and a breakdown of the integrity of the vessel lining. Endothelial damage potentially can impair important metabolic functions of the endothelial cell layer, thereby allowing exposure of the vessel wall to factors with which it normally does not come into contact. Pressure-induced changes also have the potential to alter the ability of the endothelium to release smooth muscle conditioning factors or to alter the responsiveness of the smooth muscle cells and vascular nerve terminals to substances or signals derived from endothelium.

II. EFFECT OF HYPERTENSION ON THE ENDOTHELIAL CELL BARRIER

A. Protection of Smooth Muscle from Circulating Vasoactive Agents

Although not all vessels have the same characteristics,[1] in general, it is well established that vessels with intact endothelium are much better at preventing the penetration of dyes and labeled lipids[2] into the smooth muscle layers than are vessels with damaged endothelium. Many large molecules and proteins, however, can pass readily through the endothelial cell layer into the vessel media. Albumin,[3-5] fibrinogen,[6] horseradish peroxidase, and ferritin,[8] have all been shown to pass through the endothelial layer by vesicular transport[9] and/or passage through intercellular junctions.

Endothelial cells also play a major role in controlling the presentation of smaller vasoactive compounds to the media. It has been demonstrated clearly that the endothelium is a major site of biogenic amine uptake and metabolism.[10-13] Uptake is Na-dependent, temperature-dependent, saturable, and inhibited by cocaine and imipramine. Autoradiographic studies have localized the uptake process to endothelium in both capillaries and large arteries.[12-16]

B. Effects of Hypertension on Barrier Functions

Increased blood pressure has the potential to alter many facets of blood vessel structure and function, including changes in endothelial cells. Changes in the permeability of the endothelium during hypertension are some of the best understood effects in endothelium-smooth muscle interactions. Goldby and Beilin[17] first proposed that endothelial injury resulted from an elevation in blood pressure. Subsequently, Huttner et al.[18] clearly demonstrated that endothelial permeability to horseradish peroxidase (HRP) and ferritin was increased in animals made hypertensive by either aortic coarctation or catecholamine infusion when compared to normotensive controls. In models of hypertension studied by these investigators, peroxidase products appeared earlier in the subendothelial space than in controls, suggesting that the barrier function of the endothelium was compromised. Robertson and Khairallah[19] found that acute hypertension caused by infusion of angiotensin (Ang)II led to an increase in rat aortic endothelial permeability not only to HRP, but also to ferritin, colloidal carbon, low density lipoprotein, and very low density liopoprotein. The changes in permeability were associated with structural changes in the endothelium such as opening of intercellular gaps and nuclear pinching. In chronic hypertension, similar changes in endothelial permeability and morphology have been reported.[20-24]

Alterations in endothelial permeability have implications in hypertension; as permeability increases, the access of vasoactive blood-borne substances to smooth muscle also is enhanced. The apparent sensitivity of the smooth muscle for these agents could be greater because the actual concentrations presented to the medial layer would be increased.

III. EFFECT OF HYPERTENSION ON ENDOTHELIAL METABOLISM OF VASOACTIVE SUBSTANCES

In addition to acting as a physical barrier between the blood and smooth muscle of the vessel wall and surrounding tissue, the endothelium performs important metabolic functions such as activation or inactivation of circulating autacoids, hormones, and neurotransmitters. These processes may be the most important mechanisms by which vasoactive agents are processed within the circulation.

A. Biogenic Amines

Biogenic amines such as norepinephrine (NE), phenylethylamine, and serotonin are actively taken up into endothelial cells.[13,16,25,26] These compounds are metabolized intracellularly by monoamine oxidase and the catecholamines, by catechol-*O*-methyl transferase, and the metabolic products exported out of the cell.[13,27] Cultured endothelial cells from the cow, pig, rabbit, and human[28-30] also have been shown to retain these metabolic capabilities. Pressor responses to serotonin are potentiated markedly following short periods of acute severe hypertension, comparable to alterations seen following balloon injury to the endothelium.[31,-33]

Biogenic amine metabolism is altered in hypertensive animals. Cassis et al.[34] have shown that caudal arteries from spontaneously hypertensive rats (SHR) had higher endogenous NE levels and a more active uptake mechanism than did Wistar-Kyoto normotensive controls (WKY) These investigators also found that NE metabolism by monoamine oxidase in this vessel was increased in SHR compared to WKY. In mesenteric vessels, there were no differences in NE metabolism between SHR and WKY even through the SHR vessels contained more NE.[35]

Instances where biogenic amine uptake has been studied during periods of acute pulmonary hypertension, a condition known to damage endothelium, have suggested, that serotonin and NE removal are increased.[36] In another study,[37] NE removal was decreased. A number of conditions associated with pulmonary endothelial damage also result in changes in catecholamine removal.[38] These findings suggest that hypertension, which can affect endothelial function also may alter the ability of the endothelium to take up and metabolize biogenic amines, thereby changing the amount available for interaction with smooth muscle.

B. Nucleotides

Adenosine triphosphate (ATP), adenosine diphosphate (ADP), and adenosine are very important modulators of blood vessel tone. ATP is released into the circulation by the adrenal medulla, following cell damage, and from aggregating platelets[39] and following treatment of endothelium with acetylcholine.[40] ATP and ADP are potent dilators and may act via a purine receptor (P2) distinct from the adenosine receptor (P1).[41] Circulating ATP, ADP, and adenosine monophosphate (AMP) are almost completely metabolized by the pulmonary endothelium during one passage through the lung.[42,43] These nucleotides are broken down by a series of enzymes present on endothelial plasma membranes which metabolize ATP into ADP (nucleoside triphosphatase) and ADP into AMP (nucleoside diphosphatase) and AMP into adenosine (5'-nucleotidase).[44] The large surface area of the endothelium contributes greatly to rapid adenosine uptake from the circulation. Although adenosine is taken up by both endothelium and subendothelial tissue, Nees et al.[45] have shown that when labeled adenosine is infused into the guinea pig heart, about 80% is removed by the endothelium even though the endothelium makes up less than 5% of the total cardiac mass. Recent data[46] suggest that under physiological conditions, adenosine within the vascular space is taken up and metabolized before it can reach the underlying smooth muscle. Additionally, the endothelium has an adenosine A_2 receptor which activates adenylate cyclase resulting in cAMP levels. Much of the cAMP is exported from the cell.[47]

Once taken up by the endothelium, adenosine usually is metabolized to adenine nucleotides, of which ATP is the dominant form.[44] This intracellular store of ATP can be broken down and released by the endothelium (mostly as adenosine, but also as inosine or hypoxanthine) in response to a variety of factors including hypercapnia, hypoxia, H_2O_2, or inhibition of phosphorylation.[44,45,48] The release of adenosine in response to various stimuli may be of considerable consequence since adenosine is in itself a potent vasodilator and acts directly on vascular smooth muscle via the P1 (A_2) receptor to increase cellular cAMP and to cause relaxation.

C. Peptides

1. Angiotensin I

After Ng and Vane[49] demonstrated the rapid and essentially complete conversion of Ang I to Ang II across the pulmonary vascular bed, immunohistochemical techniques were used to firmly establish that converting enzyme was localized to the lumenal surface of pulmonary vascular endothelial cells.[50] Fluorescein-labeled antibodies to converting enzyme primarily detected the enzyme in vascular endothelium of all organs examined in the rabbit.[51] The enzyme was then demonstrated in cultured endothelial cells from several species where it was concentrated in the plasma membrane.[52-54] In spite of a vast literature over the last decade regarding converting enzyme and the endothelium, almost nothing is known about mechanisms which control the synthesis and turnover of the enzyme or its enzymatic activity. There is no evidence that hypertension alters the kinetic rate or capacity of the endothelium to metabolize (convert) Ang I to Ang II.

2. Bradykinin

In 1967 Yang and Erdos[55] identified an enzyme in human plasma and hog kidney which hydrolyzed the COOH-terminal Phe-Arg dipeptide from bradykinin. They named this enzyme, kininase II. One year later, Bakhle[56] discovered that a small quantity of a crude preparation of bradykinin-potentiating factor (BPF) inhibited both converting enzyme and kininase II activities in a plasma membrane fraction of dog lung. Subsequent purification of BPF yielded several peptides many of which blocked the enzymatic hydrolysis of Ang I and bradykinin.[57] Once a homogenous converting enzyme preparation was obtained from rabbit[58,59] and hog lung,[60] it was clear that converting enzyme possessed kininase II activity.

In hypertension it has been proposed that the plasma levels of bradykinin and kallidin are decreased. However, there is no evidence that hypertension causes any change in the degradation of plasma kinins by converting enzyme in the endothelium. Inactivation of kinins by kininase I (carboxypeptidase) also appears to be normal in hypertensive animals. There have been reports that the hypotensive response to converting enzyme inhibitors in hypertensive animals and humans is dependent in part on increased plasma kinin levels.[61,62] This hypothesis does not require that hypertension be associated with accelerated rates of inactivation of the plasma kinins. In fact urinary kallikrein levels are low in hypertensive individuals and animals[63] which may suggest that the synthesis of kinins is impaired in animal models and humans with this disease.

3. Angiotensin II

Angiotensin II is eliminated rapidly when perfused through vascular beds (except the lung). All evidence indicates the Ang II is cleared from the circulation by enzymatic hydrolysis. This octapeptide also is degraded by isolated vascular strips,[64] perfused vessels, and cultured endothelial and arterial smooth muscle cells.[65] Inactivation of the peptide by the vessel wall primarily involves aminopeptidases. Ryan et al.[52] have localized and characterized an aminopeptidase in the plasma membrane of endothelial cells. Robertson and Khairallah[66] and Richardson and Beaulnes[67] have reported the uptake of Ang II by arterial endothelium. This uptake may play an important role in the delivery of Ang II to destructive peptidases. However, we found that the removal of the endothelium from rabbit aorta did not alter dose-dependent responses to Ang II,[68] suggesting a minor role for endothelium in this tissue in the elimination of the peptide. In spite of the earlier work by Leary and Ledingham,[69] there is no evidence of impaired inactivation of Ang II by endothelium in models of hypertension.

4. Other Peptides

There are several other vasoactive peptides (e.g., vasopressin, oxytocin, substance P, bombesin, parathyroid hormone, calcitonin gene-related peptide, vasoactive intestinal polypeptide, neuropeptide Y, atriopeptin, enkephalins, etc.) which have been proposed to play roles in cardiovascular regulation. Some of these peptides have even been shown to be hydrolyzed by purified preparations of converting enzyme. However, the kinetics for degradation of any of these peptides by converting enzyme are quite unimpressive. Most if not all of these peptides have short durations of action and they clearly are metabolized once they enter the circulation. Whether or not the endothelium plays a major role in clearing any of these peptides remains to be studied (as well as whether or not any modulation of catabolism occurs when blood pressure is elevated).

D. Lipids

1. Eicosanoids

a. Arachidonate

Systemic vascular endothelium synthesizes prostaglandins PGE_2, $PGF_{2\alpha}$, and prostacyclin (PGI_2[70,71]). Isolated vascular tissues also have been shown to synthesize 12-hydroxyeicosatetraenoic acid (HETE), 15-HETE, and leukotriene (LT) D_4.[72-75] In general, the vasculature synthesizes very little thromboxane (TXA_2).[76] However, the rabbit pulmonary arteries synthesize TXA_2[77,78] and epoxides,[79] and bovine aortic endothelial cell cultures (but not other species) can produce TXA_2.[80] Cultured endothelium also has been shown to produce PGI_2, PGE_2, and $PGF_{2\alpha}$.[81-86] The endothelium has been reported to contain cytochrome P450 which oxidizes arachidonic acid to unstable epoxides.[87-90]

None of the changes reported in models of hypertension for the type(s) or amount of given eicosanoids produced have been associated with any alterations in the amount of endothelial cell cyclooxygenase, lipoxygenase, or cytochrome P450 or their enzymatic activities. Increased or decreased rates of eicosanoid synthesis also could reflect changes in the activity of phospholipases (or the rates of reacylation of fatty acids into phospholipids) and thus the amount of free arachidonate available to these oxidases. Changes may occur in the kinetics of the various enzymes which catalyze conversion of PGG_2, PGH_2, HPETE, HETE, and epoxides to more biologically active compounds (e.g., PGI_2, TXA_2, PGE_2, $PGF_{2\alpha}$, LTs, diHETE, etc.). A situation also could develop where altered levels of any eicosanoid might represent enhanced or impaired rates of enzymatic catabolism.

Until about 1982, investigators who performed *in vitro* studies with vascular segments did not consider the integrity of the endothelium in their preparations. Without assessment of the endothelium, arachidonate metabolism by vessels removed from hypertensive or normotensive animals may have varied simply because of variable degrees of damage to the endothelium which occurred while preparing the vessels for study. Nevertheless, numerous investigators have proposed that eicosanoid production is altered by hypertension.[91,92] Because most of the prostaglandins undergo extensive clearance in the lung and liver, they never achieve significant circulating plasma levels and are thought to function locally at or near their site of production. The exceptions are the leukotrienes and PGI_2[93,94] which are produced at sufficient rates relative to clearance (even by lung) to function as hormones.[95]

In isolated vessels, the endothelium is responsible for a large fraction of the total PGI_2 synthesized.[70,96] Morera[97] studied the metabolism of ^{14}C-arachidonate by arterial rings from rats with two kidney, one clip Goldblatt hypertension. In all vessels studied the predominant metabolite of arachidonate was PGI_2. During the first 6 days after clipping the renal artery, synthesis of PGI_2 was increased 2.5-fold over controls. However, during the chronic phase of hypertension, PGI_2 synthesis was the same as in arterial preparations from sham-operated rats. Dusting et al.[98] reported that rat aorta only made ^{14}C-6-keto-$PGF_{1\alpha}$ when treated with labeled arachidonate. They found that aorta from rats with chronic two kidney, one clip hypertension made the same amount of PGI_2 as did control aorta. In contrast, the production of PGI_2 was increased in aorta from rats with one kidney, one clip hypertension. An earlier study[99] had found that depressor responses to exogenous arachidonate were enhanced in one kidney, one clip rats but not in the two kidney, one clip model of hypertension. In the perfused mesenteric artery, the SHR rat[100] was found to have higher basal rates of production of PGI_2 than the WKY. However, Soma et al.[101] have reported recently that synthesis of 6-keto-$PGF_{1\alpha}$, PGE_2, and TXB_2 was decreased in perfused mesenteric arteries from the SHR rat. Since synthesis of all three eicosanoids was depressed, they suggested that less free arachidonate was available in arteries from the hypertensive rat.

Early *in vivo* studies in the SHR rat reported an increased synthesis of PGI_2 vs. normotensive WKY.[102,103] Others have reported more recently no change in the urinary excretion of 6-keto-$PGF_{1\alpha}$ in the SHR[104,105] and decreased levels of this PGI_2 metabolite excreted in urine with salt loading.[106] Falardeau and Martineau[107] also have reported that PGI_2 synthesis was reduced in the

Dahl salt-sensitive rat given a high salt diet. In renovascular hypertensive rats (two kidney, one clip), urinary levels of 6-keto-PGF$_{1\alpha}$ and PGE$_2$ were not different from controls.[108]

With regard to other eicosanoids in the SHR, urinary excretion (and plasma levels) of PGE$_2$ and PGF$_{2\alpha}$ were identical in SHR vs. WKY rats.[109,104] In isolated glomeruli obtained from SHR and WKY rats, basal production of PGF$_{2\alpha}$ and 6-keto-PGF$_{1\alpha}$ were the same. However, enhanced rates of synthesis of PGE$_2$, PGF$_{2\alpha}$, and 6-keto-PGF$_{1\alpha}$ were observed in glomeruli from the SHR compared to WKY in response to arachidonate and calcium ionophore.[110] Excessive amounts of TXA$_2$ are produced by isolated glomeruli from SHR [110] as well as the isolated perfused kidney.[111,112] Urinary excretion of TXB$_2$ has been shown to be elevated in the SHR rat.[104] There is no evidence that conversion of TXA$_2$ is altered by hypertension.

In other models of hypertension in the rat (e.g., Dahl and Lyon strains), urinary excretion of PGE$_2$ was decreased when hypertensive animals were compared to normotensive ones.[113,114] During the chronic phase of hypertension in the two kidney, one clip Goldblatt dog, renal production of PGE was reported to be increased over the levels observed prior to production of hypertension.[115] Conflicting data regarding PGs also exist for mineralocorticoid/salt hypertension in the rat, rabbit, and dog.

b. PGE-9-Ketoreductase

Bovine mesenteric blood vessels contain large amounts of PGE-9-ketoreductase. This enzyme catalyzes the reduction of the 9-keto group of PGE$_2$ to yield PGF$_{2\alpha}$.[116] Bradykinin was shown to induce a two- to threefold increase in PGE-9-ketoreductase activity in bovine mesenteric vessels.[117] There is no evidence that this enzyme is localized to the endothelium or that its activity is altered in hypertension.

c. Prostaglandin 15-Hydroxydehydrogenase

PGs lose most biologic activity when acted upon by this enzyme. Both arteries and veins have been shown to contain high levels of PG 15-hyroxydehydrogenase activity.[118] This enzyme catalyzes the inactivation of PGE$_2$ and PGF$_{2\alpha}$ and the conversion of PGI$_2$ to 6,15-diketo-PGF$_{1\alpha}$.[119-121] Selective tissue uptake of certain prostaglandins in the pulmonary circulation precedes metabolism. Less than 20% of PGI$_2$ has been shown to be degraded during a single passage through the lung. This reflects the low affinity of PGI$_2$ for the tissue transport system.[122]

Decreased PG 15-hydroxydehydrogenase activity and impaired metabolism of PGs has been reported in the New Zealand genetic hypertensive rat.[123,124] The SHR rat also has been shown to have impaired catabolism of prostaglandins.[125-127] An endogenous inhibitor of PG 15-hydroxydehydrogenase has been extracted from the kidneys of the New Zealand hypertensive rat.[128] Very little is known about regulation of this enzyme.

It is not clear that reduced activity of this enzyme in hypertension in any way contributes to prolonged half-lives or elevated plasma levels of any prostaglandin.

d. 6-Keto-PGE$_1$

It has been suggested that blood vessels convert PGI$_2$ to 6-keto-PGE$_1$ which is not destroyed by the lung.[129,130] Many of the biological activities of PGI$_2$ are mimicked by 6-keto-PGE$_1$.[131] Studies related to this metabolite in models of hypertension have not been reported.

2. Platelet Activation Factor (PAF)

The role of the endothelium in the metabolism of PAF and the effects of hypertension on any interaction between the endothelium and this neutral lipid remains to be established. The endothelium has been shown to contain PAF but it is not clear how much is synthesized vs. accumulated (taken up) by endothelial cells. Since the endothelium may not be able to release PAF, uptake may account for a large percentage of the total amount of PAF extracted from this tissue. The effects of hypertension on PAF catabolism are unknown.

3. Endothelium-Derived Relaxation Factor (EDRF)

There is no reason to assume that the endothelium participates in the clearance or metabolism of EDRF. Any effect of hypertension on the half life of EDRF remains to be determined.

IV. ENDOTHELIUM-DERIVED SMOOTH MUSCLE GROWTH MODULATORS

A. Endothelium-Derived Growth Factors

The mitogens produced by cultured endothelium from a variety of species are very potent polypeptide growth factors.[132-134] Part of this activity can be explained by the fact that the endothelium is able to synthesize and release a compound indistinguishable from the platelet-derived growth factor (PDGF). PDGF is a cationic peptide which, when bound to its cell surface receptor, triggers a wide range of intracellular events resulting in cell proliferation (for review, see Ross et al.[135]). This peptide, originally isolated from platelets, has be shown to stimulate the growth of smooth muscle and other cells of mesenchymal origin in culture such that their saturation density was dependent on the concentration of PDGF.[136,137] Most of the cells that have receptors for, and respond to, PDGF were found to be connective tissue-forming cells such as smooth muscle, glia, fibroblasts, and chondrocytes.[135] However, the principal cell type lacking PDGF receptors was the arterial endothelium.[135]

The connection between endothelium and smooth muscle becomes apparent when the endothelial cell integrity is disrupted. *In vivo*, it has been proposed that sticking of platelets to the vessel wall and subsequent release of PDGF at the site of endothelial cell damage by platelets as well as endothelium results in proliferation of smooth muscle cells.[138] However, not all of the mitogenic activity secreted from endothelium is due to PDGF. Gadjusek et al.,[132] have shown that medium conditioned by cultured endothelium contains potent growth factors for nonendothelial cells which are distinct from PDGF. In fact, only about 25% of the mitogenic activity released from endothelial cells can be attributed to PDGF.[133,139,140]

B. Inhibitory Actions of Endothelium on Smooth Muscle Growth

In addition to producing smooth muscle growth promoting factors, the endothelium has been shown to release factors which inhibit smooth muscle growth.[140,141] The factor(s) responsible for the inhibition of smooth muscle proliferation *in vivo*[142] and *in vitro*[143] are heparin-like molecules produced by confluent, but not subconfluent endothelium.[144] The balance between the mitogenic and antiproliferative influences of endothelium on smooth muscle growth probably are most dependent on the state of endothelial cell replication, either *in vivo* or *in vitro*.[140] The loss of inhibitory influences from the endothelium after endothelial injury may be partially responsible for the medial hyperplasia seen after endothelial damage or denudation. In the denudation experimental injury model,[145] the endothelial cells lining the arterial wall are removed, usually by a mechanical means. At the site of injury, endothelium probably stop producing antiproliferating factors and begin to release mitogens. The injury also promotes adherence of granulocytes and monocytes which may generate mitogens. In addition, if the site of injury is large enough, exposure of the subendothelial surface to the circulation permits adherence, aggregation, and degranulation of platelets with additional PDGF release. This is followed by smooth muscle cell migration from the media into the intima and rapid smooth muscle cell proliferation. When the endothelial lining has regenerated, smooth muscle growth is diminished, probably because the confluent endothelium release smooth muscle growth inhibitors.[140]

In sustained hypertension, there is almost always a thickened vascular wall due to an increase in medial mass,[146] which may be due to smooth muscle cell hyperplasia[147,148] or hypertrophy with accompanying smooth muscle polyploidy.[149-151] Both of these processes are associated with an increase in smooth muscle DNA synthesis.[147,152] One possible explanation for the increase in medial DNA synthesis may be that the stimulus for the development of the hypertension and/ or the blood pressure increase signals the endothelium to switch off the production of the endothelium-derived antiproliferative factor. Evidence for this type of change in endothelium was first demonstrated by Schwartz and Benditt,[153] who showed that during the initial 2 to 3 weeks after the induction of renal hypertension in rats, the rate of aortic endothelial replication rose about tenfold above control levels. This increase in cell replication has been shown in several experimental models of hypertension.[154] The loss of contact inhibition and subsequent increase in endothelial cell replication might also inhibit the release of the heparin-like inhibitors of cell proliferation and potentiate the release of mitogens from the endothelium.

C. Nonmitogenic Effects of Growth Factors

In addition to its mitogenic effects, PDGF has been shown to be a potent constrictor of vascular smooth muscle. PDGF, at doses thought to be present in serum[155] and which are mitogenic for rat smooth muscle cells in culture,[156] also will cause contractions of rat aorta *in vitro*.[157] These contractions are independent of endothelial integrity and indomethacin, suggesting a direct contractile effect. Comparable results have been obtained with epidermal growth factor (EGF). The PDGF-induced contractions appeared to be associated with increases in intracellular free calcium levels as measured by increased Fura-2 fluorescence of PDGF-stimulated cultured rat aortic smooth muscle cells. These findings suggested that contractions to PDGF were mediated by processes similar to those of other vasoconstrictor substances, such as Ang II and NE, which also increase intracellular calcium.

D. Summary

The ability of the endothelium to modulate growth within the vessel wall cannot be overlooked. In hypertension, when the antiproliferative effects of the endothelium may be attenuated, the actions of mitogens to induce wall hypertrophy or hyperplasia and to directly increase the level of vascular tone could contribute significantly to increased vascular resistance and blood pressure.

V. ENDOTHELIUM-DERIVED MODULATORS OF VESSEL TONE

In addition to acting as a barrier to blood-borne vasoactive agents either as an actual physical diffusion barrier or as a metabolic barrier, the endothelium can synthesize and release compounds which can alter vessel tone directly. These compounds have the potential to increase as well as decrease blood pressure. Although the ultimate control of blood pressure is the result of a myriad of competing signals, an alteration in the synthesis, storage, release, or response to locally acting, tonically released, endothelium-derived substances could prove catastrophic to the delicate balance of feedback loops controlling vasoactive hormone release, neuronal activity levels, and central reflexes. The homeostatic mechanisms normally controlling blood pressure could be disturbed enough to produce or exacerbate hypertension.

A. Relaxing Factors

The discovery of endothlelium-dependent vasodilation at the beginning of the 1980s opened a new and rapidly expanding field of research. Furchgott and Zawadzki demonstrated in their landmark paper[158] that isolated preparations of precontracted arteries could be relaxed by a variety of agents in an endothelium-dependent manner. They found that low doses of acetylcholine (Ach, 10^{-8} to 10^{-6} M) induced relaxation of preconstricted rabbit aorta only if the endothelial layer was intact. Higher doses of Ach caused aortic contraction which was independent of the integrity of the endothelium. The endothelium-dependent relaxation with Ach was inhibited by muscarinic antagonists, although the particular muscarinic receptor subtype has yet to be elucidated. Eglen and Whiting[159] have examined the Ach muscarinic receptor subtype responsible for vasodilation and determined that the receptor profile was different from that described for gastrointestinal smooth muscle, myocardium, and the CNS.

Transfer of the EDRF was first demonstrated by "sandwiching" the intima of an intact piece of aorta against the lumenal side of an aortic strip without endothelium, which was set up to record contractions. Stimulation of the preparation with Ach-induced relaxation of the strip without endothelium only when the piece of vessel with endothelium was present, confirming the endothelial requirement for the response.[138] Transfer of EDRF from intact vascular segments with endothelium and from cultured cells under a variety of conditions also has been reported. Griffith et al.[160] reported early on that EDRF could be released from an intact segment of rabbit aorta and bioassayed by the relaxation of a denuded segment of coronary artery connected to the donor vessel by a canula. They estimated the half-life of EDRF in solution to be approximately 6 s using this technique. By decreasing the degree of oxygenation from 95% O_2 to 20% O_2, Forstermann et al.[161] demonstrated that the half-life of EDRF could be prolonged in transit to between 24 and 50 s when released from rabbit or canine arteries, respectively. EDRF also has been shown to be released from cultured endothelium,[162-168] suggesting that the compound can act as an endocrine substance.

To assay the substance under conditions where relaxation cannot be measured, a biochemical parameter which is associated with smooth muscle relaxation must be used. The most appropriate biochemical parameter appears to be the stimulation of guanylate cyclase and the subsequent accumulation of intracellular smooth muscle cyclic GMP. In fact, cyclic GMP levels have been increased in most cases in which endothelium-dependent vasodilation has been studied in concert with smooth muscle guanylate cyclase activity, and this response is very similar to that produced by the directly acting nitrovasodilators.[164,169-172] Relaxation responses which require endothelium are potentiated by selective inhibitors of cyclic nucleotide phosphodiesterase,[173,174] especially agents which impair cyclic GMP degradation. In addition compounds that are known to inhibit guanylate cyclase (e.g., methylene blue, hemoglobin, ETYA, etc.) interfere with endothelium-dependent relaxation of arterial smooth muscle.[175,176] In some studies, cultured endothelium from porcine[162] or bovine[162,164,166] sources were put into coculture with arterial smooth muscle cells. Stimulation of the cultures with agents known to release EDRF induced large increases in cyclic GMP levels, whereas stimulation of pure endothelial or smooth muscle cultures had no effect on cyclic GMP levels. These results suggested that the cyclic GMP response in cultured smooth muscle could be used as a bioassay for the presence of EDRF, and that EDRF was produced by the cultured endothelium.

Studies from a number of laboratories have shown that EDRF released from cultured endothelium grown on microcarrier beads also will relax vascular smooth muscle.[163-165,167,168,177] For these experiments, the endothelial cells grown on microcarriers were placed into a column superfused with physiological buffer. EDRF released from the cells after stimulation by agonists was bioassayed by measuring the relaxation of preconstricted, endothelium-denuded arterial segments bathed by the column effluent. Alternatively, the cell effluent could be directed onto cultured smooth muscle or arterial rings, which could then be assayed for changes in cyclic GMP content. Using this technique, Loeb et al.[164] demonstrated a very close correlation between EDRF-induced relaxation and cyclic GMP accumulation in bioassay tissues exposed to the endothelial cell column effluent.

B. Calcium Channel Activators/Ionophores/Calcium

The most potent stimulus of EDRF release discovered to date appears to be the calcium ionophore, A23187. Maximal relaxation to A23187 is always greater than with muscarinic agonists.[178,179] The response to the ionophore is reversible and sensitive to the presence of calcium in the external medium. The calcium channel activators maitotoxin and BAY K 8644 also will stimulate EDRF release, which can be inhibited by verapamil or nitrendipine pretreatment. The response to channel activators is measureable only once, due to concomitant pronounced and sustained activation of muscle contraction by these agents.[180,181] In fact almost all stimuli of EDRF release which have been examined require the presence of extracellular calcium. Several groups of investigators have shown that deletion of calcium from the bath fluid will significantly depress the release of EDRF from intact aorta in response to muscarinic agonists, ionophore (A23187), ATP, bradykinin, substance P, histamine, thrombin, etc.[179,180] Long and Stone[182] demonstrated that the decreased response was due to decreased release of EDRF from the endothelium, rather than a depression of muscle relaxation. In transfer experiments in which the intact EDRF donor vessel was exposed to zero calcium buffer while a denuded assay vessel was maintained in normal calcium buffer, they found that the EDRF response to Ach was modulated purely by changing the calcium concentration around the source of endothelium. In a further demonstration of the calcium dependence of the response, our laboratory has shown that the responses to Ach, bradykinin, maitotoxin, and A23187 could be attenuated by calcium blockers.[179,180]

The EDRF response is not dependent entirely upon the presence of extracellular calcium, however. We have found that melittin, a small polypeptide component of bee venom, will induce a transient release of EDRF even in the absence of extracellular calcium.[164] In addition, the melittin response is unaffected by verapamil pretreatment. This paradox can be explained by the fact that, in the absence of extracellular calcium, melittin causes a large increase in intracellular calcium which apparently comes from intracellular stores.[163,180,183] Other agents requiring extracellular calcium to release EDRF may depend upon receptor-activated calcium transloca- tion or, as in the case of A23187, BAY K 8644, or maitotoxin, on the direct influx of calcium to initiate the calcium-mediated release of EDRF. Melittin is not as dependent on extracellular calcium for activity since it can induce release of calcium from intracellular stores.

C. Biogenic Amines

Although the biogenic amines typically are associated with inducing contraction of smooth muscle, there have been a limited number of reports indicating a concomitant effect to induce release of a relaxing substance from endothelial cells. Cocks and Angus[32] demonstrated that NE and serotonin were much less efficacious vasoconstrictors in coronary arteries with intact endothelium than in vessels without endothelium. These investigators showed that in vessels without endothelium the dose-response curves to these two amines was shifted up and to the left. Contractions to the thromboxane analog, U46619, were unaffected and K^+ contractions were decreased by endothelium removal. They ultimately demonstrated that activation of α_2 adrener- gic- and ketanserin-insensitive serotonin receptors (S1) were responsible for endothelium- dependent modulation of tone. Since this report numerous investigators have shown potentia- tion of α_2-induced contractions following removal of the endothelium.

D. Nucleotides

The nucleotides ATP, ADP, and 5′-AMP all have been demonstrated to cause release of EDRF. Several groups of investigators have presented evidence that the relaxing properties of ATP in the dog femoral artery[184] and rabbit aorta[178] were dependent upon an intact endothelium. DeMey and Vanhoutte[184] showed that disruption of the endothelium decreased the ED_{50} of ATP and ADP for relaxation in this tissue from 10^{-5} to 10^{-4} M, a value not different from adenosine and 5′-AMP, which in the dog are endothelium-independent vasodilators. In pig aorta, Gordon and Martin[185] demonstrated that a major part of the relaxations to 5′-AMP and adenosine as well as that to ATP and ADP are endothelium dependent. In the rabbit femoral artery, ATP induced an endothelium-dependent relaxation which was correlated with a rise in cyclic GMP levels.[186] ATP-induced endothelium-dependent vasodilation in most cases results from stimualtion of a P_2 purinoceptor[187] since theophylline, a P_1 purinoceptor (adenosine antagonist), had no effect on ATP-induced relaxation of canine arteries.[184,185] The rabbit central ear artery is an exception, since 8-phenyltheophylline, a potent P_1 receptor antagonist blocked ATP-induced, endothe- lium-dependent relaxations.[187] In the rabbit femoral artery, the P_2 receptor photoaffinity antagonist ANAPP$_3$ blocked endothelium-dependent relaxation to ATP.[186]

In most vessels, adenosine-induced relaxation is endothelium-independent.[41] This nucleo- tide is believed to act directly on the smooth muscle inducing vasodilation through a cyclic AMP-mediated process.[186]

The endothelium-dependent relaxations in rabbit aorta to adenine nucleotides are greatly, but not completely, inhibited by 10^{-4} M ETYA and not inhibited at all by cyclooxygenase inhibitors. These results indicate that the endothelium-dependent response is similar to that obtained with Ach, A23187, melittin, etc. In addition to inducing endothelium-dependent relaxations, ATP stimulates increases in smooth muscle cyclic GMP levels in intact rat aorta[169] and in mixed cultures of pig or bovine endothelium and aortic smooth muscle.[162,164] There is some evidence, however, that EDRF released by ATP is different. DeMey et al.[188] reported that ETYA did not inhibit or reverse ATP-induced relaxation in the dog femoral artery. Sata et al.,[189] have presented data in both guinea pig and rat aorta, showing that endothelium-dependent relaxation and cyclic GMP accumulation induced by Ach, but not ATP, were inhibited by the spin trap reagent, phenyl-t-butylnitrone (PBN). On the basis of these findings ATP was postulated to induce relaxation via a different factor than the EDRF released by Ach.

E. Peptides

The first peptide found to release EDRF was the nonapeptide, bradykinin. Since then, a host of vasoactive peptides also has been reported to cause EDRF release. These include substance P and other tachykinins (bombesin, octa-choleycystokinin, eledoisin, kassanin, and physalaemin which function through the substance P receptor) as well as calcitonin-gene-related peptide, antidiuretic hormone, oxytocin, melittin, (and Ang II in chicken arteries and canine renal vein). These peptides appear to act via specific receptors since there is no loss of sensitivity to the relaxing ability of bradykinin after desensitization of the substance P receptor.[178] In addition, the relaxing action of bradykinin (but not other peptides) can be reversed by specific kinin receptor blockers.

Bradykinin originally was thought to cause relaxation through release of a prostaglandin since it was known to cause release of the vasodilator PGI_2, from endothelial cells. However, inhibition of PGI_2 formation did not prevent bradykinin-induced endothelium-dependent vasodilation in most muscular arteries.[178] It must be remembered that in vessels which do relax in response to PGI_2, that bradykinin probably causes dilation by the release of both PGI_2 and EDRF from the endothelial cells.

Thrombin and trypsin have both been shown to induce EDRF release[73,171,178,190] which is associated with smooth muscle cyclic GMP accumulation. The vasodilator properties of both of these serine proteases are inhibited by phospholipase A_2 blockade[171] and D-phenyl-alanyl-L-propyl-L-arginine chlormethyl ketone (PPACK), a protease inhibitor.[190] PPACK is thought to inhibit serine protease through the irreversible interaction with the histidine molecule in the enzyme active (catalytic) site.[190]

Although these agents are capable of proteolytic damage to the cell surface after prolonged exposure, repeated short exposure to either enzyme will result in tachyphylaxis to that agent alone and will not affect Ach- or ATP-induced relaxations.[190] Ku[190] also found that the action of thrombin, but not trypsin, was inhibited by heparin and antithrombin III; while trypsin (but not thrombin) relaxation was blocked by soybean trypsin inhibitor and aprotinin. These results suggest that it is the proteolytic action of thrombin and trypsin which is responsible for stimulation of EDRF release. We have found recently that plasmin specifically inhibits thrombin-induced EDRF release in rat aorta.[191]

F. Lipids

1. Platelet Activating Factor (PAF)

PAF (1-O-octadecytl-2-O-acetyl-glycero-3-phosphorylcholine) is a lipid which was first isolated from the kidney by Muirhead and colleagues.[192-194] This compound has marked blood pressure lowering properties when given either orally or intravenously to both normotensive and hypertensive rats. The compound also has been identified as a mediator of immediate hypersensitivity and is released from sensitized basophils and macrophages.[195-197] This substance stimulates the aggregation of platelets and the release of their contents, hence the name PAF. In studies designed to determine the mechanism of action of PAF, Kamitani et al.[198] and Shigenobu et al.[199] determined that the hypotensive action of PAF in isolated rat aorta was at least partially dependent upon the presence of intact endothelium. According to Kamitani et al.,[198] there were no effects of hypertension (renal or DOCA salt) on the vasodilator response to PAF *in vivo* when rats were given the drug i.v. or p.o. However, they did not examine the effects of PAF on isolated vessels from the hypertensive animals. Although PAF is present in the endothelium, it is not clear whether or not the factor is released from endothelium into the circulation.

2. Prostacyclin

One of the first chemical candidates among known compounds for the substance EDRF was PGI_2.[158] It was known that PGI_2 was a potent vasodilator[94,201] and that this eicosanoid was released from endothelial cells both *in vivo* and *in vitro*.[70,202,203] On the basis of these findings, stimulation of PGI_2 release from the endothelium could cause endothelium-dependent relaxation. In fact, Toda[204] has shown this to be true for Ang II- and histamine-stimulated relaxation of preconstricted canine arteries. Holtz et al.[205] have demonstrated that PGI_2 may have a role in the modulation of tone in some vascular beds. These investigators found that cyclooxygenase inhibition increased the basal level of tone in the coronary arteries of conscious dogs. Van Grondelle et al.[206] examined the release of PGI_2 in isolated lungs and cultured endothelial cells during alterations of flow or sheer stress, respectively, and reported that increases in these physical parameters also induced increases in PGI_2 release. These findings, taken together, suggest that PGI_2 released from endothelial cells can act as a dilator of smooth muscle in those vascular beds that respond to this eicosanoid. Vascular PGI_2 release is stimulated by many of the same stimuli that release EDRF, bradykinin, ATP, A23187[207] Ach and melittin.[96]

PGI_2 is not EDRF, however, since many vascular beds that respond to EDRF do not respond to PGI_2.[207,208] In addition, all agents that induce EDRF release do so in the presence of cyclooxygenase inhibitors[154] In summary, PGI_2 can be classified as an endothelium-derived relaxing substance which, in vascular beds sensitive to its vasodilator action, acts in concert with EDRF to modulate vascular tone. It should be noted that PGI_2 activates adenylate cyclase and causes a rise in intracellular cyclic AMP levels.

3. Fatty Acids and Triglycerides

Furchgott et al.[209] recently have found that saturated and unsaturated fatty acids of differing carbon chain lengths can cause relaxant responses which are dependent upon the presence of intact endothelium and are insensitive to cyclooxygenase inhibition. These included *cis*-4,7,10,13,16,19-docoshexanoic, oleic, elaidic, *cis*-vaccenic, and stearic acid. Data of this type suggest that exogenously added arachidonic acid, although postulated to be a precursor of EDRF, may act *in vitro* to induce the release of the factor rather than serve as a metabolic precursor of EDRF. The fatty acids mentioned above may release EDRF by displacing an endogenous lipid precursor from the plasma membrane; by enhancing the activity of endogenous phospholipase; by causing changes in membrane fluidity;[209] or by triggering ion flux across the membrane. We have found that while arachidonate does not require the presence of extracellular Ca^{2+} to release EDRF, several of the other fatty acids mentioned above do require the presence of this divalent cation for relaxing activity.[253]

4. Arachidonic Acid and Nonprostaglandin Metabolites

Although PGI_2 is not EDRF, many compounds which stimulate PGI_2 synthesis and release also promote the release of EDRF. This finding suggested to many that EDRF may be arachidonic acid, which is liberated prior to PGI_2 formation, or some other noncyclooxygenase metabolite of arachidonic acid.

Exogenous arachidonic acid (AA) applied to a preconstricted intact aortic ring will induce relaxation which is dependent on the endothelium. This was first demonstrated by Singer and Peach.[208] These investigators found that high doses (1 to 100 μM) of AA could relax preconstricted rings of rabbit aorta. The relaxation was potentiated when cyclooxygenase inhibitors were present, suggesting the concomitant production by the vessel segment of eicosanoids, some of which may be vasoconstrictor prostaglandins. Rings without endothelium responded to exogenous AA with a small contraction which also was blocked by cyclooxygenase inhibition. In the absence of tone in rabbit aorta, AA induced endothelium-dependent vasoconstriction which was blocked by indomethacin. Cherry and co-workers[210] have reported similar relaxation responses in canine femoral arteries treated with AA with doses of 10 to 100 μM. Lower doses (<1 μM) produced dilation which was blocked by cyclooxygenase inhibitors, findings similar to those reported by DeMey and Vanhoutte.[73] The relaxations induced by the lower AA concentrations were probably due to PGI_2.[73] Arachidonate also induces endothelium-dependent relaxation of rat aorta.[169]

Ignarro et al.[211] have examined the effects of both high (micromolar) and low (submicromolar) concentrations of exogenous AA on bovine intrapulmonary arteries and veins. They found that indomethacin inhibited relaxations of the arteries to low doses of AA and potentiated relaxations at doses of AA greater than 10 μM. Indomethacin pretreatment prevented the concomitant rise in intracellular cAMP levels, but not the rise in tissue cGMP concentrations. In arteries without endothelium, and in veins with or without endothelium, exogenous AA induced constriction. In these tissues indomethacin prevented the contractions, suggesting a constrictor eicosanoid was being produced from AA by cyclooxygenase.

Several investigators recently have utilized agents thought to mobilize endogenous AA in order to examine the role of this fatty acid in the elaboration of EDRF. For this purpose, studies have relied on phospholipases or on the direct phospholipase A_2 activator, melittin, a polypeptide derived from bee venom,[212] to release AA from tissues or cells. Forstermann and Neufang[96] and Loeb et al.[164] have shown that melittin induces endothelium-dependent relaxation which is not affected by cyclooxygenase inhibition. The relaxation response to melittin was inhibited by ETYA, NDGA, mepacrine, p-bromophenacyl bromide, BW 755C, and hydroquinone, agents which block EDRF-dependent relaxation. Melittin, like other compounds which release EDRF, induced an increase in cyclic GMP levels within the tissue. Repetitive exposures to melittin will induce reproducible relaxation responses if the concentration of peptide does not exceed 3 or 4 $\mu g/ml$. Concentration of melittin of 5 $\mu g/ml$ or greater are toxic and cause cell lysis.[213]

Melittin has been shown to release endogenous AA and one of its metabolites, PGI_2 from endothelium.[214-217] In fact, melittin may act to liberate AA from membranes which then acts on its own to release EDRF. Studies from our laboratory have shown that melittin will induce a (dose-dependent) release of ^3H-AA from cultured endothelium of up to 40% of the total releasable ^3H-AA pool. In addition, both melittin and AA have similar relaxation profiles—there is a delay of 60 to 90 s after either agent is added to a tissue bath before the beginning of relaxation. Other agents typically induce relaxation with little delay (i.e., than that time necessary for mixing). Another important similarity between melittin and exogenous AA is the lack of a requirement for extracellular Ca^{2+} for full peak relaxant action. These agents are the only two endothelium-dependent dilators studied to date which do not require extracellular Ca^{2+} for their activity (164). Other vasodilators such as Ach, and A23187, do require Ca^{2+} for their actions.[172,182,208]

Forstermann et al.[168] have used thimerosal, an agent which inhibits acyl-CoA, and lysolecithin acyltransferase (LAT), an enzyme which resynthesizes diacylphospholipids from their component parts, to stimulate EDRF release. Inhibition of LAT would prevent the incorporation of AA into phospholipids and therefore increase the amount of AA available for metabolism. They found that thimerosal was able to release EDRF on its own, and in subthreshold concentrations, could significantly potentiate the actions of other endothelium-dependent vasodilators. This is another approach which implicates endogenous release of AA in the formation of EDRF.

Although AA itself is not EDRF, the possibility remains that AA may be a precursor to EDRF, as described above. This hypothesis has been based on the observations that inhibitors of nonprostaglandin metabolites of AA also will inhibit EDRF-induced relaxation. The other routes of AA metabolism described in endothelial cells or the vessel wall to date are through the lipoxygenase[218,219] and cytochrome P 450[88,90] pathways.

5. *Lipoxygenase*

Several inhibitors of the lipoxygenase system were among the first compounds shown to antagonize EDRF-mediated relaxation. These compounds include ETYA, BW755C, NDGA, nafazatrom, and phenidone.[158,208,220]

Because these inhibitors block the EDRF response, the products of the lipoxygenase pathway have been considered to be potential candidates for EDRF although none has been so identified. It may be, however, that these agents possess nonspecific actions which result in antagonism of EDRF. The doses of ETYA (>100 μM) and NDGA (>25 μM) necessary to block EDRF responses are in great excess of the reported K_i values for inhibition of lipoxygenase.[172] At these high concentrations, both compounds are potent antioxidants which could act to inhibit the guanylate cyclase response in smooth muscle[176,221] and/or to inactivate EDRF in solution.[222] At high concentrations, both ETYA and NDGA have been reported to attenuate the SNP-stimulated rise in cyclic GMP levels in smooth muscle.[169,254] These and other lipoxygenase inhibitors with antioxidant activity also have been reported to inactivate EDRF in solution. Using a transfer system in which the inhibitor never came into contact with the endothelial source of EDRF, Griffith et al.[222] demonstrated that these agents were able to completely inactivate EDRF after a short period of interaction. Since other free radical scavengers and antioxidants (butylated hydroxytoluene, vitamin E, KBH_4, hydroquinone, phenidone, cysteine, DTT) also will block the EDRF response,[222,223] it has been suggested that EDRF might be a free radical. This view is consistent with the observations that hemoglobin and methylene blue (both free radical scavengers) can block the EDRF response.[209,224] However, not all antioxidants and free radical scavengers will inhibit EDRF.[222] Recently, several groups[177,225] have shown that superoxide dismutase, a radical scavenger, will actually prolong the half life of EDRF.

6. *Cytochrome P450*

The metabolism of AA by cytochrome P450 monooxygenase enzymes to produce hydroxy- and hydroperoxy-eicosatetranoic acids, which are then further metabolized into vasoactive compounds, perhaps via free radical steps, is now under intense study. The suggestion that cytochrome P450 might be involved in the production of EDRF was first proposed by Singer et al.,[89] who demonstrated that two inhibitors of this enzyme, SK525A and metyrapone, were each able to block the endothelium-dependent relaxation responses to Ach, A23187, and exogenously added AA in rabbit aorta. Recently, Pinto et al.[79] reported that the concentration-dependent relaxations to AA could be increased tenfold in the aorta of rabbits treated for 3 days with agents known to induce the P450 enzyme system. These AA-induced relaxations were inhibited by treatment with $CoCl_2$, an agent known to deplete cytochrome P450 enzymes. Another interesting feature of the P450 hypothesis is that at high doses (100 μM), ETYA and NDGA also block P450 enzyme activity.[226,227] Indeed, treatment of rat liver microsomes with NDGA (100 μM) caused a shift in the P450 spectra to that of the denatured enzyme.[228]

There is some recent evidence suggesting that EDRF may not be a metabolite of AA, however. Cocks et al.[165] have found that EDRF released from cultured cells would pass over a C^{18} column at neutral pH, but was retained or destroyed on an ion exchange column. Their data suggest that EDRF may not be lipophilic, as one would expect an AA metabolite to be. However, hydrophilic metabolites like LT D_4 would not be retained by a C_{18} resin at neutral pH. The discovery that EDRF can be produced in large quantity by cultured cells[164,177] should allow a more exacting search for the identity of the factor.

VI. EFFECTS OF HYPERTENSION ON RELAXING FACTORS

Konishi and Su[229] first reported that *in vitro* responses to vasodilators which require the endothelium were diminished in arteries from the spontaneously hypertensive rat (SHR) compared to relaxation observed in vessels from normotensive (WKY) rats. Impaired endothelium-dependent relaxation responses to Ach in SHR vs. WKY thoracic aorta also were observed by Luscher and Vanhoutte[230] and Van de Voorde and Leusen.[231] Winquist et al.[232] studied the New Zealand strain of rats with genetic hypertension and found marked attenuation of aortic responses to endothelium-dependent vasodilators. In each of these studies, responses to directly acting (e.g., sodium nitroprusside, isoproterenol, papaverine) vasodilators were not changed in the hypertensive rats. Lockette and colleagues[233] have evaluated relaxation responses in the thoracic aortae from rats using three experimental models of hypertension: (1) renovascular; (2) mineralocorticoid-sodium chloride; and (3) co-arctation of the aorta. They found that responses to sodium nitroprusside were reduced slightly in vessels from these hypertensive rats regardless of the model. Endothelium-dependent relaxation was strikingly decreased in aorta from all three models of hypertension vs. controls. When hypertension was reversed in these models by either removing the clip on the aorta or renal artery or by discontinuation of the mineralocorticoid, relaxation of aortic preparations to directly and indirectly acting vasodilators were identical to controls. In general, in all models of chronic hypertension with different etiologies in the rat, vasodilators which act via the endothelium are less efficacious.

It was not clear from any of these studies just discussed whether chronic hypertension decreased receptors for agonists on the endothelium, or impaired the production/release of relaxing factor(s) by the endothelium or interfered with the capacity of arterial smooth muscle to respond to endothelium-derived substances such as EDRF or PGI_2. When intact aortic segments from hypertensive rats were perfused and the perfusate was bioassayed for relaxing factor using an arterial ring, denuded of endothelium, from normotensive rats, the endothelium of the hypertensive rat produced dilator factors in response to agents such as Ach, A23187, and histamine.[231] In contrast, aortic rings from hypertensive animals failed to detect the presence of relaxing substance(s) in the perfusate from normal donor endothelium. Therefore, hypertension does not impair responses of the endothelium to stimuli or the release of relaxing factor(s) by the endothelium, but rather the arterial smooth muscle has a decreased capacity to relax in response to substances released from the endothelium.

Several laboratories also have studied the effects of an acute, severe elevation in blood pressure on endothelium-dependent vasodilation. Responses to agents such as Ach and A23187 are severely diminished or completely absent in the cerebral circulation,[234] coronary,[33] and skeletal muscle[236] vascular beds of rats and dogs following an acute increase in blood pressure of 75 to 100 mmHg for a period of 20 to 30 min. The pressure threshold(s) and time course for changes in endothelium-dependent responses associated with acute hypertension remains to be determined. It also is not known if the lesion with acute hypertension involves decreased production of or response to EDRF.

In models of chronic atherosclerosis (cholesterol-fed rabbits), responses induced by endothelium-dependent vasodilators are markedly decreased.[235-237] There appeared to be a good correlation between the magnitude of the atherosclerotic lesion in the aortic media and the degree to which relaxation produced by Ach and A23187 was attenuated. The endothelial cells of an atherosclerotic segment of aorta produced EDRF in response to Ach, but the muscle of the aortic wall failed to relax. In part the impaired response to EDRF may be due to a diffusion barrier to EDRF created by the atheroma in the aorta. On the other hand, the muscle cells simply may not respond much like the lesion seen with chronic hypertension.

A. Modulation

In the early 1980s we observed that anoxia caused a constriction in rings of rabbit aorta which contained endothelium[238] but not when the intima had been denuded of endothelium. We found that the occurrence and the magnitude of this endothelium-dependent contractile response to anoxia in the rabbit aorta required and were proportional to the amount of tone present.[239] Thus, the endothelium in this artery would appear to respond to anoxia by releasing a substance which modulates responses to pressor agents. The modulator, however, was not a directly acting constrictor substance. The identity of this endothelium-derived modulator remains to be determined.

B. Constrictor Substances

In isolated canine femoral artery, DeMey and Vanhoutte[240] found that anoxia induced endothelium-dependent contractions. Subsequent studies from this laboratory[241] showed that hypoxia released a vasoconstrictor substance from canine vascular endothelium. Contractile responses induced in these canine vessels by decreasing the pO_2 were not dependent on preexisting tone in the artery. Endothelium-dependent, hypoxia-induced vasoconstriction also has been of considerable interest to individuals studying the pulmonary circulation.[242,243] Part of the pulmonary arterial response to hypoxia may actually reflect reduced production of EDRF at low pO_2 in addition to production of a constrictor substance or a modulator by the endothelium.

C. Eicosanoids

In 1983 Singer and Peach[208] reported that AA caused endothelium-dependent vasoconstriction of the rabbit aorta. The contraction induced by AA was blocked by indomethacin pretreatment. Holden and McCall[242] reported that hypoxia-induced release of a vasoconstrictor also was blocked by inhibitors of cyclooxygenase. Altiere et al.[78] found that the endothelium contributed significantly to Ach-induced, thromboxane A_2-mediated constriction of rabbit intrapulmonary arteries. Cultured bovine aortic endothelial cells produce TXA_2[80] but synthesis has not been observed with endothelium from other species. Clearly, the endothelium can produce other cyclooxygenase products of AA which are vasoconstrictors. In the aorta of SHR (but not WKY) rats with no induced tone, Ach caused an endothelium-dependent contraction. This response to Ach in the SHR was blocked by inhibitors of cyclooxygenase and appears to be due to some non-TXA_2 eicosanoid.[244] Comparable responses have not been evaluated in other species or different models of hypertension.

Other studies have suggested that hypoxia-induced pulmonary hypertension may be mediated by leukotrienes[245] and/or the absence of epoxides.[79] Arterial endothelium contains lipoxygenase and can convert AA to HPETE and HETE which are precursors of leukotrienes.[72,73,77] Leukotrienes C_4 and D_4 are vasoconstrictors in the pulmonary circulation and have been shown to be released during hypoxia. Blood vessels are known to contain cytochrome P450[87] which only recently has been localized to the endothelium.[90] Singer et al.[89] reported that inhibitors of cytochrome P450 blocked endothelium-dependent relaxation in response to AA. Cultured endothelial cells produce a variety of hydroxy and epoxy derivatives of AA[214] and such eicosanoids could arise from cytochrome P450 and lipoxygenase. In the rabbit pulmonary artery, AA metabolites formed by P450 appear to mediate relaxation.[79] Hypoxia may decrease the rate of formation of P450 metabolites in the lung.

In 1983 Cocks and Angus[32] reported that response in canine and swine coronary arteries to epinephrine and serotonin was potentiated markedly when the endothelium had been removed. Responses to K^+ and a TXA_2 mimetic, however, were not changed by disruption of the endothelium. They interpreted their studies to indicate that epinephrine and serotonin act via alpha 2 adrenoceptors and S_2 serotonergic receptors, respectively, and stimulate the release of a dilator substance (e.g. EDRF) from the endothelium. This dilator in turn compromises the direct constrictor actions of these biogenic amines. Several investigators[31,33,235] have observed potentiation of vasoconstrictor responses to serotonin following mechanical disruption of the endothelium or damage caused by brief periods of acute hypertension.

In isolated arteries of the rat, several investigators[246-248,225] have shown that alpha 2 adrenergic agonists (e.g., clonidine, guanabenz, BHT-920, BHT-933) are constrictor substances only when the endothelium has been removed. In intact arteries, treatment with methylene blue unmasked pressor responses to α_2-agonist presumably by blocking guanylate cyclase[248] We recently have found that the response to α_2-agonists in arteries denuded of endothelium was blocked by indomethacin and that production of this constrictor eicosanoid by smooth muscle was suppressed by the endothelium.[249] In studies with cultured endothelial cells, clonidine stimulated the release of a relaxing factor (bioassay). However, this factor did not activate guanylate cyclase in smooth muscle so it probably was not EDRF.[164]

D. Peptides

In 1984 two laboratories reported that endothelial cell cultures produced a substance which constricted isolated arteries.[242,250] Hickey et al.[251] found that cultured bovine aortic endothelial cells produced a heat-stable, trypsin-sensitive contractile substance. They estimated the molecular weight of this putative peptide to be 8500. Gillespie et al.[252] confirmed the presence of a constrictor peptide in culture media of bovine aortic endothelium. Contractions of the coronary artery by this factor were not altered by blockade of α–adrenergic, serotonergic or histaminergic receptors or inhibition of cyclooxygenase and lipoxygenase. Both laboratories[251,252] found that the substance induced a sustained contraction of smooth muscle. The term endothelium-derived constrictor factor (EDCF) has been proposed for this substance produced by cultured bovine aortic endothelial cells.[252] No studies have been performed to determine if any drugs (hormones, neurotransmitters) or conditions (e.g, hypoxia) enhance or reduce the amount of EDCF elaborated by cultures of bovine endothelium. It also is not known if this peptide is made by other species or types of endothelium and whether or not all arteries and veins contract when exposed to the factor. The relationship of EDCF(s) to hypertension and vascular spasms remains to be determined.

VII. CONCLUSIONS

The endothelium and smooth muscle interact in a great many ways to influence each others exposure to and metabolism of vasoactive and nonvasoactive substances, growth, and vascular tone. These interactions are extremely important for normal vascular functioning. Thus, malfunction of either endothelium or smooth muscle can have dire consequences. Hypertension has been shown to alter many of the properties of both smooth muscle and endothelium. In spite of what is now known, much remains to be elucidated. We are just beginning to understand many of the smooth muscle-endothelium interactions mediating cell metabolism growth and vascular tone. The consequences of hypertension on the delicate balance is largely unknown. We expect that during the next decade many of these relationships will be clarified and lead to a more unified picture of how the vasculature is affected by high blood pressure. One should also expect a better appreciation of the benefits of therapeutic interventions in maintaining integrity and function of vascular endothelium.

REFERENCES

1. **Thorgirsson, G. and Robertson, A. L.,** The vascular endothelium-Pathobiologic significance, *Am. J. Pathol.,* 93, 802, 1978.
2. **Bondjers, G. and Bjorkerud, S.,** Arterial repair and atherosclerosis after mechanical injury. III. Cholesterol accumulation and removal in morphologically defined regions of aortic atherosclerotic lesions in the rabbit, *Atherosclerosis,* 17, 71, 1983.

3. **Bell, F. P., Adamson, I. L., and Schwartz, C. J.,** Aortic endothelial permeability to albumin: focal and regional patterns of uptake and transmural distribution of ^{131}I-albumin in the young pig, *Exp. Mol. Pathol.,* 20, 281, 1974.

4. **Shasby, D. M., Lind, S. E., Shasby, S. S., Goldsmith, J. C., and Hunninghake, G. W.,** Reversible oxidant-induced increases in albumin transfer across cultured endothelium: alterations in cell shape and calcium homeostasis, *Blood,* 63, 605, 1985.

5. **Tedgui, A. and Lever, M. J.,** Filtration through damaged and undamaged rabbit thoracic aorta, *Am. J. Physiol.,* 247, H784, 1984.

6. **Bell, F. P., Gallus, A., and Schwartz, C. J.,** Focal and regional patterns of uptake and transmural distribution of ^{131}I-fibrinogen in the pig aorta, *in vivo, Exp. Mol. Pathol.,* 20, 293, 1974.

7. **Florey, L. and Sheppard, B. L.,** The permeability of arterial endothelium to horseradish peroxidase, *Proc. R. Soc. London,* 174, 435, 1970.

8. **Huttner, I., Boutet, M., and More, R.,** Studies on protein passage through arterial endothelium. II. Regional differences in permeability to fine structural protein tracers in arterial endothelium of normotensive rat, *Lab. Invest.,* 28, 678, 1973.

9. **Tagami, M., Kubota, A., Sunaga, T., Fugino, H., Maezawa, H., Kihara, M., Nara, Y., and Yamori, Y.,** Increased transendothelial transport of cerebral capillary endothelium in stroke-prone SHR, *Stroke,* 14, 591, 1983.

10. **Gaddum, J. H., Hebb, C. D., Silver, A., and Swan, A. A. B.,** 5-Hydroxytryptamine. Pharmacological action and destruction in perfused lung, *Q. J. Exp. Physiol.,* 38, 255, 1953.

11. **Ginn, R. W. and Vane, J. R.,** Disappearance of catecholamines from the circulation, *Nature (London),* 219, 740, 1968.

12. **Junod, A. F.,** Uptake, metabolism, and efflux of [14]c-5-hydroxytryptamine in isolated perfused rat lungs, *J. Pharmacol. Exp. Ther.,* 183, 341, 1972.

13. **Hughes, J., Gillis, C. N., and Bloom, F. L.,** Uptake and disposition of norepinephrine in perfused rat lung, *J. Pharmacol. Exp. Ther.,* 169, 237, 1969.

14. **Iwasawa, Y., Gillis, C. N., and Aghajanian, G.,** Hypothermic inhibition of 5-hydroxytryptamine and norepinephrine uptake by lung: cellular localization of amines after uptake, *J. Pharmacol. Exp. Ther.,* 186, 98, 1973.

15. **Shepro, D., Batbouta, J. C., Robllee, L. S., Carson, M. P., and Belamarich, F. A.,** Serotonin transported by cultured bovine aortic endothelium, *Circ. Res.,* 36, 799, 1975.

16. **Strum, J. and Junod, A. F.,** Radioautographic demonstration of 5-hydroxytryptamine-^{3}H uptake by pulmonary endothelial cells, *J. Cell Biol.,* 54, 456, 1972.

17. **Goldby, F. S. and Beilin, L. S.,** Relationship between arterial pressure and the permeability of arterioles to carbon particles in acute hypertension in the rat, *Cardiovasc. Res.,* 6, 384, 1972.

18. **Huttner, I., Boutet, M., Rona, G., and More, R. H.,** Studies on protein passage through arterial endothelium. III. Effect of blood pressure levels on the passage of fine structural protein tracers through rat arterial endothelium, *Lab. Invest.,* 29, 536, 1973.

19. **Robertson, A. L. and Khairallah, P. A.,** Arterial endothelial permeability and vascular disease: the "trapdoor" effect, *Exp. Mol. Pathol.,* 18, 241, 1973.

20. **Giacomelli, F., Weiner, J., and Spiro, D.,** The cellular pathology of experimental hypertension. V. Increased permeability of cerebral arterial vessels, *Am. J. Pathol.,* 59, 133, 1970.

21. **Gabbiani, G., Badonnel, M. C., and Rona, G.,** Cytoplasmic contractile apparatus in aortic endothelial cells of hypertensive rats, *Lab. Invest.,* 32, 227, 1975.

22. **Jellinck, H., Nagy, Z., Huttner, I., Balint, A., Koczi, A., and Kerenyi, T.,** Investigations of the permeability changes of the vascular wall in experimental malignant hypertension by means of a colloidal iron preparation, *Br. J. Exp. Pathol.,* 56, 13, 1969.

23. **Majack, R. A. and Bhalla, R. C.,** Endothelial alterations and colloidal carbon permeability in the peripheral vasculature of the spontaneously hypertensive rat, *Exp. Mol. Pathol.,* 32, 201, 1980.

24. **Still, W. S. S. and Dannison, S.,** The arterial endothelium of the hypertensive rat, *Arch. Pathol.,* 97, 337, 1974.

25. **Gillis, C. N. and Roth, J. A.,** Pulmonary disposition of circulating vasoactive hormones, *Biochem. Pharmacol.,* 25, 2547, 1976.

26. **Pitt, B. R., Hammond, G. L., and Gillis, C. N.,** Comparison of pulmonary and extrapulmonary extraction of biogenic amines, *J. Appl. Physiol.,* 52, 1545, 1982.

27. **Rorie, D. K. and Tyce, G. M.,** Uptake and metabolism of norepinephrine by endothelium of dog pulmonary artery, *Am. J. Physiol.,* 248, H193, 1985.

28. **Small, R., Macarak, E., and Fisher, A. B.,** Production of 5-hydroxyindoleacetic acid from serotonin by cultured endothelial cells, *J. Cell Physiol.,* 90, 225, 1977.

29. **Roth, J. A. and Ventner, J. C.,** Predominance of the B form of monoamine oxidase in cultured vascular intimal endothelial cells, *Biochem. Pharmacol.,* 27, 2371, 1978.

30. **Trevethick, M. A., Olverman, H. J., Pearson, J. D., Gordon, J. L., Lyles, G. A., and Callingham, B. A.,** Monoamine oxidase activities of porcine vascular endothelial and smooth muscle cells, *Biochem. Pharmacol.,* 30, 2209, 1981.

31.   **Brum, J. M., Sufun, Q., Lane, G., and Bore, A. A.,** Increased vasoconstrictor activity of proximal coronary arteries with endothelial damage in intact dogs, *Circulation,* 70, 1066, 1984.

32.   **Cocks, T. M. and Angus, J. A.,** Endothelium-dependent relaxation of coronary arteries by noradrenaline and serotonin, *Nature (London),* 305, 627, 1983.

33.   **Lamping, K. G., Marcus, M. L., and Dole, W. P.,** Removal of the endothelium potentiates canine large coronary artery constrictor responses to 5-hydroxytryptamine *in vivo, Circ. Res.,* 57, 46, 1985.

34.   **Cassis, L. A., Stitzel, R. E., and Head, R. J.,** Hypernoradrenergic innervation of the caudal artery of the spontaneously hypertensive rat: an influence upon neuroeffector mechanisms, *J. Pharmacol. Exp. Ther.,* 234, 792, 1985.

35.   **Head, R. J., Cassis, L. A., Barone, S., Stitzel, and DeLaLande, I. S.,** Neuronal deamination of endogenous and exogenous norepinephrine in the mesenteric artery of the spontaneously hypertensive rat, *J. Pharm. Pharmacol.,* 36, 382, 1984.

36.   **Gillis, C. N., Cronau, H. L., Green, N., and Hammond, G. L.,** Removal of 5-hydroxytryptamine and norepinephrine from the pulmonary vascular space in man: influence of cardiopulmonary bypass and pulmonary arterial pressure on these processes, *Surgery,* 76, 608, 1974.

37.   **Sole, M. J., Drobac, M., Schwartz, L. O., Hussain, M. N., and Vaughan-Neil, E. F.,** The extraction of circulating catecholamines by the lungs in normal man and in patients with pulmonary hypertension, *Circulation,* 60, 160, 1979.

38.   **Gillis, C. N. and Pitt, B. R.,** The fate of circulating amines within the pulmonary circulation. *Annu. Rev. Physiol.,* 44, 269, 1982.

39.   **Pearson, J. D. and Gordon, J. L.,** Vascular endothelial and smooth muscle cells in culture selectively release adenine nucleotides, *Nature (London),* 281, 384, 1979.

40.   **Schrader, J., Thompson, C. I., Hindlmayer, G., and Gerlach, E.,** Role of purines in acetylcholine-induced coronary vasodilation, *J. Mol. Cell Cardiol.,* 14, 427, 1982.

41.   **Burnstock, G. and Kennedy, C.,** A dual function for adenosine 5¢-triphosphate in the regulation of vascular tone: excitatory cotransmitter with noradrenaline from perivascular nerves and locally released inhibitory intravascular agent, *Circ. Res.,* 319, 1986.

42.   **Ryan, J. W. and Ryan, U.,** Pulmonary endothelial cells, *Fed. Proc.,* 36, 2683, 1977.

43.   **Crutchley, D. J., Eling, T. E., and Anderson, M. W.,** ADPase activity of isolated perfused rat lung, *Life Sci.,* 22, 1413, 1978.

44.   **Pearson, J. D. and Gordon, J. L.,** Nucleotide metabolism by endothelium, *Annu. Rev. Physiol.,* 47, 617, 1985.

45.   **Nees, S. and Gerlach, E.,** Adenosine nucleotide and adenosine metabolism in cultured coronary endothelial cells: formation and release of adenine compounds and functional implications, in *Regulatory Function of Adenosine,* Berne, R. M., Rall, T. W., and Rubio, R., Eds., Martinus Nijhoff, Boston, 1983, 347.

46.   **Nees, S., Herzog, V., Becker, B. F., Bock, M., DesRosiers, C., and Gerlach, E.,** The coronary endothelium: a highly active metabolic barrier for adenosine, *Basic Res. Cardiol.,* 80, 515, 1985.

47.   **Goldman, S. J., Dickenson, E. S., and Slakey, L. L.,** Effect of adenosine on synthesis and release of cyclic AMP by cultured vascular cells from swine, *J. Cyclic Nucleotide Protein Phosphor. Res.,* 9, 69, 1983.

48.   **Ager, A. and Gordon, J. L.,** Differential effects of hydrogen peroxide on indices of endothelial cell function, *J. Exp. Med.,* 159, 592, 1984.

49.   **Ng, K. K. F. and Vane, J.,** Fate of angiotensin I in the circulation, *Nature (London),* 218, 144, 1968.

50.   **Ryan, J. W., Ryan, U. S., Schultz, D. R., Whitaker, C., Chung, A., and Dorer, F. E.,** Subcellular localization of pulmonary angiotensin converting enzyme (kininase II), *Biochem. J.,* 146, 497, 1975.

51.   **Caldwell, P. R. P., Seegal, B. C., Hsu, K. C., Das, M., and Soffer, R. L.,** Angiotensin-converting enzyme: vascular endothelial localization, *Science,* 191, 1050, 1976.

52.   **Ryan, U. S., Ryan, J. W., and Chiu, A.,** Kininase II (angiotensin converting enzyme) and endothelial cells in culture, *Adv. Exp. Med. Biol.,* 70, 217, 1976

53.   **Hagyes, L. W., Goguen, C. A., and Slakey, L.** Angiotensin converting enzyme: accumulation in medium from cultured endothelial cells, *Biochem. Biophys. Res. Commun.,* 82, 1147, 1978.

54.   **Johnson, A. R. and Erdos, E. G.,** Metabolism of vasoactive peptides by human endothelial cells in culture. Angiotensin I converting enzyme (kininase II) and angiotensinase, *J. Clin. Invest.,* 59, 684, 1977.

55.   **Yang, H. Y. T. and Erdos, E. G.,** Second kininase in human blood plasma, *Nature (London),* 215, 1402, 1967.

56.   **Bakhle, Y. S.,** Conversion of angiotensin I to angiotensin II by cell-free extracts of dog lung, *Nature (London),* 220, 919, 1968.

57.   **Ferreira, S. H., Greene, L. J., Alabaster, V. A., Bakhle, Y. S., and Vane, J. R.,** Activity of various fractions of bradykinin potentiating factor against angiotensin I converting enzyme, *Nature (London),* 225, 379, 1970.

58.   **Soffer, R. L., Reza, R., and Caldwell, P. R. B.,** Angiotensin-converting enzyme from rabbit pulmonary particles, *Proc. Natl. Acad. Sci. U.S.A.,* 71, 1720, 1974.

59.   **Tsai, B. S. and Peach, M. J.,** Angiotensin homologs and analogs as inhibitors of rabbit pulmonary angiotensin-converting enzyme, *J. Biol. Chem.,* 252, 4674, 1977.

60.   **Dorer, F. E., Kahn, J. R., Lentz, K. E., Levine, M., and Skeggs, L. T.,** Hydrolysis of bradykinin by angiotensin-converting enzyme, *Circ. Res.,* 34, 824, 1974.

61. **Thurston, H. and Swales, J. D.,** Converting enzyme inhibitor and saralasin infusion in rats, *Circ. Res.,* 42, 588, 1978.

62. **Williams, G. H. and Hollenberg, N. K.,** Accentuated vascular and endocrine response to SQ20881 in hypertension, *N. Engl. J. Med.,* 297, 184, 1977.

63. **Margolius, H.S.,** The kallikrein-kinin system and the kidney, *Annu. Rev. Physiol.,* 46, 303, 1984.

64. **Regoli, D., Park, W. K., and Rioux, F.,** Pharmacology of angiotensin, *Pharmacol. Rev.,* 26, 69, 1974.

65. **Peach, M. J.,** Renin-angiotensin system: biochemistry and mechanisms of action, *Physiol. Rev.,* 57, 313, 1977.

66. **Robertson, A. L. and Khairallah, P. A.,** Effects of angiotensin II and some analogs on vascular permeability in the rabbit, *Circ. Res.,* 31, 923, 1972.

67. **Richardson, J. B. and Beaulnes, A.,** The cellular site of action of angiotensin, *J. Cell Biol.,* 51,4 19, 1971.

68. **Saye, J. A., Singer, H. A., and Peach, M. J.,** Role of endothelium in converstion of angiotensin I to angiotensin II in rabbit aorta, *Hypertension,* 6, 216, 1984.

69. **Leary, W. P. P. and Ledingham, J. G.,** Renal and hepatic inactivation of angiotensin in rats. Influence of sodium balance and renal artery compression, *Clin. Sci.,* 38, 573, 1970.

70. **Moncada, S., Herman, A. G., Higgs, E. A., and Vane, J. R.,** Differential formation of prostacyclin (PGX or PGI$_2$) by layers of the arterial wall. An explanation for the anti-thrombotic properties of vascular endothelium, *Thromb. Res.,* 11, 323, 1977.

71. **Terragno, D. A., Crowshaw, K., Terragno, N. A., and McGiff, J. C.,** Prostaglandin synthesis by bovine mesenteric arteries and veins, *Circ. Res.,* 36 and, 37 (Suppl. I), 76, 1975.

72. **Greenwald, J. E., Bianchine, J. R., and Wong, L. K.,** The production of the arachidonate metabolite HETE in vascular tissue, *Nature (London),* 281, 588, 1979.

73. **DeMey, J. G. and Vanhoutte, P. M.,** Endothelium-dependent inhibitory effects of acetylcholine, adenosine triphosphate, thrombin, and arachidonic acid in the canine femoral artery, *J. Pharmacol. Exp. Ther.,* 222, 166, 1982.

74. **Hamberg, M.,** On the formation of thromboxane B$_2$ and 12L-hydroxy-5,8,10,14-eicosatetraenoic acid (12 ho-20:4) in tissue from the guinea pig, *Biochem. Biophys. Acta,* 431, 651, 1976.

75. **Piper, P. J., Letts, L. G., and Galton, S. A.,** Generation of a leukotriene-like substance from porcine vascular and other tissues, *Prostaglandins,* 25, 591, 1983.

76. **Hamberg, M. and Samuelsson, B.,** Prostaglandin endoperoxides. Novel transformations of arachidonic acid in human platelets, *Proc. Natl. Acad. Sci. U.S.A.,* 71, 3400, 1974.

77. **Salzman, P.M., Salmon, J., and Moncada, S.,** Prostacyclin and thromboxane A$_2$ synthesis by rabbit pulmonary artery, *J. Pharmacol. Exp. Ther.,* 215, 240, 1980.

78. **Altiere, R. J., Kiritsy-Roy, J. A., and Catravas, J. D.,** Acetylcholine-induced contractions in isolated pulmonary arteries. Role of thromboxane A$_2$, *J. Pharmacol. Exp. Ther.,* 236, 535, 1986.

79. **Pinto, A., Abraham, N. G., and Mullane, K. M.,** Cytochrome P450-dependent monooxygenase activity and endothelium-dependent relaxations induced by arachidonic acid, *J. Pharmacol. Exp. Ther.,* 236, 445, 1986.

80. **Ingerman-Wojenski, C., Silver, M. J., Smith, J. B., and Macarak, E.,** Bovine endothelial cells in culture produce thromboxane as well as prostacyclin, *J. Clin. Invest.,* 67, 1292, 1981.

81. **Gimbrone, M. and Alexander, R. W.,** Angiotensin II stimulation of prostaglandin production in cultured human vascular endothelium, *Science,* 198, 219, 1975.

82. **Weksler, B. B., Ley, C. W., and Jaffe, E. A.,** Stimulation of endothelial cell prostacylin production by thrombin, trypsin, and A23187, *J. Clin. Invest.,* 62, 923, 1978.

83. **Remuzzi, G., Mecca, G., Livio, M., De Gaetano, G., Donati, M. B., Pearson, J. D., and Gordon, J. L.,** Prostacyclin generation by cultured endothelial cells in haemolytic uraemic syndrome, *Lancet,* 1, 656, 1980.

84. **Ager, A., Gordon, J. L., Moncada, S., Pearson, J. D., Salmon, J. A., and Trevethick, M. A.,** Effects of isolation and culture on prostaglandin synthesis by porcine aortic endothelial and smooth muscle cells, *J. Cell Physiol.,* 110, 9, 1982.

85. **Wherton, A. R., Young, S. L., Data, J. L., Barchowsky, A., and Kent, R. S.,** Mechanism of bradykinin-stimulated prostacyclin synthesis in porcine aortic endothelial cells, *Biochim. Biophys. Acta,* 712, 79, 1982.

86. **Gerritsen, M. E. and Cheli, C. D.,** Arachidonic acid and prostaglandin endoperoxide metabolism in isolated rabbit and coronary microvessels and isolated and cultivated coronary microvessel endothelial cells, *J. Clin. Invest.,* 72,1658, 1983.

87. **Juchau, M. , Bond, J. A., and Benditt, E. P.,** Aryl-4-monooxygenase and cytochrome-P450 in the aorta: possible role in atherosclerosis, *Proc. Natl. Acad. Sci. U.S.A.,* 73, 3723, 1976.

88. **Baird, W. M., Chemerys, R., Grinspan, J. B., Mueller, S. N. and Levine, E. M.,** Benzo(a)pyrene metabolism in bovine aortic endothelial and bovine lung fibroblast-like-cell cultures, *Cancer Res.,* 40, 1781, 1980.

89. **Singer, H. A., Saye, J. A., and Peach, M. J.,** Effects of cytochrome P450 inhibitors on endothelium dependent relaxation in rabbit aorta, *Blood Vessels,* 21, 223, 1984.

90. **Abraham, N. G., Pinto, A., Mullane, K. M., Levere, R. D., and Spokas E.,** Presence of cytochrome P-450-dependent monooxygenase in intimal cells of the hog aorta, *Hypertension,* 7, 899, 1985.

91. **Watson, M. L.,** Prostanoids and the development of hypertension, in *Essential Hypertension as an Endocrine Disease,* Edwards, C. R. W. and Carey, R. M., Eds., Butterworths, London, 1985, chap. 9.

92. **Dunn, M. J.,** The relationship of prostaglandins and thromboxane to the pathophysiology of renal disease and hypertension, in *Kidney Hormone, Vol. 3,* Fisher, J. W., Ed., Academic Press, London, 1986, 398.

93. **Gryglewski, R., Korbut, R., and Ocetkiewcz, A.,** Generation of prostacyclin by lungs, *in vivo* and its release into the arterial circulation, *Nature (London),* 273, 765, 1978.

94. **Moncada, S., Korbut, R., Bunting, S., and Vane, J. R.,** Prostacyclin is a circulating hormone, *Nature (London),* 273, 767, 1978.

95. **Fitzgerald, G. A., Brash, A. R., Falardeau, P., and Oates, J. A.,** Estimated role of prostacyclin secretion into the circulation of normal man, *J. Clin. Invest.,* 68, 1272, 1978.

96. **Forstermann, U. and Neufang, B.,** Endothelium-dependent vasodilation by melittin: are lipoxygenase products involved?, *Am. J. Physiol.,* 249, H14, 1985.

97. **Morera, S., Santoro, F. M., Roson, M. I., and DeLa Riva, I. J.,** Prostacyclin (PGI$_2$) synthesis in the vascular wall of rats with bilateral renal artery stenosis, *Hypertension,* 5 (Suppl. 5), 38, 1983.

98. **Dusting, G. J., Dickens, P. A., Di Nicolantonio, R., and Doyle, A. E.,** Vascular prostacyclin and Goldblatt hypertensive rats, *J. Hypertension,* 2, 31, 1984.

99. **Dusting, G. J., Drysdale, T., Veroni, M., and Doyle, A. E.,** Differences in arachidonic acid metabolism and effects of aspirin between one- and two-kidney Goldblatt hypertensive rats, *Clin. Exp. Pharmacol. Physiol.,* 10, 355, 1983.

100. **Pipili, E. and Poyser, N. L.,** Release of prostaglandins I$_2$ and E$_2$ from the perfused mesenteric arterial bed of normotensive and hypertensive rats. Effects of sympathetic nerve stimulation and norepinephrine administration. *Prostaglandins,* 23, 543, 1982.

101. **Soma, M., Manku, M. S., Jenkins, D. K., and Horrobin, D. F.,** Prostaglandins and thromboxane outflow from the perfused mesenteric vascular bed in spontaneously hypertensive rats. *Prostaglandins,* 29, 323, 1985.

102. **Limas, C. J. and Limas C.,** Vascular prostaglandin synthesis in the spontaneously hypertensive rat, *Am. J. Physiol.,* 233, H493, 1977.

103. **Pace-Asciak, C. R., Carrara, M. C., Rangaraj, G., and Nicolaou, K. C.,** Enhanced formation of PGI$_2$, a potent hypotensive substance, by aortic rings and homogenates of the spontaneously hypetensive rat, *Prostaglandins,* 15, 1005, 1978.

104. **Shibouta, Y., Terashita, Z., Inada, Y., Kato, K., and Nishikawa, K.,** Renal effects of pinane-thromboxane A$_2$ and indomethacin in saline volume-expanded spontaneously hypertensive rats, *Eur. J. Pharmacol.,* 85, 51, 1982.

105. **Falardeau, P., Robillard, M., and Martineau, A.,** Urinary levels of 2,3-dinor-6-oxo-PGF$_{2a}$: a reliable index of the production of PGI$_2$: in the SHR, *Prostaglandins,* 29, 621, 1985.

106. **Martineau, A., Robillard, M., and Falardeau, P.,** Defective synthesis of vasodilator prostaglandins in the SHR, *Hypertension,* 6 (Suppl. I), 161, 1984.

107. **Falardeau, P. and Martineau, A.** , *In vivo* production of prostaglandin I$_2$ in Dahl salt-sensitive and salt-resistant rats, *Hypertension,* 5, 701, 1983.

108. **Vandongen, R. and O'Dwyer, J.,** Urinary 6-keto PGF$_{1\alpha}$ and PGE$_2$ in two kidney-one clip hypertension in the rat, in *Rat Prostaglandin Leukotr. Med.,* 13, 289, 1984.

109. **Dunn, M. J.,** Renal prostaglandin production in the Japanese (Kyoto) spontaneously hypertensive rat, *Clin. Sci. Mol. Med.,* 55 (Suppl.), 191s, 1978.

110. **Konieczkowski, M., Dunn, M. J., Stork, J. E., and Hassid, A.,** Glomerular synthesis of prostaglandins and thromboxanes in spontaneously hypertensive rats, *Hypertension,* 5, 446, 1983.

111. **Shibouta, Y., Inada, Y., Terashita, Z., Nishikawa, K., Kikuchi, S., and Shimamoto, K.,** Angiotensin II-stimulated release of thromboxane A$_2$ and prostacyclin (PGI$_2$) in isolated perfused kidneys of spontaneously hypertensive rats, *Biochem. Pharmacol.,* 28, 3601, 1979.

112. **Shibouta, Y., Terashita, Z., Inada, Y., Nishikawa, K., and Kikuchi, S.,** Enhanced thromboxane A$_2$ biosynthesis in the kidney of SHR during development of hypertension, *Eur. J. Pharmacol.,* 70, 247, 1981.

113. **Sustarsic, D. L., McPartland, R. P. and Rapp, J. P.,** Developmental patterns of blood pressure and urinary protein, kallikrein, and prostaglandin E$_2$ in Dahl salt-hypertension-susceptible rats, *J. Lab. Clin. Med.,* 98, 599, 1981.

114. **Benzoni, D., Vincent, M., and Sussard, J.,** Urinary prostaglandins in the Lyon strains of hypertensive, normotensive, and low blood pressure rats, *Hypertension,* 4, 325, 1982.

115. **Watson, M. L., McCormick, J., and Ungar, A.,** Angiotensin sensitivity and prostaglandins in dogs with renal hypertension, *J. Hypertension,* 2, 479, 1984.

116. **Leslie, C. A. and Levine, L.,** Evidence for the presence of a prostaglandin E$_2$-9-keto reductase in rat organs, *Biochem. Biophys. Res. Commun.,* 52, 717, 1973.

117. **Wong, P. Y. -K., Terragno, D. A., Terragno, N. A., and McGiff, J. C.,** Dual effects of bradykinin on prostaglandin metabolism: relationship to the dissimilar vascular actions of kinins, *Prostaglandins,* 13, 1113, 1977.

118. **Wong, P. Y. -K. and McGiff, J. C.,** Detection of 15-hydroxyprostaglandin dehydrogenase in bovine mesenteric blood vessels, *Biochim. Biophys. Acta,* 500, 436, 1977.

119. **Anggard, E., Larsson, C., and Samuelsson, B.,** The distribution of 15-hydroxy prostaglandin dehydrogenase and prostaglandin-Δ^{13}-reductase in tissues of the swine. *Acta Physiol. Scand.,* 81, 396, 1971.

120. **Sun, F. F. and Taylor, B. M.,** Metabolism of prostacyclin in the rat, *Biochemistry,* 17, 4096, 1978.

121. **Wong, P. Y. -K., Sun, F. F., and McGiff, J. C.,** Metabolism of prostacyclin in blood vessels, *J. Biol. Chem.,* 253, 5555, 1978.

122. **Wong, P. Y. -K., McGiff, J. C., Sun, F. F., and Malik, K. U.** Pulmonary metabolism of prostacyclin (PGI_2) in the rabbit, *Biochem. Biophys. Res. Commun.,* 83, 731, 1978.

123. **Armstrong, J. M., Blackwell, G. J., Flower, R. J., McGiff, J. C., Mullane, K. M. and Vane, J. M.,** Genetic hypertension in rats is accompanied by a defect in renal prostaglandin catabolism, *Nature (London),* 260, 528, 1976.

124. **Armstrong, J. M., Bell, C., Lattimer, N., McGiff, J. C., and Mullane, K. M.,** Contribution of prostaglandins to the renal vascular supersensitivity to vasoconstrictor agents exhibited by New Zealand genetic hypertensive rats, *Clin. Sci. Mol. Med.,* 51 (Suppl.), 275s, 1976.

125. **Dunn, M. J.,** Renal prostaglandin synthesis in the spontaneously hypertensine rat, *J. Clin. Invest.,* 58, 862, 1976.

126. **Limas, C. J. and Limas, C.,** Prostaglandin metabolism in the kidneys of spontaneously hypertensive rats, *Am. J. Physiol.,* 233, H87, 1977.

127. **Pace-Asciak, C. R.,** Decreased renal prostaglandin metabolism precedes onset of hypertension in the developing spontaneously hypertensive rat, *Nature (London),* 263, 10, 1976.

128. **Wong, P. Y, Baer, P. G., and McGiff, J. C.,** Evidence for an endogenous inhibitor of 15-hydroxyprostaglandin dehydrogenase in New Zealand genetically hypertensive rats, *Jpn. Heart J.,* 20 (Suppl. 1), 186, 1979.

129. **Wong, P. Y. -K., Lee, W. H., and McGiff, J. C.,** Metabolism of prostacyclin (PG_2) by the 9-hydroxyprostaglandin dehydrogenase (9-OHPGDH) in human platelets, *Circulation,* 60, (Suppl. II), 269, 1979.

130. **Quilley, C. P., Wong, P. Y. -K., and McGiff, J. C.,** Hypotensive and novascular actions of 6-keto-prostaglandin E_1, a metabolite of prostacyclin, *Eur. J. Pharmacol.,* 57, 273, 1979.

131. **Wong, P. Y.-K., McGiff, J. C., Sun, F. F., and Lee, W. H.,** 6-Keto-prostaglandin E_1 inhibits the aggregation of human platelets, *Eur. J. Pharmacol.,* 60, 245, 1979.

132. **Gajdusek, C. M., DiCorletto, P. E., Ross, R., and Schwartz, S.,** An endothelial cell-derived growth factor, *J. Cell Biol.,* 85, 467, 1980.

133. **DiCorletto, P. E., Gajdusec, C. M., Schwartz, S. M., and Ross, R.,** Biochemical properties of the endothelium-derived growth factor: comparison to other growth factors, *J. Cell Physiol.,* 114, 339, 1983.

134. **DiCorletto, P. E. and Bowen-Pope, D. F.,** Cultured cells produce a platelet-derived growth factor-like protein, *Proc. Natl. Acad. Sci. U.S.A.,* 80, 1919, 1983.

135. **Ross, R., Bowen-Pope, D. F., and Raines, E. W.,** Platelets, macrophages, endothelium, and growth factors, *Ann. N.Y. Acad. Sci.,* 454, 254, 1985.

136. **Vogel, A., Raines, E., Kariya, B., Rivest, M. J., and Ross, R.,** Coordinate control of 3T3 cell proliferation by platelet-derived growth factor and plasma components, *Proc. Natl. Acad. Sci. U.S.A.,* 75, 2810, 1980.

137. **Schwartz, S. M., Gajdusek, C. M., and Owens, G. K.,** Vessel wall growth control, in *Pathology of the Endothelial Cell,* Nossel, H. L. and Vogel, H. J., Eds., Academic Press, New York, 1982, 63.

138. **Ross, R. and Harker, L.,** Hyperlipidemia and atherosclerosis, *Science,* 193, 1094, 1976.

139. **DiCorletto, P. E.,** Cultured endothelial cells produce multiple growth factors for connective tissue cells, *Exp. Cell Res.,* 153,167, 1984.

140. **Campbell, J. H. and Campbell, G. R.,** Endothelial cell influences on vascular smooth muscle phenotype, *Annu. Rev. Physiol.,* 48, 295, 1986.

141. **Davies, P. F.,** Vascular cell interactions with special reference to the pathogenesis of atherosclerosis, *Lab. Invest.,* 55, 5, 1986.

142. **Clowes, A. W. and Karnovsky, M. J.,** Suppression by heparin of smooth muscle cell proliferation in injured arteries, *Nature (London),* 265, 625, 1977.

143. **Hoover, R. L., Rosenberg, R. D., Haering, W., and Karnovsky, M. J.,** Inhibition of rat arterial smooth muscle cell proliferation by heparin. II. *In vitro* studies, *Circ. Res.,* 47, 578, 1980.

144. **Castellot, J. J., Rosenberg, R. D., and Karnovsky, M. J.,** Endothelium, heparin, and the regulation of cell growth, in *Biology of Endothelial Cells,* Jaffe, E., Ed. Martinus Nijhoff, Boston, 1984, 118.

145. **Ross, R.,** The arterial wall and atherosclerosis, *Annu. Rev. Med.,* 30, 1, 1979.

146. **Folkow, B.,** Cardiovascular structural adaptation: its role in the intiation and maintenance of primary hypertension, *Clin. Sci. Mol. Med.,* 55 (Suppl. 4), 3, 1978.

147. **Carlier, P.G., Rorive, G.L., and Barbason, H.,** Kinetics of proliferation of rat aortic smooth muscle cells in Goldblatt one-kidney, one-clip hypertension, *Clin. Sci.,* 65, 351, 1983.

148. **Lee, R. M. K. W., Garfield, R. E., and Daniel, E. E.,** Morphometric study of structural changes in the mesenteric blood vessels of spontaneously hypertensive rats, *Blood Vessels,* 20, 57, 1983.

149. **Olivetti, G., Anversa, P., Melissari, M., and Loud, A. V.,** Morphometry of medial hypertrophy in the rat thoracic aorta, *Lab. Invest.,* 42, 559, 1980.

150. **Owens, G. K. and Schwartz, S. M.,** Alterations in vascular smooth muscle mass in the spontaneously hypertensive rat: role of cellular hypertrophy, hyperploidy, and hyperplasmia, *Circ. Res.,* 51, 280, 1982.

151. **Owens, G. K. and Schwartz, S. M.,** Vascular smooth muscle cell hypertrophy and hyperploidy in the Goldblatt hypertensive rat, *Circ. Res.,* 53, 491, 1983.

152. **Loeb, A. L., Mandel, H. G., Straw, J. A., and Bean, B. L.,** Increased aortic DNA synthesis precedes renal hypertension in rats. An obligatory step?, *Hypertension,* 8, 54, 1986.

153. **Schwartz, S. M. and Benditt, D.,** Aortic endothelial cell replication. I. Effects of age and hypertension in the rat, *Circ. Res.,* 41, 248, 1977.

154. **Peach, M. J. and Singer, H. A.,** The endothelium in hypertension, in *Essential Hypertension as an Endocrine Disease,* Edwards, C. R. W. and Carey, R. M., Eds., Butterworths, London, 1985, chap. 8.

155. **Schwartz, S. M. and Ross, R.,** Cellular proliferation in atherosclerosis and hypertension, *Prog. Cardiovasc. Dis.,* 26, 355, 1984.

156. **Raines, E. and Ross, R.,** Platelet-derived growth factor. I. High yield purification and evidence for multiple forms, *J. Biol. Chem.,* 54, 5754, 1982.

157. **Berk, B. C., Alexander, R. W., Brock, T. A., Gimbrone, M. A., and Webb, R. C.,** Vasoconstriction: a new activity for platelet-derived growth factor, *Science,* 232, 87, 1986.

158. **Furchgott, R. and Zawadzki, D.,** The obligatory role of endothelial cells in the relaxation of arterial smooth muscle by acetylcholine, *Nature (London),* 288, 373, 1980.

159. **Eglen, R. M. and Whiting, R. L.,** Determination of the muscarinic receptor subtype mediating vasodilatation, *Br. J. Pharmacol.,* 84, 3, 1985.

160. **Griffith, T., Edwards, D., Lewis, M., Newley, A., and Henderson, A.,** The nature of endothelium-derived vascular relaxant factor, *Nature (London),* 308, 645, 1984.

161. **Forstermann, U., Trogisch, G. ,and Busse, R.,** Species-dependent differences in the nature of endothelium-derived vascular relaxing factor, *Eur. J. Pharmacol.,* 106, 639, 1985.

162. **Loeb, A. L., Owens, G. K., and Peach, M. J.,** Evidence for endothelium-derived relaxing factor in cultured cells, *Hypertension,* 7, 804, 1985.

163. **Loeb, A. L., Johns, R. A., and Peach, M. J.,** Extracellular calcium is not required for melittin induced endothelium-dependent relaxation, in *Proceeding of Mechanisms of Vasodilatation,* Vanhoutte, P. M., Ed., Raven Press, New York, 1987, in press.

164. **Loeb, A. L., Johns, R. A., Milner, P., and Peach, M. J.,** Studies on endothelium-derived relaxing factor from cultured cells, *Hypertension,* 1987, in press.

165. **Cocks, T. M., Angus, J. A., Campbell, J. H., and Campbell, G. R.,** Release and properties of endothelium-derived relaxing factor (EDRF) from endothelial cells in culture, *J. Cell Physiol.,* 123, 310, 1985.

166. **Ganz, P., Davies, P. F., Leopold, J. A., Gimbrone, M. A., and Alexander, R. W.,** Short- and long-term interactions of endothelium and vascular smooth muscle in co-culture: effects on cyclic GMP production, *Proc. Natl. Acad. Sci. U.S.A.,* 83, 3552, 1986.

167. **Gryglewski, R. J., Moncada, S., and Palmer, R. M. J.,** Bioassay of prostacyclin and endothelium-derived relaxing factor (EDRF) from porcine aortic endothelial cells, *Br. J. Pharmacol.,* 87, 685, 1986.

168. **Forstermann, U., Goppelt-Strube, M., Frolich, J. C., and Busse, R.,** Inhibitors of acyl-coenzyme A: lysolecithin acyltransferase activate the production of endothelium-derived vascular relaxing factor, *J. Pharmacol. Exp. Ther.,* 238, 352, 1986.

169. **Rapoport, R. and Murad, F.,** Endothelium-dependent and nitrovasodilator-induced relaxation of vascular smooth muscle: role of cyclic GMP, *J. Cyclic Nucleotide Prot. Phos. Res.,* 9, 281, 1983.

170. **Furchgott, R. and Jothianandan, D.,** Relation of cyclic GMP levels to endothelium-dependent relaxation by acetylcholine in rabbit aorta, *Fed. Proc.,* 42, (Abstr.), 619, 1983.

171. **Rapoport, R. M., Draznin, M. B., and Murad, F.,** Mechanisms of adenosine triphosphate-, thrombin-, and trypsin-induced relaxation of rat thoracic aorta, *Circ. Res.,* 55,468, 1984.

172. **Peach, M. J., Loeb, A. L., Singer, H. A., and Saye, J. A.,** Endothelium-derived vascular relaxing factor, *Hypertension,* 7 (Suppl. I), 94, 1985.

173. **Martin, W., Furchgott, R. F., Villani, G. M., and Jothianandan, D.,** Phosphodiesterase inhibitors induce endothelium-dependent relaxation of rat and rabbit aorta by potentiating the effects of spontaneously released endothelium-derived relaxing factor, *J. Pharmacol. Exp. Ther.,* 237, 539, 1986.

174. **Ignarro, L. J. and Kadowitz, P. J.,** The pharmacological and physiological role of cyclic GMP in vascular smooth muscle relaxation, *Annu. Rev. Pharmacol. Toxicol.,* 25, 171, 1985.

175. **Rapoport, R. M., Waldman, S. A., Schwartz, K., Winquist, R. J., and Murad, F.,** Effects of atrial natriuretic factor, sodium nitroprusside, and acetylcholine on cyclic GMP levels and relaxation in rat aorta, *Eur. J. Pharmacol.,* 115, 219, 1985.

176. **Clark, D. L. and Linden, J.,** Modulation of guanylate cyclase by lipoxygenase inhibitors, *Hypertension,* 8, 947, 1986.

177. **Gryglewski, R. J., Palmer, R. M., and Moncada, S.,** Superoxide anion is involved in the breakdown of endothelium-derived vascular relaxing factor, *Nature (London),* 320, 454, 1986.

178. **Furchgott, R.,** Role of endothelium in responses of vascular smooth muscle, *Circ. Res.,* 53, 557, 1983.

179. **Singer, H. A. and Peach, M. J.,** Calcium- and endothelial-mediated vascular smooth muscle relaxation in rabbit aorta. *Hypertension,* 4 (Suppl. II), 19, 1982.

180. **Peach, M. J., Singer, H. A., Izzo, N. J., and Loeb, A. L.,** Role of calcium in endothelium-dependent relaxation of arterial smooth muscle, *Am. J. Cardiol.,* 59, 35A, 1987.

181. **Vagy, P. L., Williams, J. S., and Schwartz, A.,** Receptor pharmacology of calcium entry blocking agents. *Am. J. Cardiol.,* 59, 9A, 1987.

182. **Long, C. J. and Stone, T. W.,** The release of endothelium-derived relaxant factor is calcium dependent, *Blood Vessels,* 22, 205, 1985.

183. **Mix, L. L., Dinerstein, R. J., and Villereal, M. L.,** Mitogens and melittin stimulate an increase in intracellular free calcium concentration in human fibroblasts, *Biochem. Biophys. Res. Commun.,* 119, 69, 1984.

184. **DeMey, J. and Vanhoutte, P.,** Role of the intima in cholinergic and purinergic relaxation of isolated canine femoral arteries, *J. Physiol. (London),* 316, 347, 1981.

185. **Gordon, J. L. and Martin, W.,** Endothelium-dependent relaxation of the pig aorta: relationship to stimulation of ^{86}Rb efflux from isolated endothelial cells, *Br. J. Pharmacol.,* 79, 531, 1983.

186. **Cassis, L. A., Loeb, A. L., and Peach, M. J.,** Mechanisms of adenosine- and ATP-induced relaxation in rabbit femoral artery: role of the endothelium and cyclic nucleotides, in *Proceedings of the 3rd International Symposium on Adenosine,* Springer-Verlag, Berlin, in press.

187. **Kennedy, C. and Burnstock, G.,** ATP produces vasodilation via P_1 purinoceptors and vasoconstriction via P_2-purinoceptors in the isolated rabbit central ear artery, *Blood Vessels,* 22, 145, 1985.

188. **DeMey, J. G., Claeys, M., and Vanhoutte, P. M.,** Endothelium-dependent inhibitory effects of acetylcholine, adenosine triphosphate, thrombin, and arachidonic acid in the canine femoral artery, *J. Pharmacol. Exp. Ther.,* 222, 166, 1983.

189. **Sata, T., Misra, H. P., Linden, J. M., Lin, L. W., Kubota, E., and Said, S. I.,** A carbon-centered free radical mediates acetylcholine-induced relaxation of rabbit aorta and guinea pig pulmonary artery, *Clin. Res.,* 34, 10A, 1986.

190. **Ku, D. D.,** Mechanism of thrombin-induced endothelium-dependent coronary vasodilation in dogs: Role of proteolytic enzymatic activity, *J. Cardiovasc. Pharmacol.,* 8, 29, 1986.

191. **Milner, P. G., Loeb, A .L., and Peach, M.J .,** Plasmin inhibits thrombin induced endothelial dependent vasodilation, *Circulation,* 74 (Suppl. II), 413, 1986.

192. **Muirhead, E. E., Leach, B. E., Byers, L. W., Brooks, B., Daniels, E. G., and Hinman, J. W.,** Antihypertensive neutral renomedullary lipid (ANRL), in *Kidney Hormones,* Fisher, J. W., Ed., Academic Press, London, 1970, 485.

193. **Muirhead, E.E.,** Antihypertensive functions of the kidney, *Hypertension,* 2, 444, 1980.

194. **Prewitt, R. L., Leach, B. E., Byers, L. W., Brooks, B., Lands, W. E. M., and Muirhead, E. E.,** Antihypertensive polar renomedullary lipid, a semisynthetic vasodilator, *Hypertension,* 1, 299, 1979.

195. **Demopoulos, C. A., Pinckard, R. N., and Hanahan, D. J.,** Platelet activating factor. Evidence for 1-O-alkyl-2-acetyl-sn-glyceryl-3-phosphorylcholine as the active component (a new class of lipid chemical mediators), *J. Biol. Chem.,* 254, 9355, 1979.

196. **Benveniste, J., Henson, P. M., and Cochrane, C. G.,** Leukocyte-dependent histamine release from rabbit platelets: the role of Ig E$_1$ basophils, and a platelet-activating factor, *J. Exp. Med.,* 136, 1356, 1972.

197. **Mencia-Huerta, J. M. and Benveniste, J.,** Platelet-activating factor and macrophages. I. Evidence for the release from rat and mouse peritoneal macrophages and not from mastocytes, *Eur. J. Immunol.,* 9, 409, 1979.

198. **Kamitani, T., Katamoto, M., Tatsumi, M., Katsuta, K., Ono, T., Kikuchi, H., and Kumada, S.,** Mechanisms of the hypotensive effect of synthetic 1-O-octadecyl-2-O-acetyl-glycero-3-phosphorylcholine, *Eur. J. Pharmacol.,* 98, 357, 1984.

199. **Shigenobu, K., Masuda, Y., Tanaka, Y., and Kasuya, Y.,** Platelet activating factor analogues: lack of correlation between their activities to produce hypotension and endothelium-mediated vasodilation, *J. Pharmacobiodyn.,* 8, 128, 1985.

201. **Needleman, P., Marshall, G. R. and Sobel, B. E.,** Hormone interactions in the isolated rabbit heart: synthesis and coronary vasomotor effects of prostaglandins, angiotensin, and bradykinin, *Circ. Res.,* 37, 302, 1975.

202. **McIntire, D. E., Pearson, J. D., and Gordon, J. L.,** Localization and stimulation of prostacyclin production in vascular cells, *Nature (London),* 271, 549, 1978.

203. **Weksler, B. B., Marcus, A. J., and Jaffe, E. A.** Synthesis of prostaglandin I$_2$ (prostacyclin) by cultured human and bovine endothelial cells. *Proc. Natl. Acad. Sci. U.S.A.,* 74, 3922, 1977.

204. **Toda, N.,** Endothelium-dependent relaxation induced by angiotensin II and histamine in isolated arteries of dog, *Br. J. Pharmacol.,* 81, 301, 1984.

205. **Holtz, J., Forstermann, U., Pohl, U., Giesler, M., and Bassenge, E.,** Flow-dependent, endothelium-mediated dilation of epicardial coronary arteries in conscious dogs: effects of cyclooxygenase inhibition, *J. Cardiovasc. Pharmacol.,* 6, 1161, 1984.

206. **Van Grondelle, A., Worthen, G. S., Ellis, D., Mathias, M. M., Murphy, R. C., Strife, R. J., Reeves, J. T., and Voelkel, N. F.,** Altering hydrodynamic variables influences PGI$_2$ production by isolated lungs and endothelial cells. *J. Appl. Physiol.,* 57, 388, 1984.

207. **Gordon, J. L. and Martin, W.,** Stimulation of endothelial prostacyclin production plays no role in endothelium-dependent-relaxation of the pig aorta, *Br. J. Pharmacol.,* 80, 179, 1983.

208. **Singer, H. A. and Peach, M. J.,** Endothelium-dependent relaxation of rabbit aorta. I. Relaxation stimulated by arachidonic acid *J. Pharmacol. Exp. Ther.,* 266, 790, 1983.

209. **Furchgott, R., Cherry, P., Zawadzki, J., and Jothianandan, D.,** Endothelial cells as mediators of vasodilation of arteries, *J. Cardiovasc. Pharmacol.,* 6 (Suppl. 2) S336, 1984.

210. **Cherry, P. D., Furchgott, R. and Zawadzki, J.,** The endothelium-dependent relaxation of vascular smooth muscle by unsaturated fatty acids, *Fed. Proc.,* 42, 619, 1983.

211. **Ignarro, L. J., Harbison R. G., Wood, K. S., Wolin, M. S., McNamara, D. B., Nyman, A. L., and Kadowitz, P. J.,** Differences in responsiveness of intrapulmonary artery and vein to guanosine 3',5'mono-phosphate and cyclic adenosine 3',5'-monophospahte, *J. Pharmacol. Exp. Ther.,* 233, 560, 1985.

212. **Habermann, E.,** Bee and wasp venoms, *Science,* 177, 314, 1972.

213. **Johnson, A. R., Revtyak, G., and Campbell, W. B.,** Arachidonic acid metabolites and endothelial injury: studies with cultures of human endothelial cells, *Fed. Proc.,* 44, 19, 1985.

214. **Johnson, A. R., Callahan, K. S., Tsai, S. C., and Campbell, W. B.,** Prostacyclin and prostaglandin biosynthesis in human pulmonary endothelial cells, *Bull. Eur. Physiopathol. Respir.,* 17, 531, 1981.

215. **Shier, W. T.,** Activation of high levels of endogenous phospholipase A$_2$ in cultured cells, *Proc. Natl. Acad. Sci. U.S.A.,* 76, 195, 1979.

216. **Rice, R. H. and Levine, L.,** Melittin-stimulated arachidonate metabolism by cultured malignant human epidermal keratinocytes, *Biochem. Biophys. Res. Commun.,* 124, 303, 1984.

217. **Milner, P. M., Loeb, A. L., and Peach, M. J.,** Endothelium-dependent vasodilation is not altered by steroid treatment, *Circulation,* 74 (Suppl. II), 414, 1986.

218. **Gorman, R. R., Oglesby, T. D., Bundy, G. L., and Hopkins, A. K.,** Evidence for 15-HETE synthesis by human umbilical vein endothelial cells, *Circulation,* 72, 708, 1985.

219. **Buchanan, M. R., Batt, R. W., Magas, Z., Van Ryan, J., Hirsh, J., and Nazir, D. J.,** Endothelial cells produce a lipoxygenase-derived chemo-repellant which influences platelet-endothelial cell interactions — effect of aspirin and salycilate, *Thromb. Haemostasis,* 53, 306, 1985.

220. **Forstermann, U. and Neufang, B.,** The endothelium-dependent vasodilator effect of acetylcholine: charac-terization of the endothelial relaxing factor with inhibitors of arachidonic acid metabolism, *Eur. J. Pharmacol.,* 103, 65, 1984.

221. **Spies, C., Schultz, K. D. and Schultz, G.,** Inhibitory effects of mepacrine and eicosatetraynoic acid on cyclic GMP elevations caused by calcium and hormonal factors in rat ductus deferens, *Naunyn Schmiedebergs Arch. Pharmacol.,* 311, 71, 1980.

222. **Griffith, T. M., Edwards, D. H., Lewis, M. J., and Henderson, A. H.,** Evidence that cyclic guanosine monophosphate (cGMP) mediates endothelium-dependent relaxation, *Eur. J. Pharmacol.,* 112, 195, 1985.

223. **Forstermann, U. and Neufang, B.,** The endothelium-dependent relaxation of rabbit aorta: effects of antioxidants and hydroxylated eicosatetraenoic acids, *Br. J. Pharmacol.,* 82, 765, 1984.

224. **Martin, W., Villani, G. M., Jothianandan, D., and Furchgott, R. F.,** Selective blockade of endothelium-dependent and glyceryl trinitrate-induced relaxation by hemoglobin and by methylene blue in the rabbit aorta, *J. Pharmacol. Exp. Ther.,* 708, 708, 1985.

225. **Rubanyi, G. M. and Vanhoutte, P. M.,** Superoxide anions and hypoxia inactivate endothelium-derived relaxing factor, *Am. J. Physiol.,* 250, H822, 1986.

226. **Morrison, A. R. and Pascoe, N.,** Metabolism of arachidonate through NADPH-dependent oxygenase of renal cortex, *Proc. Natl. Acad. Sci. U.S.A.,* 78, 7375, 1981.

227. **Snyder, G. D., Capdevila, J., Chacos, N., Mauna, S., and Falck, J. R.,** Action of luteinizing hormone-releasing hormone: involvement of novel arachidonate metabolites, *Proc. Natl. Acad. Sci. U.S.A.,* 80, 3504, 1983.

228. **Izzo, N. J., Singer, H. A., Saye, J. A., and Peach, M. J.,** Cytochrome P450 inhibitors block endothelium-dependent aortic relaxation responses, *Fed. Proc.,* 42, 651, 1983.

229. **Konishi, M., Su, C.,** Role of endothelium in dilator responses of spontaneously hypertensive rat arteries, *Hypertension,* 5, 881, 1983.

230. **Luscher, T. F. and Vanhoutte, P. M.,** Endothelium-dependent responses to platelets and serotonin in spontaneously hypertensive rats, *Hypertension,* 8(Suppl. II) 55, 1986.

231. **Van De Voorde, J. and Leusen, I.,** Endothelium-dependent and independent relaxation of aortic rings from hypertensive rats, *Am. J. Physiol.,* 250, H711, 1986.

232. **Winquist, R. J., Bunting, P. B., Baskin, E. P., and Wallace, A. A.,** Decreased endothelium-dependent relaxation in New Zealand genetic hypertensive rats, *J. Hypertension,* 2, 541, 1984.

233. **Lockette, W., Otsuka, Y., and Carretero, O.,** The loss of endothelium-dependent vascular relaxation in hypertension, *Hypertension,* 8 (Suppl. II), 61, 1986.

234. **Kontos, H. A.,** Oxygen radicals in cerebral vascular injury, *Circ. Res.,* 57, 508, 1985.
235. **Harrison, D. G., Freiman, P. C., Armstrong, M. L., and Heistad, D. D.,** Improvement of receptor mediated endothelium-dependent vascular relaxation following regression of atherosclerosis, *Circulation,* 74 (Suppl. II), 286, 1986.
236. **Habib, J. B., Bossaller, C., Wells, S., Williams, C., Morrisett, J. D., and Henry, P. D.,** Preservation of endothelium-dependent vascular relaxation in cholesterol-fed rabbits by treatment with the calcium blocker PN200110, *Circ. Res.,* 58, 305, 1986.
237. **Verbeuren, T. J., Jordaens, F. H., Zonnekeyn, L. L., VanHove, C. E., Coene, M. C., and Herman, A. G.,** Effect of hypercholesterolemia on vascular reactivity in the rabbit. I. Endothelium-dependent and endothelium-independent contractions and relaxations in isolated arteries of control and hypercholesterolemic rabbits, *Circ. Res.,* 58, 552, 1986.
238. **Singer, H. A., Wagner, J. D., Duling, B., and Peach, M. .,** Endothelial-smooth muscle in rabbit thoracic aorta: muscarinic relaxation and hypoxic-induced contraction, *Fed. Proc.,* 40, 689, 1981.
239. **Peach, M. J., Singer, H. A., and Loeb, A. L.,** Mechanisms of endothelium-dependent vascular smooth muscle relaxation, *Biochem. Pharmacol.,* 34, 1867, 1985.
240. **DeMey, J. and Vanhoutte, P.M.,** Anoxia and endothelium dependent reactivity of the canine femoral artery, *J. Physiol.,* 335, 65, 1983.
241. **Rubanyi, G. M. and Vanhoutte, P. M.,** Hypoxia releases vasoconstrictor substance(s) from the coronary endothelium, *J. Physiol.,* 364, 45, 1985.
242. **Holden, W. E. and McCall, E.,** Hypoxia-induced contractions of porcine pulmonary artery strips depends on an intact endothelium, *Exp. Lung Res.,* 8, 101, 1984.
243. **Madden, J., Dawson, C., Gradall, K., and Harder, D.,** Effect of endothelium removal on hypoxic constriction in cat isolated pulmonary arteries, *Fed. Proc.,* 45, 277, 1986.
244. **Luscher, T. F. and Vanhoutte, P. M.,** Endothelium-dependent contractions to acetylcholine in the aorta of the spontaneously hypertensive rat, *Hypertension,* 8, 344, 1986.
245. **Morganroth, M. L., Reeves, J. T., Murphy, R. C., and Voelkel, N. F.,** Leukotriene synthesis and receptor-blockers block hypoxic pulmonary vasoconstriction, *J. Appl. Physiol.,* 56, 1340, 1984.
246. **Egleme, C., Godfraind, T., and Miller, R.,** Enhanced responsiveness of rat isolated aorta to clonidine after removal of the endothelial cells. *Br. J. Pharmacol.,* 81, 16, 1984.
247. **Biguad, M., Schoeffter, P., Stoclet, J., and Miller, R.,** Dissociation between endothelium-mediated increase in tissue cyclic GMP levels and modulation of aortic contractile responses, *Naunyn Schmeidebergs Arch. Pharmacol.,* 328, 221, 1984
248. **Miller, R., Mony, M., Schini, V., Schoeffter, P., and Stoclet, J.,** Endothelial mediated inhibition of contraction and increase in cyclic GMP levels evoked by the åa-adrenoceptor agonist BHT-920 in rat isolated aorta, *Br. J. Pharmacol.,* 83, 903, 1984.
249. **Cassis, L. A. and Peach, M. J.,** Enhanced responses of denuded rat aortic rings to the alpha-2 agonist BHT-920 involves the production of a prostanoid, *Br. J. Pharmacol.,* 1987, in press.
250. **O'Brien, R. F. and McMurtry, I. F.,** Endothelial cell supernates contract bovine pulmonary artery rings, *Am. Rev. Respir. Dis.,* 129, A337, 1984.
251. **Hickey, K. A., Rubanyi, G., Paul, R. J., and Highsmith, R. F.,** Characterization of a coronary vasoconstrictor produced by cultured endothelial cells, *Am. J. Physiol.,* 248, C550, 1985.
252. **Gillespie, M. N., Owasoyo, J. O., McMurtry, I. F., and O'Brien, R .F.,** Sustained coronary vasoconstriction provoked by a peptidergic substance released from endothelial cells in culture, *J. Pharmacol., Exp. Ther.,* 236, 339, 1986.
253. **Peach, M. J.,** unpublished research.
254. **Peach, M. J.,** unpublished research.

Chapter 4

STRUCTURAL AND FUNCTIONAL RAREFACTION OF MICROVESSELS
IN HYPERTENSION

R. L. Prewitt, H. Hashimoto, and D. L. Stacy

TABLE OF CONTENTS

I. CONTRIBUTION OF SMALL ARTERIOLES TO VASCULAR RESISTANCE

A. Microvascular Pressure Profiles

A primary question when considering increased vascular resistance in hypertension is the site of that resistance. Pressure profiles throughout the systemic circulation indicate that the major site of pressure dissipation, and therefore vascular resistance, is the arteriolar bed. Recently, however, greater emphasis has been placed on the role of the smallest arteries in regulating vascular resistance. Although it is well established that the large and medium arteries contribute little resistance to blood flow, the point where significant resistance begins is presently unclear and appears to differ among vascular beds. In the tenuissimus muscle of the cat, for example, systemic arterial pressure is reduced by only 15% in vessels larger than 115 μm internal diameter.[1] In 70 μm arterioles, 79% of the arterial pressure head remains, and then it falls with increased steepness as the capillaries are approached. Although the profile of the pressure drop is different in the cat mesentery, the total resistance contribution of the arteriolar bed is similar to that in the tenuissimus muscle.[1,2] Measurements in the rat cremaster[3] and spinotrapezius[4] muscles, however, show a pressure reduction of approximately 40% in vessels proximal to the feeding arterioles, the point at which the microcirculation begins. Despite these demonstrations of large pressure drops prior to the microcirculation, they should not as yet be accepted as a general rule. The cremaster and spinotrapezius muscles may represent examples of low pressure microcirculatory beds because of the structural arrangement of their feeding vessels. They receive their arterial supply at the far end of small feeding arteries, while other muscles, such as the rat gracilis, receive their supply directly from a large artery by way of a short feeding artery. This latter type of vascular arrangement should result in a higher pressure bed similar to that in the cat tenuissimus muscle.

The location of elevated vascular resistance in hypertension can vary with the type of hypertension. In the spontaneously hypertensive rat (SHR), vascular resistance is proportionally elevated throughout the microcirculation in skeletal muscle, implying that arterioles contribute significantly to the rise.[3,4] In established renal and deoxycorticosterone-salt (DOCA-salt) hypertension the elevated arterial blood pressure is almost normalized at the level of the feeding or first-order arteriole of the cremaster.[5] This observation indicates that the small arteries play the dominant role in maintaining elevated vascular resistance and the exchange area under such conditions is almost normotensive.

Other tissues like the brain[6] and intestine,[7] on the other hand, have their own distinct vascular structure and distribution of resistance. Over 50% of the vascular resistance is above the first-order arteriole of the normal pial circulation, but these vessels have a resting internal diameter of only 51 mm.[6] Pressure in the first-order arteriole of the normotensive rat intestine is 78% of systemic pressure,[8] which, for these 86 μm vessels, is much closer to values in the cat tenuissimus than to those in rat cremaster or spinotrapezius. Thus, the exact nature of the microvascular alterations in hypertension can vary between vascular beds, but the arteriolar segments of the microvasculature always contain a significant portion of total vascular resistance.

The site of increased resistance also changes during the development of hypertension. Meininger et al.[9] have shown that the smaller arterioles constrict during the first 3 h of 2-kidney, 1-clip (2K-1C) hypertension in rats, while the larger arterioles either remain unchanged or actually increase in diameter. Thus, the contribution to increased vascular resistance is disproportionally centered at the terminal section of the vascular bed in the acute stages of 2K-1C hypertension. After 4 weeks, however, the locus of most of the elevated resistance in this model shifts above the level of the microcirculation.[5] Such a shift does not seem to occur in young SHR,[4] possibly due to the more gradual onset of hypertension in this model. In older SHR the resistance might shift upstream as hypertension becomes fully developed. Although there are many variations in the distribution of vascular resistance, the smallest arteries and arterioles

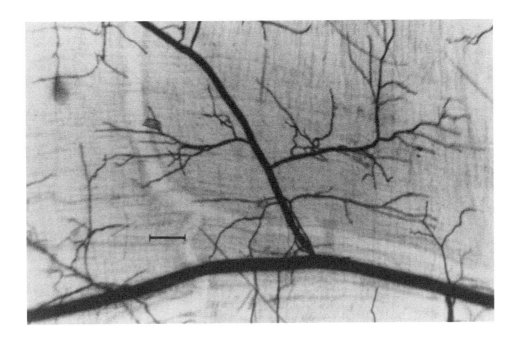

FIGURE 1. Light micrograph of the arteriolar bed in a cremaster muscle of a normotensive Wistar rat. The vessels were perfused-fixed, injected with Microfil, and cleared in glycerine. The first-order arteriole runs horizontally near the bottom of the micrograph. A second-order arteriole branches diagonally upward near the center, and third-order branches can be seen branching from the second-order at right angles. Fourth-order and fifth-order branches also appear. The calibration bar represents 250 mm.

appear to be the most appropriate sites at which to study elevated vascular resistance in hypertension.

B. Arteriolar Branching Patterns

Since this chapter reviews structural changes in the microvasculature, especially that of skeletal muscle, it is necessary to first describe the anatomy of the microcirculation and the numbering system used by many investigators. The most popular means of microvessel classification in hypertensive studies has been the numbering system used by Hutchins and Darnell.[10] In this system the major feeding vessel entering the rat cremaster muscle is designated as the first-order arteriole or 1A (Figure 1). Branches from this vessel are termed second-order arterioles (2A), and so on, to fourth- or fifth-order arterioles, which in turn give rise to capillaries. Paired venules follow the same numbering system. Although this system appears simple, it is not always applicable in its strictest sense. For example, a vessel branching from a 2A may be another 2A, a 3A, or even a 4A. To correctly identify the vessel one must recognize its branching pattern, size, and destination. Another nomenclature widely used[1,4] names the arterioles according to function. In the tenuissimus muscle of the cat for example, the central artery gives rise to arterioles branching at near right angles and which run transverse to the muscle fibers.[1] These have been called transverse arterioles and they give rise to terminal arterioles. This anatomical arrangement of a central artery and vein giving rise to transverse arterioles and venules is described by Myrhage[11] as the "basic unit" in skeletal muscle which is replicated in large muscles. A more recent classification published by Engelson et al.[12] for the rat spinotrapezius divides the arterioles into arcade arterioles which form a network spanning the entire muscle, and transverse arterioles which branch from the arcade arterioles and supply a highly localized area of muscle. Observations of the branching pattern in the rat gracilis have shown

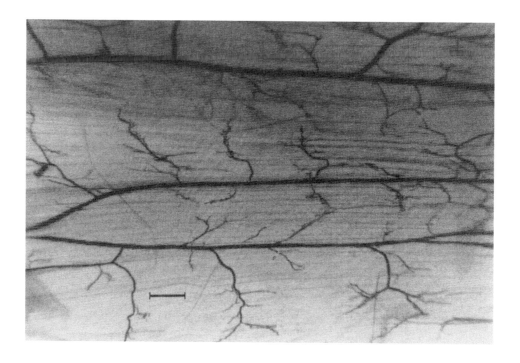

FIGURE 2.   Light micrograph of the arteriolar bed in a gracilis muscle of a normotensive Wistar rat. The vessels were perfused-fixed, injected with Microfil, and cleared in glycerine. Three second-order arterioles run horizontally, giving rise to third-order arterioles which run transverse to the muscle fibers. The calibration bar represents 500 mm.

how all of these classifications can be combined into one uniform schema. In a young rat the gracilis muscle resembles two tenuissimus muscles side by side. There are two central arteries and veins running the length of the muscle giving off transverse arterioles and venules, i.e., two basic units. By young adulthood, growth of the muscle has usually resulted in the addition of a third basic vascular unit (Figure 2). These central arteries connect at various points to form a network of arcading arterioles. Although it is not obvious in a cremaster preparation because of the incision required to open the muscle and lay it flat, the second-order arterioles also form an arcading network. Thus, the central artery of Myrhage,[11] the arcading arteriole of Engelson et al.,[12] and the second-order arteriole of Hutchins and Darnell[10] all serve the same function of distributing blood flow throughout the muscle and preventing the interruption of blood flow upon injury.[12] These arterioles also give rise to the transverse arterioles which are identical to third-order arterioles and provide an unmistakable landmark[4] from which to start classifying vessels. The third-order arteriole branches tree-like into fourth-order arterioles (Figures 1 and 2) which then give rise to a surrounding capillary bed. Thus, the third-order arteriole is in the center of the tissue which it serves, an ideal location for autoregulatory control. In the rat gracilis muscle some of the third-order arterioles form arcades especially along the margins of the muscle. These arcades, however, are narrower than those in the second-order arteriolar network and are easily distinguished from them.

All of the classification systems can be combined if one recognizes that the basic unit described by Myrhage[11] is a second-order arteriole giving rise to third-order arterioles at near right angles. If there is more than one basic unit in a muscle, the second-order arterioles interconnect to form an arcade. If the muscle fibers are arranged in a single direction, as in the gracilis, the basic units usually run parallel with the muscle fibers. In the cremaster muscle there are two layers of muscle fibers oblique to each other and the basic units are oriented in various directions between the two layers of muscle. From the fourth-order arteriole down to the capillary bed, the microvascular network is quite similar in these various muscles. All capillaries run parallel to the muscle fibers except the short branches which circumscribe the muscle fibers.

For microvascular beds in other tissues such as the brain[6] and intestine,[7,8] a similar numbering system often is used, but the microvascular network, pressure profiles, and function of the individual branches usually differ from those in skeletal muscle. Nevertheless, the numbering system remains quite useful for comparison of data obtained from similar tissues.

C. Mechanisms of Increased Vascular Resistance

1. Vasoconstriction

The most obvious mechanism increasing resistance to blood flow in arteries is vasoconstriction. This is a very powerful means by which blood flow and blood pressure are controlled throughout the circulatory system. Because resistance through a vessel is inversely proportional to the fourth power of the vessel radius, only small changes in lumen size are required to make large adjustments in flow and pressure. Vasoconstriction plays a continuous role in the moment-to-moment regulation of blood pressure through baroreceptor feedback acting via the sympathetic nervous system. In hypertension, all aspects of vasoconstriction seem to be enhanced, especially during the initial stages of experimental hypertension where arterial pressure rises rapidly and structural changes have not yet taken place. Meininger et al.[9] have shown that third- and fourth-order arterioles in the rat cremaster constrict significantly during the onset of 2K-1C hypertension. Protection of the hindquarters from the pressure rise reduces the amount of vasoconstriction, indicating that autoregulatory mechanisms mediate part of the increase in vascular tone. In young SHR, Bohlen[13] has shown increased sensitivity to norepinephrine applied directly to arterioles in the cremaster, and several investigators have indicated increased sympathetic nerve activity in SHR.[14-17] In the 1-kidney, 1-clip (1K-1C) hypertensive rat, vasoconstriction was significantly greater than control levels in gracilis arterioles 4 to 6 weeks after renal artery stenosis, but this effect was not apparent after 8 to 10 weeks, despite an increased level of hypertension.[18] The reasons for this change appear twofold. First, structural increases in vascular resistance develop with time and become responsible for a greater proportion of the total increase in resistance. Second, autoregulatory mechanisms may shift their operating point to higher pressure levels with time, as they do in SHR,[6] so that their contribution to elevated vascular resistance is diminished. Although more data on long-term hypertension are needed before definite conclusions can be drawn, the present data suggest that vasoconstriction plays a dominant role early in the hypertensive process, and this role diminishes as structural mechanisms assume the maintenance of elevated vascular resistance.

2. Wall-to-Lumen Ratio

Hypertrophy of the vascular wall resulting in decreased lumen size, increased vasodilated vascular resistance, and increased maximal response to vasoconstrictors is a major hypothesis in the field of hypertension.[19,20] Although such structural changes have been shown in vessels from large[21] and small arteries[21,22] to small arterioles,[23] recent studies indicate that there are several variations in the findings predicted by this hypothesis. In skeletal muscle arterioles of SHR there appears to be little difference in vasodilated diameter or wall-to-lumen ratio.[24,25] Coronary arterial vessels of all sizes in the 1K-1C hypertensive dog show no increases in wall-to-lumen ratio because hypertrophy of the vascular wall is accompanied by increases in lumen size.[26] This variation may result from demands for more blood flow due to the increased work load of the hypertensive myocardium. Intestinal arteries of human hypertensives[27,28] and skeletal muscle arterioles of renal hypertensive rats[18,29] develop increases in vasodilated wall-to-lumen ratio without hypertrophy, when measured as cross-sectional wall area. Although DOCA-salt hypertensive rats show hypertrophy of the wall of arteries and arterioles after 8 weeks of hypertension, there is a reduction in lumen size without hypertrophy of the vascular wall after 4 months of metacorticoid hypertension.[30] In all of these examples of increased wall-to-lumen ratio without hypertrophy, the vasodilated circumference of the vessels is structurally reduced. Interestingly, these same structural changes take place in cremaster arterioles of aortic-coarctation hypertensive rats where there is no increase in intraluminal pressure of the studied vessels.[19] Thus, many different structural alterations occur in the walls of resistance vessels depending upon the type of hypertension, its duration, and the tissue in which the vessels are found.

3. Rarefaction

A second alteration of resistance vessels in hypertension is rarefaction, a reduction in the number or density of vessels. Rarefaction can be either functional, where it is due to vasoconstriction to the point of nonperfusion of the vessel, or structural, in which case the vessels are absent. Functional rarefaction of the capillary bed in skeletal muscle of normotensive animals has been known for a long time.[31] Some of the capillaries are not perfused during resting conditions, but they are recruited during functional hyperemia. Because capillaries themselves cannot constrict, it is generally thought that a terminal portion of an arteriole, sometimes called the precapillary sphincter, controls functional capillary density. However, functional rarefaction of arterioles has been shown in normotensive animals in vessels as large as third-order arterioles.[13,18,25] This finding suggests that all the smaller arterioles and most of the capillaries fed by a closed third-order vessel would be unperfused. Some of the capillaries could possibly receive blood through interconnections with capillaries fed by other arterioles. Functional rarefaction has not been reported for skeletal muscle arterioles larger than third-order, which is consistent with the function of first- and second-order arterioles as supply vessels for the whole muscle. In hypertension both functional and structural rarefaction of microvessels are greatly enhanced. Arterioles appear to go through a period of increased functional rarefaction, followed by structural rarefaction during the development of hypertension in SHR.[25] Functional rarefaction remains elevated in the capillary bed for up to 18 weeks of age in SHR, the oldest rats in which this parameter has been measured. Thus, the decrease in total cross-sectional area of the microvascular bed causes a structural increase in vascular resistance. This could account, at least in part, for the increased vasodilated resistance of hypertensive animals, and allow the remaining vessels to control blood flow with less vasoconstriction.

4. Variation of Microvascular Alterations in Hypertension

Although every model of experimental hypertension involves an increase in peripheral vascular resistance, each model seems to have its own unique combination of mechanisms for increasing resistance, especially during the development of hypertension. The initial changes which occur in the microcirculation depend upon the factors first responsible for elevating arterial pressure. Since these factors include changes in blood volume, cardiac output, sympathetic drive, the renin-angiotensin system, receptor sensitivity, membrane potentials, and many other alterations, it is not surprising that initial changes in the microcirculation reflect these different mechanisms of onset. Although there is not complete agreement in the literature, the young SHR can be characterized as having vasoconstriction,[25,32] rarefaction,[10,25,33-35] no structural decreases in arteriolar lumen, no hypertrophy of the arteriolar wall,[24,25] and no structural increase in wall-to-lumen ratio.[24,25] The renal hypertensive rat shows vasoconstriction,[9,18] rarefaction,[8,18] structural decreases in arteriolar lumen,[18,36] and increases in wall-to-lumen ratio without hypertrophy.[18,29] The DOCA-salt hypertensive rat has vasoconstriction,[5,37] no structural rarefaction[37] (after 4 weeks of hypertension), structural decreases in arteriolar lumen[30] and hypertrophy of the vascular wall early, but not after long-term hypertension.[30] It is not surprising that the microvascular pressure profile also differs in the cremaster of these three models of experimental hypertension.[3-5] The changes in microvascular structure and function in the later stages of hypertension are more likely to include secondary changes in response to the long-standing high pressure and thus show more similarities among the various hypertensive models. As yet there is little microcirculatory data from animals with long-term hypertension.

II. RAREFACTION OF MICROVESSELS IN HYPERTENSION

A. Human Data

The earliest suggestion of microvascular rarefaction came from clinical studies of hypertensive patients. In 1933, Ruedemann[38] reported a decrease in the number of capillaries in the conjunctiva of patients with essential hypertension. Intracutaneous injections of histamine did not increase the number of capillaries, and the venules appeared congested and tortuous. Malignant hypertension was reported to involve a loss in the number of vessels, a narrowing of their lumens, and an increase in venous tortuosity. A sparseness of the conjunctival capillary bed in hypertensive subjects was reported again by Lack et al.[39] in 1949. Other capillary abnormalities in these subjects included narrowing and increased looping. A correlation between narrowing of conjunctival capillaries and nail fold capillaries of hypertensives was observed by Landau and Davis.[40] In a more quantitative study, Jackson[41] found that in hypertensive patients: (1) vasomotor rates were higher in conjunctival vessels than in those of controls; (2) stellate ganglionic block by local xylocaine anesthesia eliminated vasomotor activity; (3) sensitivity of the conjunctival bed to epinephrine was increased relative to control values; and (4) severe vascular spasm resulted in a preponderance of nonperfusion over perfusion of the capillary bed.

Recent studies on the conjunctiva of hypertensive subjects have again shown rarefaction of capillaries and arterioles.[42,43] Patients with high-cardiac-output borderline hypertension had reduced conjunctival capillary and venular density.[42] Arteriolar density showed a tendency toward reduction, but the difference was not statistically significant. Capillary density was inversely correlated with cardiac output in controls as well as in borderline hypertensives, suggesting the operation of an autoregulatory mechanism. In established hypertension, arteriolar density and diameter were reduced compared to age-matched controls.[43] This sequence of capillary rarefaction followed by arteriolar rarefaction in established hypertension is similar to results obtained in studies using SHR gracilis muscle.[25] In these studies, capillary density was reduced in 6- to 8-week-old SHR but no arteriolar rarefaction or vasoconstriction was observed. By 16 to 18 weeks of age, however, both arteriolar rarefaction and vasoconstriction were evident in the SHR. The progression of rarefaction from the capillary bed to larger arterioles observed in these studies may reflect vasoconstriction of increasing severity as blood pressure rises. Vasoconstriction will diminish later as structural changes are established.

An excellent documentation of arteriolar rarefaction in the intestinal circulation of human hypertensives was published by Short.[27,28,44] In this study, the superior mesenteric artery was injected with radiopaque bismuth oxychloride-gelatin suspension at pressures of 150 to 250 mmHg. The arteries and arterioles were fixed in the vasodilated state, as indicated by a smooth internal elastic lamina. Segments of intestine were opened along the mesenteric line, laid flat, and arteriograms were made. Counts of arteries and arterioles crossing a test line indicated that vessels with inside diameters of 70 to 200 μm were decreased in number by approximately 50% whereas vessels of 30 to 70 μm diameter were reduced by about 35% in chronic hypertension. Histological studies of these vessels showed an increase in wall-to-lumen ratio, no hypertrophy of the vascular wall, and a structurally-reduced lumen size compared to vessels in normotensive control subjects. In one of these six cases of established hypertension, there was a stenosis of the superior mesenteric artery which probably lowered the arterial pressure in more distal vessels. No rarefaction of the arterial bed nor structural changes of the vascular wall was noted in this subject. Short and Thomson[27] concluded from this observation that the elevated pressure leads to arterial constriction which produces structural changes in the arterial wall over long periods. This in turn renders the vessel wall less distensible. Thus, changes in the structure of the vessel wall and rarefaction would appear to be long-term autoregulatory mechanisms. It would have been beneficial to have data from other vascular beds in this same patient, since experiments on coarctation of the aorta in rats showed the same structural changes in normotensive arterioles as in renovascular hypertensive arterioles.[29]

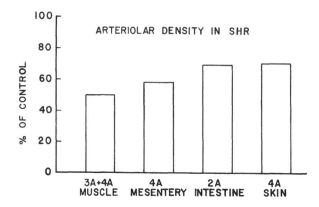

FIGURE 3.   Arteriolar density in various tissues of SHR shown as a percent of their respective control values. Data were taken from the following references: muscle,[10] mesentery,[24] intestine,[7] and skin.[35]

The most recent study of microvascular rarefaction in humans indicates that capillary density is reduced in pectoralis muscle, quadriceps muscle, myocardium, and stomach in patients with primary hypertension when compared to values in normotensive controls.[45] Rarefaction is not seen in the diaphragm or zona granulosa of the cerebellum. Because this type of data is difficult to obtain from human subjects, it is fortunate that there are many similarities in microvascular alterations between human hypertensives and hypertensive animals. As will be discussed below, microvascular rarefaction has been found in SHR muscle,[10] intestine,[7] and myocardium,[46] but not in cerebrum.[6] Although no model of experimental hypertension is exactly the same as human hypertensive disease, similarities in the data from animals and man suggest that at least some of the basic mechanisms are shared, and that the animal data can be used as a guide to fruitful measurements in man.

B. SHR

Arteriolar rarefaction in SHR cremaster muscle was reported first by Hutchins and Darnell[10] in 1974. By counting the number of each order of arterioles, they found that third- and fourth-order arterioles were reduced in SHR by approximately 50% compared to normotensive controls (Figure 3). Fourth-order venules in SHR were found to be approximately double the normal number. In a later publication, Hutchins et al.[47] reported that arteriolar rarefaction in the SHR cremaster is greatest at 6 weeks of age and absent at 3, 12, and 30 weeks. Experiments by Bohlen[13] on 18- to 20-week-old animals showed significantly more functional rarefaction of third-order arterioles in SHR than in WKY and indicated that increased responsiveness to norepinephrine may be responsible for the closure of arterioles in SHR. Chen et al.[33] confirmed the findings of Hutchins and Darnell[10] on arteriolar rarefaction using stereological methods in 4- to 6-week-old SHR. These workers also found a 32% structural rarefaction of capillaries in the hypertensive rats. Functional rarefaction of capillaries in SHR was even greater, with only 39% of existing capillaries perfused in the resting state, vs. 70% in WKY. This strong functional capillary rarefaction indicates that terminal arteriolar vascular tone is elevated in SHR even though arteriolar diameters do not always show a significant difference between SHR and WKY.[4,10,24,25,33] By measuring intrajunctional arteriolar lengths, Roy and Mayrovitz[48] determined that there are fewer small arterioles in SHR cremaster of 7 to 8 weeks of age.

Similar changes, but delayed in time, occur in SHR gracilis muscle.[25,49] At 6 to 8 weeks of age there was significant functional and structural rarefaction of capillaries in SHR, but no difference from WKY in arteriolar density.[25] At 12 to 14 weeks of age there was significant functional rarefaction of arterioles and capillaries in SHR, but no structural rarefaction. That is, under resting conditions fewer arterioles and capillaries were perfused in the SHR gracilis, but

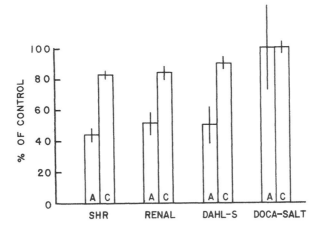

FIGURE 4. Microvascular density in gracilis muscles of various models of experimental hypertension expressed as a percent of their respective control values. Data were taken from the following references: SHR,[25] renal,[18] Dahl-S,[58] and DOCA-salt.[37] Arteriolar density is designated by an A and capillary density is designated by a C.

after vasodilation there were no significant differences between SHR and WKY. In SHR, 24 out of 60 arterioles were not perfused under resting conditions vs. 5 out of 62 in WKY. All but two of the closed arterioles were less than 20 μm in diameter after vasodilation with sodium nitroprusside. By 16 to 18 weeks of age functional and structural rarefaction of arterioles as well as capillaries (Figure 4) was present in SHR gracilis muscle. A frequency distribution of arteriolar sizes indicated that the loss of arterioles occurred in the range that was functionally rarefied at 12 to 14 weeks of age. Capillary rarefaction in SHR gracilis muscle was noted also by Henrich and Hertel[49] in 16- to 17-week-old animals. Although it seems that microvascular rarefaction in SHR cremaster muscle is fairly well established, it should be pointed out that some investigators have found neither arteriolar[50] nor capillary[51] rarefaction in SHR spinotrapezius muscle. It may be that the spinotrapezius muscle does not develop microvascular rarefaction, or a more likely possibility is that the animals studied were not old enough to have developed structural rarefaction.

In an extensive study of the mesentery, Henrich et al.[34] found only 58% as many fourth-order arterioles in SHR as in WKY (Figure 3) and a severe reduction in SHR capillary density. In the SHR mesentery, however, there were many more A-V shunts than in the WKY mesentery, and so the calculated hindrance to blood flow through the capillary bed was not elevated. Arteriolar diameters were not reduced in the SHR, either under resting conditions or when relaxed with verapamil and phenoxybenzamine. Thus, increased resistance to blood flow in SHR was provided by reduction in parallel conductance channels. In the intestinal wall of 18- to 21-week-old SHR, Bohlen[7] found 69% as many second-order arterioles per milligram tissue as in WKY (Figure 3). There was significant functional rarefaction of SHR third-order arterioles, but after vasodilation the difference between SHR and WKY was not statistically significant. None of these changes was evident in rats of 4 to 5 weeks of age, a time when rarefaction was well developed in the cremaster muscle. This again supports the idea that microvascular alterations develop at different rates in different tissues.

In a study of fixed tissues, Haack et al.[35] found 30% fewer small arterioles in the cutaneous microcirculation of SHR in comparison to WKY of 5 to 10 weeks of age (Figure 3). Vessels with and without blood cells in their lumen were counted, so rarefaction was probably structural. The inside diameters of these arterioles were 22% larger in SHR than in WKY, but it is difficult to judge the meaning of this measurement because the vessels were not perfusion fixed. Another interesting finding in this study is that there were no differences between SHR and WKY in the number of fourth-order venules. This is quite different from the cremaster muscle where SHR have twice as many fourth-order venules as WKY.[10]

Arterioles on the surface of the cerebral cortex of 18- to 21-week-old SHR showed no rarefaction, but first-, second-, and fourth-order arterioles of SHR had smaller resting diameters than comparable arterioles of WKY.[6] Passive diameters of these arterioles did not differ between SHR and WKY, which implies that the cerebral microcirculatory bed relies on vasoconstriction rather than rarefaction to increase its vascular resistance. In the brainstem, however, rarefaction of vessels from 6 to 15 μm was found in SHR, whereas the normal number of capillaries was present.[52] Thus, different parts of the brain show different microvascular alterations in hypertension.

Rarefaction of capillaries in the ciliary processes and choroid in the eyes of SHR was observed by Funk and Rohen.[53] This effect in the ciliary processes, together with a reduction in the number of fenestrations in their capillary endothelia, and hyalinization of the connective tissue surrounding the ciliary body may be the cause of the decreased aqueous formation and the low ocular pressure found in SHR. As in other vascular beds showing rarefaction, diameters of arterioles measured from resin casts were larger in SHR than in WKY.

Rarefaction may occur in the coronary circulation of SHR. Capillary density is decreased in the left ventricle of the SHR,[46] and minimal coronary vascular resistance, expressed for 100 g of tissue is increased.[54] Myocardial hypertrophy with no change in the vasculature would lower capillary density and thus increase vascular resistance per 100 g of tissue.[55] Although this would be a type of rarefaction, it is not the same as the decrease in the number of vessels seen in other tissues. However, increases in minimal coronary vascular resistance are seen in SHR right ventricles which are exposed to increased perfusion pressure but do not have after-load-induced hypertrophy.[54,56] Also treatment with hydralazine lowers arterial pressure and returns coronary vascular resistance to normal in SHR, but does not alleviate cardiac hypertrophy.[54] Thus, hypertrophy alone does not explain all of the decrease in coronary total cross-sectional area. A structural decrease in the lumen of the coronary arterioles is an alternate hypothesis for the increase in coronary minimal resistance. More data on arteriolar structure and density in the SHR is needed before this question can be resolved.

C. Renovascular Hypertension

Microvascular rarefaction is seen in the gracilis muscle of 1K-1C hypertensive rats 8 to 10 weeks after renal artery stenosis.[18] Similar to SHR gracilis, arteriolar density was reduced by approximately 50% (Figure 4) and capillary density was reduced 16% compared to age-matched controls. The difference in capillary density between hypertensives and controls was greatest under resting conditions, indicating that the terminal arteriolar segments of the 1K-1C rats had increased vascular tone. Eight out of 19 arterioles observed in 1K-1C rats were closed under resting conditions, whereas only 3 out of 32 arterioles were closed in the controls. Thus, there was significant functional rarefaction as well as structural rarefaction. These results are significant because they show that microvascular rarefaction occurs in a nongenetic form of hypertension. The arterioles of the hypertensive rats had smaller lumens and increased wall-to-lumen ratios, but no increases in wall cross-sectional area. Similar results were obtained recently in the cremaster muscle of 1K-1C and coarctation hypertensive rats by Plunkett and Overbeck.[29] In both of these hypertensive models, fourth- and fifth-order arterioles had increased wall-to-lumen ratios in the relaxed state, without a significant increase in wall cross-sectional area, compared to arterioles of their respective controls. The results were very similar in the two different models of hypertension even though the arterioles in the coarctation hypertensive rats were not exposed to the hypertensive pressures. Although the experiments were not designed to measure the density of the microvessels, the authors did note functional rarefaction of arterioles that seemed to be greater in the hypertensive rats. The closed arterioles opened upon application of sodium nitroprusside. A true demonstration of rarefaction in the aortic coarctation model would be strong evidence against the long-term autoregulation mechanism for loss of vessels.

Meininger et al.,[8] using a unique approach, have obtained evidence for arteriolar rarefaction in the intestinal wall of 2K-1C hypertensive rats. By measuring red cell velocity and internal diameters of the various branches of arterioles, one can calculate the flow in each vessel. The ratio of the flows in each order of branching allows the calculation of the number of the smaller vessels needed to carry the flow in the larger. Using this approach, Meininger et al.[8] calculated that the number of third-order arterioles in the 2K-1C hypertensive rat intestine was reduced to 38% of control values. Fourth-order arterioles were not measured. Although calculation of blood flow from red cell velocity is potentially erroneous, it is reassuring that this method provides functional data in agreement with data obtained by the anatomical approach used by most investigators.

Alexandrova et al.[52] found rarefaction of brainstem arterioles with diameters between 6 and 15 μm in Grollman hypertensive rats, but the density of vessels smaller than 5 μm in diameter was unchanged. According to Sokolova et al.,[57] the third-, fourth-, and fifth-order pial arterioles are also rarefied in the Grollman hypertensive rat. Because these measurements were made on preparations filled with gelatin in India ink, it is not clear whether this was structural or only functional rarefaction. These investigators also found arteriolar density reductions 24 h after compression of the kidney, which almost certainly was functional rarefaction.

D. DOCA-Salt Hypertension

In the gracilis muscle of the DOCA-salt hypertensive rat, neither functional nor structural arteriolar rarefaction (Figure 4) was observed after 4 to 6 weeks of hypertension.[37] Rarefaction may simply take longer than 4 to 6 weeks to develop in the DOCA-salt hypertensive rat, since it takes that long in the 1K-1C hypertensive rat,[18] and blood pressure rises more slowly in the DOCA-salt model. Functional but not structural rarefaction of the capillaries was found in the gracilis muscle of DOCA-salt hypertensive rats compared to controls given either salt water or tap water to drink. Less arteriolar vasoconstriction was noted in this model of hypertension than in SHR or 1K-1C hypertensive rats, which supports the idea that DOCA-salt treatment induces volume-dependent hypertension. Sokolova et al.[57] found rarefaction of the pial arterioles and brainstem capillaries of the DOCA-salt hypertensive rats, but again, it was not determined whether this was functional or structural rarefaction.

E. Dahl-S Hypertension

Arteriolar but not capillary rarefaction (Figure 4) was reported for gracilis muscle of the Dahl-S hypertensive rat.[58] In these experiments Dahl-S and Dahl-R rats were fed a diet containing 8% sodium chloride from 6 weeks of age and the microvascular measurements were made 3 to 4 weeks later. The results resemble a combination of those obtained from SHR and DOCA-salt hypertensive rats. There was structural but not functional rarefaction of arterioles and functional but not structural rarefaction of capillaries in the Dahl-S compared to the Dahl-R. Because hypertension develops rapidly when the Dahl-S rat is placed on the high sodium diet, functional rarefaction of arterioles, which was seen in SHR gracilis at 12 to 14 weeks of age, may have occurred before the measurements were made. In any case, the quick development of arteriolar rarefaction implies that, in skeletal muscle, the Dahl-S hypertensive rat is probably more vasoconstricted than the DOCA-salt rat during the development of hypertension. A remote possibility is that Dahl-S rats have fewer arterioles from birth.

F. Pulmonary Hypertension

Although this review primarily concerns systemic hypertension, for the sake of complete-ness, microvascular alterations in pulmonary hypertension should be discussed. In both primary pulmonary hypertension and cystic fibrosis, patients with increased pulmonary artery pressure have right ventricular hypertrophy, increased thickness of the arterial wall, and rarefaction of arterioles in the lung.[59] Patients with primary pulmonary hypertension have increased muscularity of arteries of all sizes[59] and fewer arterioles less than 40 μm in diameter.[60] Exposure of humans or animals to high altitude or chronic hypoxia results in pulmonary hypertension and changes in the pulmonary arterial bed similar to those seen in primary pulmonary hypertension. In subjects native to high altitude, pulmonary arteries (mean outside diameter 246 μm) were found to have increased wall-to-lumen ratios and increased cross-sectional area of the media compared to vessels from subjects at sea level, whereas arterioles (mean outside diameter 69 μm) did not differ significantly between the two groups.[61] Rats maintained in a hypobaric chamber at 380 mmHg ambient pressure developed right ventricular hypertrophy, increased arterial wall thickness, and a loss of arterial vessels as large as 200 μm.[62] Although lung volume increased in these animals, there was a true reduction in arterial number as determined by the ratio of alveoli to vessels. The loss of vessels was very rapid with a 20% reduction by 7 days of exposure and a 40% reduction by 14 days. Thus, microvascular changes in the pulmonary circulation are similar, whether pulmonary hypertension is primary, or secondary to hypoxia. In either case structural changes may be linked to the elevated pressure or chronic vasoconstriction. It is of interest that arteriolar rarefaction and increases in arterial wall thickness occur in pulmonary hypertension because this syndrome may be very different from systemic hypertension in the role of the sympathetic nervous system, the renin-angiotensin system, blood volume regulation, and many other factors. It appears that the common findings in both diseases are an elevation in intraluminal pressure and chronic vasoconstriction.

III. POSSIBLE MECHANISMS LEADING TO RAREFACTION

A. Vasoconstrictors

As yet there have been no direct experiments on the causes of microvascular rarefaction. Haack et al.[35] suggested that rarefaction may be due to genetic factors unrelated to hypertension. This hypothesis is refuted, however, by the development of rarefaction in the renal hypertensive rat,[18] the Dahl-S hypertensive rat,[58] which differs genetically from the SHR, and of course, from data on human hypertensive subjects.[27,38,42,43,45] Alternatively, rarefaction may be the result of chronic vasoconstriction. According to the mechanisms outlined in Figure 5, which are derived primarily from experiments on the SHR gracilis muscle,[25] chronic vasoconstriction may lead to functional rarefaction. This is essentially an upstream extension of closure of the terminal portion of the precapillary resistance vessels, a phenomenon which is already well established as the regulator of functional capillary density. Why functional rarefaction leads to the loss of some vessels and not others, and what chemical mediators are involved in the process have not been addressed as yet. Somehow the closure of the arteriole becomes irreversible and the vessel apparently atrophies. In early cases of pulmonary hypertension remnants of such atrophied arterioles, termed "ghost arteries", were visible.[59,60] "Ghost arteries" had concentric layers of cells with elongated nuclei either partly or completely obliterating the lumen.

Regardless of the mechanisms responsible for the development of structural rarefaction, functional rarefaction may be initiated by chronic vasoconstriction in response to vasoconstrictive agents or autoregulatory mechanisms. Activity of the sympathetic nervous system is heightened in hypertension[14-17] and arterioles of hypertensive animals have increased sensitivity[13] and reactivity[19,20] to norepinephrine and other vasoactive agents.[63] Experiments on the cremaster muscle conducted by Bohlen[13] showed that doses of norepinephrine that caused minimal responses in WKY resulted in complete closure of arterioles in SHR. In addition, functional rarefaction of third-order arterioles was reversed by transection of the sympathetic nerve supplying the cremaster arterioles. Further evidence comes from the experiments of Dusseau and Hutchins[64] who showed that chronic treatment with the β₂ agonist, salbutamol, increases the number of arterioles in SHR cremaster without lowering blood pressure. Acute

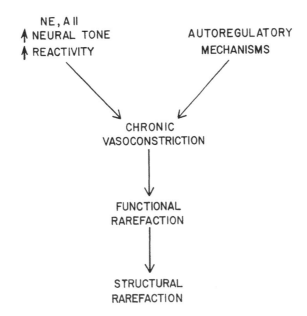

FIGURE 5. Outline of possible steps in the development of microvascular rarefaction in hypertension. NE = norepinephrine, AII = angiotensin II.

administration of salbutamol, as expected, causes vasodilatation of arterioles in the cremaster muscle of SHR and WKY.[65] Rarefaction in the cutaneous circulation[35] supports a role for sympathetic neural innervation over autoregulatory mechanisms in the initiation of rarefaction, because the cutaneous circulation is primarily controlled by neural mechanisms.

B. Autoregulation

Hutchins and Darnell[10] first suggested that arteriolar rarefaction may be a mechanism for long-term autoregulation of blood flow. The rising blood pressure during the development of hypertension could initiate both myogenic and metabolic autoregulatory mechanisms to increase resistance to blood flow. An autoregulatory increase in resistance has been suggested as a major factor in the development of hypertension.[66] Meininger et al.[9] have shown that autoregulatory mechanisms do indeed contribute to vasoconstriction of rat cremaster arterioles in the acute phase of 2K-1C renal hypertension. Lombard et al.[67] found that arterioles in the SHR cremaster constricted more strongly in response to increases in local oxygen tension than arterioles of WKY. In experiments on normotensive rats, Hogan and Hirschmann[68] showed that lowering the perfusion pressure of the cremaster muscle for 3 weeks by ligating its arterial supply resulted in an increase in the number of arterioles. Although hypertension is not simply the opposite of this type of pressure drop, it is of interest to recall that the single patient studied by Short[28] that did not have arteriolar rarefaction of the intestinal wall had a severe stenosis of the mesenteric artery which probably lowered pressure distal to that point.

Additional experiments are needed to determine the relative contribution of vasoconstrictive agents and autoregulatory mechanisms to chronic vasoconstriction and functional rarefaction. It may be that both mechanisms are operable, and when vascular wall tension is high enough, for whatever reason, the vessel closes.

C. Aging

According to the results obtained by Hutchins et al.,[47] arteriolar rarefaction was no longer present in SHR cremaster muscle of animals 12 and 30 weeks old. This age dependency has led to the hypothesis that rarefaction is a temporary phenomenon of the growth process.[49] Capillary density decreases in skeletal muscle of growing rats but capillary-to-fiber ratio increases.[69] Because the number of muscle fibers does not change, this means that new capillaries are developing. Capillary density falls because cross-sectional area of the muscle fibers increases at a faster rate than new capillaries are added. If capillaries and arterioles develop more slowly in SHR than in WKY, an age-dependent rarefaction would result. But with time, continued formation of blood vessels in SHR might remove any difference between SHR and WKY. This very sequence has been documented in the SHR coronary circulation.[70] As myocardial hypertrophy developed to a peak at 7 months of age in the SHR, capillary density decreased to its lowest point. During the next 8 months capillary density in SHR increased to WKY levels, whereas cardiocyte diameter remained unchanged. Although this hypothesis would not account for the functional rarefaction that precedes structural rarefaction,[25] it cannot be ruled out completely. The aging hypothesis would not be supported if rarefaction were shown to develop in renal hypertensive rats where hypertension was initiated in adult animals.

IV. FUNCTIONAL IMPLICATIONS OF RAREFACTION

A. Increased Vascular Resistance

Although microvascular rarefaction appears to be a result rather than a primary cause of hypertension, it develops soon enough to assist in the rise in blood pressure and certainly provides a structural basis for maintenance of hypertension. Through a reduction in parallel conductance pathways, rarefaction increases vascular resistance in a linear manner. The hemodynamic consequences of arteriolar rarefaction were demonstrated by Hallback et al.[71] in experiments where rarefaction was simulated by injecting 50-μm microspheres into the hindquarters of normotensive rats. A 50% increase in vasodilated vascular resistance was produced by this blockage of arterioles. When these "rarefied" hindquarters were subjected to constant-flow perfusion with increasing concentrations of norepinephrine only a small upward shift in the pressure response was observed. This was quite different from the large increase in maximum pressor response seen in SHR hindquarters.[19] Thus, structural rarefaction should contribute to increased minimal resistance, but not to increased reactivity to vasoactive agents.

Rarefaction provides a mechanism by which the capillary bed may contribute to elevated vascular resistance in hypertension. Because capillaries cannot constrict and their diameter changes little in hypertension, resistance through the capillary bed can only change by varying the number of perfused capillaries. Chen and Prewitt[72] found that capillary red cell velocity was 24% higher in SHR than in WKY, whereas capillary diameter and hematocrit were similar in both groups. Capillary pressure gradients calculated from these data showed a 42% elevation in SHR, whereas mean blood pressure was elevated 39%. Thus, it appears that rarefaction proportionally increases resistance through the hypertensive capillary bed by forcing blood through fewer channels at a higher velocity. Direct measurements of microvascular pressures by Bohlen et al.[3] also indicate that the pressure drop over the SHR capillary bed is increased in proportion to the rise in systemic blood pressure.

Arteriolar vasoconstriction can be underestimated in intravital studies based on diameter measurements when functional rarefaction is present. As shown in the 12- to 14-week-old SHR gracilis muscle,[25] functionally rarefied arterioles tend to be the smaller vessels. Since these nonperfused arterioles cannot be located by intravital microscopy, they are not included in measurements of mean resting arteriolar diameter. Although the resting diameters of perfused arterioles are similar in 12- to 14-week-old SHR and WKY gracilis muscles,[25] inclusion of the nonperfused arterioles demonstrates that the mean resting diameter is actually 35% lower in SHR compared to WKY ($p < 0.05$). Functional arteriolar rarefaction is vasoconstriction to closure of the arteriole. Since this is more prevalent at certain stages of hypertension, it must be taken into account when comparing vasoconstriction between normotensive and hypertensive animals.

B. Transcapillary Exchange

Transcapillary escape rate of albumin is higher in human hypertensive subjects[73] and SHR[74] than it is in controls. By decreasing surface area for exchange, capillary rarefaction should reduce the effects of increases in permeability. Edwards and Diana[75] found evidence that capillary surface area was reduced in SHR hindquarters, but a more recent study by Korthuis et al.[76] showed no difference between SHR and WKY hindquarters in permeability or surface area. They suggested that any decreases in capillary density in the SHR may be offset by increases in small-venular density as reported by Hutchins and Darnell.[10] Rippe and Folkow[77] also found no increase in permeability of SHR hindquarters and they proposed, as did Korthuis et al.,[76] that the increased transcapillary escape rate was due to elevated capillary pressure in the SHR. Laine and Granger[78] found increased intestinal microvascular permeability to macromolecules in the 1K-1C hypertensive dog. Permeability may be increased only in certain vascular beds of hypertensive animals, not including skeletal muscle, and these beds may account for the increase in the whole-body transcapillary escape rate of albumin. Structural and functional rarefaction of the capillary bed should oppose increases in fluid and macromolecular escape, whether such increases are due to elevations in permeability or capillary pressure.

C. Diffusion Distance

Capillary rarefaction increases diffusion distance, which in turn could limit the exchange of gases and nutrients in the microcirculation. Calculations based on capillary density measurements in gracilis muscles of 16- to 18-week-old rats yielded half-intercapillary distances of 50.5 μm for SHR and 34.2 μm for WKY under resting conditions.[25] To supply oxygen to the midpoint between capillaries without falling below a critical value near zero, capillary oxygen tension would have to be 12.85 mmHg higher in SHR than in WKY. The combination of higher capillary red cell velocity in SHR[72] and normal blood flow to SHR skeletal muscle[79,80] may allow for a higher capillary oxygen tension and normal oxygen delivery. An increase in small venular density[10] may also assist in these exchange functions. Capillary reserve is higher in SHR than in WKY,[25,33] and recruitment of these capillaries during exercise would maintain performance in the face of increased demand for nutrient exchange.

V. CONCLUSIONS AND FUTURE TRENDS

Intravital studies of the microcirculation in hypertension have made valuable and unique contributions to understanding the different ways in which vascular resistance is increased. Direct observations have shown that the small arterioles, which play a critical role in control of blood pressure and flow, undergo a variety of structural alterations in hypertension. These include increases in wall-to-lumen ratio with or without hypertrophy of the media, no increase in wall-to-lumen ratio in some instances, and rarefaction of arterioles and capillaries. In whole organ studies, it is not possible to differentiate among these various changes in the resistance vessels. Maximal responses to vasoconstrictors are apt to involve responses of large and medium arteries that have little to do with regulation of blood pressure and flow in normotensive or hypertensive animals. Larger arteries usually increase their wall-to-lumen ratio in hypertension, and their resultant increased reactivity to vasoconstrictors in a whole organ experiment may obscure the responses of the arterioles. Microvascular alterations vary with the type of hypertension, its duration, and the tissue in which the vessels are found. Vasoconstriction appears to dominate at the onset of hypertension and to be gradually replaced by structural increases in vascular resistance. More studies are needed on microvascular alterations in different models of experimental hypertension to fully document the variety of possible responses. Chronic studies especially are needed to establish the time frame in which the different alterations take place. Many of the results in the literature are seemingly contradictory, probably because studies were initiated at various times during the development of hypertension when mechanisms and structures were changing.

Mechanisms responsible for microvascular rarefaction are incompletely understood, but appear to be multifactorial, possibly involving responses to pressure, flow, circulating vasoconstrictors, autoregulatory mechanisms, and sympathetic innervation. Additional experiments are needed to determine if rarefaction is (1) produced by chronic vasoconstriction due to elevated sympathetic tone or circulating vasoactive agents, (2) a mechanism of long-term regulation of blood flow that matches vascular density with blood pressure, or (3) a failure of vessels to develop as rapidly in growing hypertensive animals as in normotensive ones.

ACKNOWLEDGMENTS

Writing of this review was supported in part by NIH Grants HL 36551 and HL 36448. R.L. Prewitt is a recipient of NIH Research Career Development Award HL 01778.

REFERENCES

1. **Fronek, K. and Zweifach, B. W.,** Microvascular pressure distribution in skeletal muscle and the effect of vasodilation, *Am. J. Physiol.,* 228, 791, 1975.
2. **Gore, R. W.,** Pressures in cat mesenteric arterioles and capillaries during changes in systemic arterial blood pressure, *Circ. Res.,* 34, 581, 1974.
3. **Bohlen, H. G., Gore, R. W., and Hutchins, P. M.,** Comparison of microvascular pressure in normal and spontaneously hypertensive rats, *Microvasc. Res.,* 13, 125, 1977.
4. **Zweifach, B. W., Kovalcheck, S., DeLano, F., and Chen, P.,** Micropressure-flow relationships in a skeletal muscle of spontaneously hypertensive rats, *Hypertension,* 3, 601, 1981.
5. **Meininger, G. A., Harris, P. D., and Joshua, I. G.,** Distributions of microvascular pressure in skeletal muscle of one-kidney, one clip, two-kidney, one clip, and deoxycorticosterone-salt hypertensive rats, *Hypertension,* 6, 27, 1984.
6. **Harper, S. L. and Bohlen, H. G.,** Microvascular adaptation in the cerebral cortex of adult spontaneously hypertensive rats, *Hypertension,* 6, 408, 1984.
7. **Bohlen, H. G.,** Intestinal microvascular adaptation during maturation of spontaneously hypertensive rats, *Hypertension,* 5, 739, 1983.
8. **Meininger, G. A., Fehr, K. L., Yates, M. B., Borders, J. L., and Granger, H. J.,** Hemodynamic characteristics of the intestinal microcirculation in renal hypertension, *Hypertension,* 8, 66, 1986.
9. **Meininger, G. A., Lubrano, V. M., and Granger, H. J.,** Hemodynamic and microvascular responses in the hindquarters during the development of renal hypertension in rats. Evidence for the involvement of an autoregulatory component, *Circ. Res.,* 55, 609, 1984.
10. **Hutchins, P. M. and Darnell, A. E.,** Observations of a decreased number of small arterioles in spontaneously hypertensive rats, *Circ. Res.,* 34 (Suppl 1), 161, 1974.
11. **Myrhage, R.,** Microvascular supply of skeletal muscle fibers, *Acta Orthop. Scand.,* Suppl. 168, 1, 1977.
12. **Engelson, E. T., Skalak, T. C. and Schmid-Schonbein, G. W.,** The microvasculature in skeletal muscle. 1. Arteriolar network in rat spinotrapezius muscle, *Microvasc. Res.,* 30, 29, 1985.
13. **Bohlen, H. G.,** Arteriolar closure mediated by hyperresponsiveness to norepinephrine in hypertensive rats, *Am. J. Physiol.,* 236, H157, 1979.
14. **Henrich, H.,** Sympathetic-adrenergic regulation of the hypertensive microvasculature, in *Microvascular Aspects of Spontaneous Hypertension,* Henrich, H., Ed., Hans Huber, Bern, 1982, 91.
15. **Judy, W. V., Watanabe, A. M., Henry, D. P., Besch, H. R., Jr., Murphy, W. R., and Hockel, G. M.,** Sympathetic nerve activity, role in regulation of blood pressure in the spontaneously hypertensive rat, *Circ. Res.,* 38 (Suppl. II), 21, 1976.
16. **Mueller, S. M. and Ertel, P. J.,** Association between sympathetic nerve activity and cerebrovascular protection in young spontaneously hypertensive rats, *Stroke,* 14, 88, 1983.
17. **Smith, P. G., Poston, C. W., and Mills, E.,** Ontogeny of neural and non-neural contributions to arterial blood pressure in spontaneously hypertensive rats, *Hypertension,* 6, 54, 1984.
18. **Prewitt, R. L., Chen, I. I. H., and Dowell, R. F.,** Microvascular alterations in the one-kidney, one-clip renal hypertensive rat, *Am. J. Physiol.,* 246, H728, 1984.

19. **Folkow, B., Hallback, M., Lundgren, Y., and Weiss, L.,** Background of increased flow resistance and vascular reactivity in spontaneously hypertensive rats, *Acta Physiol. Scand.,* 80, 93, 1970.

20. **Folkow, B., Hallback, M., Lundgren, Y., Sivertsson, R., and Weiss, L.,** Importance of adaptive changes in vascular design for establishment of primary hypertension, studied in man and in spontaneously hypertensive rats, *Circ. Res.,* 32 (Suppl. I), 2, 1973.

21. **Furuyama, M.,** Histometrical investigations of arteries in reference to arterial hypertension, *Tohoku J. Exp. Med.,* 76, 388, 1962.

22. **Mulvany, M. J., Hansen, P. K., and Aalkjaer, C.,** Direct evidence that the greater contractility of resistance vessels in spontaneously hypertensive rats is associated with a narrowed lumen, a thickened media, and an increased number of smooth muscle cell layers, *Circ. Res.,* 43, 854, 1978.

23. **Hart M. N., Heistad, D. D., and Brody, M. J.,** Effect of chronic hypertension and sympathetic denervation on wall/lumen ratio of cerebral vessels, *Hypertension,* 2, 419, 1980.

24. **Bohlen, H. G. and Lobach, D.,** *In vivo* study of microvascular wall characteristics and resting control in young and mature spontaneously hypertensive rats, *Blood Vessels,* 15, 322, 1978.

25. **Prewitt, R. L., Chen, I. I. H., and Dowell, R.,** Development of microvascular rarefaction in the spontaneously hypertensive rat, *Am. J. Physiol.,* 243, H243, 1982.

26. **Tomanek, R. J., Palmer, P. J., Peiffer, G. L., Schreiber, K. L., Eastham, C. L., and Marcus, M. L.,** Morphometry of canine coronary arteries, arterioles, and capillaries during hypertension and left ventricular hypertrophy, *Circ. Res.,* 58, 38, l986.

27. **Short, D. S. and Thomson, A. D.,** The arteries of the small intestine is systemic hypertension, *J. Pathol. Bacteriol.,* 78, 321, 1959.

28. **Short, D. S.,** Morphology of the intestinal arterioles in chronic human hypertension, *Br. Heart J.,* 28, 184, 1966.

29. **Plunkett, W. C. and Overbeck, H. W.,** Increased arteriolar wall-to-lumen ratio in a normotensive vascular bed in coarctation hypertension, *Am. J. Physiol.,* 249, H859, 1985.

30. **Friedman, S. M., Nakashima, M., and Mar, M. A.,** Morphological assessment of vasoconstriction and vascular hypertrophy in sustained hypertension in the rat, *Microvasc. Res.,* 3, 416, 1971.

31. **Krogh, A.,** The supply of oxygen to the tissues and the regulation of the capillary circulation, *J. Physiol. (London),* 52, 457, 1919.

32. **Roy, J. W., and Mayrovitz, H. N.,** Microvascular pressure, flow, and resistance in spontaneously hypertensive rats, *Hypertension,* 6, 877, 1984.

33. **Chen, I. I. H., Prewitt, R. L., and Dowell, R. F.,** Microvascular rarefaction in spontaneously hypertensive rat cremaster muscle, *Am. J. Physiol.,* 241, H306, 1981.

34. **Henrich, H., Hertel, R., and Assmann, R.,** Structural differences in the mesentery microcirculation between normotensive and spontaneously hypertensive rats, *Pfluegers Arch.,* 375, 153, 1978.

35. **Haack, D. W., Schaffer, J. J., and Simpson, J. G.,** Comparisons of cutaneous microvessels from spontaneously hypertensive, normotensive Wistar-Kyoto and normal Wistar rats, *Proc. Soc. Exp. Biol. Med.,* 164, 453, 1980.

36. **Joshua, I. G., Wiegman, D. L., Harris, P. D., and Miller, F. N.,** Progressive microvascular alterations with the development of renovascular hypertension, *Hypertension,* 6, 61, 1984.

37. **Prewitt, R. L., Hashimoto, H., and Stacy, D. L.,** Microvascular alterations in hypertension, in *Microvascular Perfusion and Transport in Health and Disease,* S. Karger, Basel, 1987, 31.

38. **Ruedemann, A. D.,** Conjunctival vessels, *JAMA,* 101, 1477, 1933.

39. **Lack, A., Adolph, W., Ralston, W., Leiby, G., Winsor, T., and Griffith, G.,** Biomicroscopy of conjunctival vessels in hypertension, *Am. Heart. J.,* 38, 654, 1949.

40. **Landau, J. and Davis, E.,** Capillary thinning and high capillary blood-pressure in hypertension, *Lancet,* 1, 1327, l957.

41. **Jackson, W. B.,** The functional activity of the human conjunctival capillary bed in hypertensive and normotensive subjects, *Am. Heart J.,* 56, 222, 1958.

42. **Sullivan, J. M., Prewitt, R. L., and Josephs, J. A.,** Attenuation of the microcirculation in young patients with high-output borderline hypertension, *Hypertension,* 5, 844, 1983.

43. **Harper, R. N., Moore, M. A., Marr, M. C., Watts, L. E. and Hutchins, P. M.,** Arteriolar rarefaction in the conjunctiva of human essential hypertensives, *Microvasc. Res.,* 16, 369, 1978.

44. **Short, D. S.,** Arteries of intestinal wall in systemic hypertension, *Lancet,* 2, 1261, 1958.

45. **Fischer, P., Heimgartner, W., Hartung, E., and Henrich, H. A.,** Capillary rarefication in different organ tissues of hypertensive patients, *Int. J. Microcirc. Clin. Exp.,* 4 (Abstr.), 106, 1985.

46. **Lund, D. D. and Tomanek, R. J.,** Myocardial morphology in spontaneously hypertensive and aortic-constricted rats, *Am. J. Anat.,* 152, 141, 1978.

47. **Hutchins, P. M., Dusseau, J. W., Marr, M. C., and Greene, A. W.,** The role of arteriolar structural changes in hypertension, in *Microvascular Aspects of Spontaneous Hypertension,* Henrich, H., Ed., Hans Huber, Bern, 1982, 41.

48. **Roy, J. W. and Mayrovitz, H. N.,** Microvascular blood flow in the normotensive and spontaneously hypertensive rat, *Hypertension,* 4, 264, 1982.

49. **Henrich, H. and Hertel, R.F.,** Microvascular hemodynamics in spontaneous hypertension, in *Microvascular Aspects of Spontaneous Hypertension,* Henrich, H., Ed., Hans Huber, Bern 1982, 21.

50. **Schmid-Schoenbein, G. W., Firestone, G., and Zweifach, B. W.,** The arterial network for the spinotrapezius muscle of normotensive and spontaneously hypertensive rats (SHR), *Microvasc. Res.,* 29 (Abstr.), 218, 1985.

51. **Gray, S. D.,** Morphometric analysis of skeletal muscle capillaries in early spontaneous hypertension, *Microvasc. Res.,* 27, 39, 1984.

52. **Alexandrova, T. B., Rodionov, I. M., and Shinkarenko, V. S.,** Variation of the morphometric parameters of brain microvessels in experimental hypertension, *Bull. Exp. Biol. Med.,* 98, 366, 1984.

53. **Funk, R. and Rohen, J. W.,** Comparative morphological studies on blood vessels in eyes of normotensive and spontaneously hypertensive rats, *Exp. Eye Res.,* 40, 191, 1985.

54. **Tomanek, R. J., Wangler, R. D., and Bauer, C. A.,** Prevention of coronary vasodilator reserve decrement in spontaneously hypertensive rats, *Hypertension,* 7, 533, 1985.

55. **Mueller, T. M., Marcus, M. L., Kerber, R. E., Yound, J. A., Barnes, R. W., and Abboud, F. M.,** Effect of renal hypertension and left ventricular hypertrophy on the coronary circulation in dogs, *Circ. Res.,* 42, 543, 1978.

56. **Wangler, R. D., Peters, K. G., Marcus, M. L., and Tomanck, R. J.,** Effects of duration and severity of arterial hypertension and cardiac hypertrophy on coronary vasodilator reserve, *Circ. Res.,* 51, 10, 1982.

57. **Sokolova, I. A., Manukhina, E. B., Blinkov, S. M., Koshelev, V. B., Pinelis, V. G., and Rodionov, I. M.,** Rarefication of the arterioles and capillary network in the brain of rats with different forms of hypertension, *Microvasc. Res.,* 30, 1, 1985.

58. **Prewitt, R. L. and Rapp, J. P.,** Rarefaction of arterioles in Dahl-S hypertensive rat gracilis muscle, *Microvasc. Res.,* 27 (Abstr.), 259, 1984.

59. **Reid, L. M.,** The pulmonary circulation: remodeling in growth and disease, *Am. Rev. Respir. Dis.,* 119, 531, 1979.

60. **Anderson, E. G., Simon, G., and Reid, L.,** Primary and thrombo-embolic pulmonary hypertension: a quantitative pathological study, *J. Pathol.,* 110, 273, 1973.

61. **Arias-Stella, J. and Saldana, M.,** The terminal portion of the pulmonary arterial tree in people native to high altitudes, *Circulation,* 28, 915, 1963.

62. **Hislop, A. and Reid, L.,** New findings in pulmonary arteries of rats with hypoxia-induced pulmonary hypertension, *Br. J. Exp. Pathol.,* 57, 542, 1976.

63. **Berecek, K. H., Stocker, M., and Gross, F.,** Changes in renal vascular reactivity at various stages of deoxycorticosterone hypertension in rats, *Circ. Res.,* 46, 619, 1980.

64. **Dusseau, J. W. and Hutchins, P. M.,** Stimulation of arteriolar number by salbutamol in spontaneously hypertensive rats, *Am. J. Physiol.,* 236, H134, 1979.

65. **Dusseau, J., Smith, T. L., and Hutchins, P. M.,** Acute microvascular and blood pressure responses to salbutamol in WKY and SHR rats, *Microvasc. Res.,* 15, 263, 1978.

66. **Coleman, T. G., Granger, H. J., and Guyton, A. C.,** Whole-body circulatory autoregulation and hypertension, *Circ. Res.,* 28 (Suppl. II), 76, 1971.

67. **Lombard, J. H., Hess, M. E., and Stekiel, W. J.,** Neural and local control of arterioles in SHR, *Hypertension,* 6, 530, 1984.

68. **Hogan, R. D. and Hirschmann, L.,** Arteriolar proliferation in the rat cremaster muscle as a long-term autoregulatory response to reduced perfusion, *Microvasc. Res.,* 27, 290, 1984.

69. **Banchero, N.,** Long term adaptation of skeletal muscle capillarity, *The Physiologist,* 25, 385, 1982.

70. **Tomanek, R. J., Searls, J. C., and Lachenbruch, P. A.,** Quantitative changes in the capillary bed during developing, peak, and stabilized cardiac hypertrophy in the spontaneously hypertensive rat, *Circ. Res.,* 51, 295, 1982.

71. **Hallback, M., Gothberg, G., Lundin, S., Ricksten, S.-E., and Folkow, B.,** Hemodynamic consequences of resistance vessel rarefication and of changes in smooth muscle sensitivity, *Acta Physiol. Scand.,* 97, 233, 1976.

72. **Chen, I. I. H., and Prewitt, R. L.,** Capillary pressure gradients in cremaster muscle of normotensive and spontaneously hypertensive rats, *Microvasc. Res.,* 25, 145, 1983.

73. **Parving, H. H. and Gyntelberg, F.,** Transcapillary escape rate of albumin and plasma volume in essential hypertension, *Circ. Res.,* 32, 643, 1973.

74. **Rippe, B., Lundin, S., and Folkow, B.,** Plasma volume, blood volume and transcapillary escape rate (TER) of albumin in young spontaneously hypertensive rats (SHR) compares with controls (NCR), *Acta Physiol. Scand.,* 102 (Abstr.), 55A, 1978.

75. **Edwards, M. T. and Diana, J. N.,** Pre- and postcapillary resistance capillary pressure and filtration coefficients in spontaneously hypertensive rats, in Spontaneous Hypertension its Pathogenesis and Complications II, Bumpus, F. and Okamoto, K., Eds., U.S. Government Printing Office, Washington, D. C., 1976, 70.

76. **Korthuis, R. J., Kerr, C. R., Townsley, M. I., and Taylor, A. E.,** Microvascular pressure, surface area, and permeability in isolated hindquarters of SHR, *Am. J. Physiol.,* 249, H498, 1985.

77. **Rippe, B. and Folkow, B.,** Capillary permeability to albumin in normotensive and spontaneously hyperten-sive rats, *Acta Physiol. Scand.,* 101, 72, 1977.
78. **Laine, G. A. and Granger, H. J.,** Permeability of intestinal microvessels in chronic arterial hypertension, *Hypertension,* 5, 722, 1983.
79. **Nishiyama, K., Nishiyama, A., and Frohlich, E. D.,** Regional blood flow in normotensive and spontaneously hypertensive rats, *Am. J. Physiol.,* 230, 691, 1976.
80. **Tobia, A. J., Walsh, G. M., Tadepalli, A. S., and Lee, J. Y.,** Unaltered distribution of cardiac output in the conscious young spontaneously hypertensive rat: evidence for uniform elevation of regional vascular resistances, *Blood Vessels,* 11, 287, 1974.

Chapter 5

NEURAL AND LOCAL CONTROL OF THE MICROCIRCULATION IN HYPERTENSION

Julian H. Lombard

I. MICROCIRCULATORY ALTERATIONS IN HYPERTENSION

A. Introduction

The microcirculation is importantly involved in the development and maintenance of hypertension. In addition, microcirculatory alterations which occur in response to the initial elevation of arterial pressure could limit the effectiveness of therapeutic interventions and eventually undermine tissue perfusion and exchange.[1] Since the arterioles are the primary source of resistance in the terminal vasculature, direct studies of the microcirculation in major vascular beds of hypertensive animals can provide vital insight into the mechanisms of the increased total peripheral resistance in hypertension and the effects of this elevated resistance upon tissue perfusion and organ function.

The increased resistance to blood flow which occurs in the microcirculation in hypertension may result either from constriction of arterioles[2-7] or vessel rarefaction, i.e., a reduction in the number of arterioles open for flow.[8-12] The constriction of arterioles in hypertension may reflect an elevated active vascular smooth muscle tone[2,5,6] or a structural narrowing of the vessel due to wall thickening and an increased wall/lumen ratio.[13] Vessel rarefaction may occur as a result of active closure of arterioles (functional rarefaction) or an actual absence (structural or anatomic rarefaction) of microvessels.[9-12] The increases in arteriolar tone which contribute to constriction or active closure of arterioles may result from several factors, including increased sympathetic nervous activity,[14-16] increased levels of circulating vasoconstrictor agents,[17] an altered vascular smooth muscle sensitivity to neurotransmitters or other vasoactive agents,[4,9,18,19] alterations in the intrinsic membrane properties of the vascular smooth muscle cells of hypertensive vessels,[20] or the activity of local metabolic and myogenic autoregulatory mechanisms.[17,21-25]

B. Constriction of Arterioles

Narrowing of flowing arterioles has been observed in many forms of hypertension. However, in some cases, e.g., the spontaneously hypertensive rat (SHR) genetic model of hypertension, the contribution of arteriolar constriction to the elevated peripheral vascular resistance remains controversial. For example, several authors have reported that arteriolar constriction does not contribute substantially to an elevated skeletal muscle microvascular resistance in SHR, especially in the early stages of hypertension.[8,10,11,26] These studies seem to favor functional or anatomic rarefaction of arterioles as the primary source of the elevated microvascular resistance in this model of hypertension. However, other studies[2,22,27] have indicated that some orders of arterioles are constricted in the skeletal muscle microcirculation of SHR relative to normotensive controls. For example, Zweifach et al.[27] reported a narrowing of the second-, third-, and fourth-order arterioles in the spinotrapezius muscle of young SHR, suggesting a role for increased smooth muscle tone in contributing to an elevated vascular resistance in these animals. These authors proposed that the increased precapillary resistance in SHR initially involves the smaller arterioles (less than 20 μm), while larger arterioles (30 to 40 μm) become involved as the disease progresses.

The contribution of arteriolar constriction to an increased microvascular resistance in hypertension may differ between vascular beds, or between different branching orders within a vascular bed. For example, some studies have suggested that mesenteric arterioles of SHR are not constricted, relative to those of normotensive Wistar-Kyoto (WKY) controls.[28] However, Bohlen[29] reported that the largest and smallest arterioles supplying the intestine of SHR were smaller than those of WKY, while other branching orders of SHR were similar to or larger than those of WKY. In contrast, Harper and Bohlen[3] observed a significant reduction in the resting lumenal diameters of first- to fourth-order arterioles in the cerebral circulation of SHR. Finally, variations in diameter along the length of individual microvessels may make comparisons of arteriolar diameters in hypertensive and normotensive animals difficult, unless all measurements are made in the same general location on the arteriolar tree.[2]

Arteriolar constriction seems to be more prominent in renal hypertension than in SHR. In 1942, Abell and Page[5] reported that ear arterioles constrict following the development of one-kidney, one-clip (1K-1C) or one-kidney one-wrapped renal hypertension in the rabbit. In hamsters with bilateral Grollman hypertension, i.e., figure-8 ligatures around both kidneys, large arterioles of the cheek pouch exhibit a reduced diameter relative to those of sham-operated normotensive controls.[30] However, the luminal diameters of the smaller arterioles are not significantly different in hypertensive hamsters and sham-operated controls.[18] The larger (first- and second-order) arterioles are also constricted in rats with 1K-1C renal hypertension relative to those of normotensive controls.[4,7,31] Prewitt et al.[12] reported that the decrease in arteriolar conductance due to vasoconstriction (percent reduction from the conductance in the vasodilated state) was significantly greater in the gracilis muscle of 1K-1C renal hypertensive rats 4 to 6 weeks after clipping than in uninephrectomized, unclipped controls. However, constriction in the hypertensive animals 8 to 10 weeks after clipping was not significantly different from that in control animals. In 2K-1C renal hypertension, first- and second-order arterioles are constricted in hypertensive animals relative to normotensive controls, whereas first- to third-order arterioles are constricted in DOCA-salt hypertension.[7] Finally, cremasteric arterioles of rats with reduced renal mass hypertension produced by infusion of 145 mM NaCl for 36 h following recovery from a 75% reduction of renal mass exhibit intense constriction and very high frequencies of vasomotion relative to noninfused normotensive controls subjected to similar surgical procedures.[6]

In human hypertensives, the diameters of conjunctival arterioles of borderline hypertensive patients are similar to those of normotensive controls,[32] while those of untreated human essential hypertensives are smaller than those of age- and sex-matched normotensive controls.[33] Autopsy specimens of intestine from human hypertensives also exhibit a diffuse narrowing of submucosal arteries.[34]

C. Microvessel Sensitivity to Vasoactive Agents

A number of studies suggest that the sensitivity of microvessels to various vasoconstrictor agents is increased in hypertension. For example, Bohlen[9] reported that closure of arterioles in the cremaster muscle of SHR was mediated by hyperresponsiveness of the vessels to norepinephrine. Click et al.[18] observed that the sensitivity of cheek pouch arterioles to norepinephrine was increased in the early (15 days) and late (70 days) phases of bilateral Grollman hypertension in the hamster. These authors also reported that venular sensitivity to norepinephrine was increased in the late stage of hypertension.[18] In another study, this group reported that the vasoconstrictor sensitivity of arterioles to K$^+$, norepinephrine, and angiotensin were all increased in hamsters which developed sustained Grollman hypertension, relative to sham-operated controls or animals whose hypertension was transient.[19] A particularly interesting finding of the latter study was that the sensitivity of arterioles to elevated K$^+$ (22.2 mM) was transiently increased in the animals which developed a sustained hypertension, but not in normotensive animals or in animals whose hypertension was transient. Based upon this observation, these authors hypothesized that the transient increase in the K$^+$ sensitivity of arterioles of the hypertensive hamsters might be indicative of a fundamental ionic and/or electrogenic alteration, which could lead to changes in vascular smooth muscle E_m, and a subsequent potentiation of arteriolar responses to other vasoactive agents.[19]

However, the finding of an enhanced sensitivity of microvessels to vasoactive agents is not universal in hypertension. For example, some authors[31] have reported that there is no change in the sensitivity of small cremasteric arteries and veins to norepinephrine in SHR, whereas small arteries in the cremaster muscle of 1K-1C renal hypertensive rats actually exhibit a decreased sensitivity to norepinephrine relative to normotensive controls.

D. Structural Factors and Vessel Rarefaction

Considerable evidence had been accumulated to indicate that structural factors e.g., an increased wall to lumen ratio[13] or an actual disappearance of microvessels, (i.e., anatomical or structural rarefaction [see Chapter 4]) can contribute to the increased vascular resistance in hypertension. Although wall/lumen ratios of arterioles are not increased in the cremaster muscle of SHR,[11,26] increased wall to lumen ratios have been reported in third-order intestinal mesenteric arterioles of SHR,[29] and in first- to fourth-order cerebral arterioles of SHR.[3] In hamsters with bilateral Grollman hypertension, arteriolar wall/lumen ratios are significantly increased after 70 days of hypertension, but not after 15 days of hypertension.[18] This increase in wall/lumen ratio persists after antihypertensive therapy with propranolol. In 1K-1C renal hypertensive rats, Prewitt et al.[12] have reported that wall/lumen ratio is increased in arterioles of the gracilis muscle 4 to 6 weeks and 8 to 10 weeks after clipping. Finally, Wiegman et al.[31] proposed that the reduction in the diameters of first- and second-order arterioles which they observed in the cremaster muscle of 1K-1C renal hypertensive rats involved structural changes, since it could not be eliminated with vasodilator agents.[31]

A reduced density of arterioles and/or capillaries has been reported in spontaneously hypertensive rats,[8-11] in 1K-1C renal hypertensive rats,[12] in the conjunctival microcirculation of human borderline hypertensive[32] and untreated essential hypertensive patients,[33] and in autopsy specimens of the intestine taken from human hypertensives.[34] In SHR[9-11] and in 1K-1C renal hypertension,[12] active closure of arterioles (functional rarefaction) seems to precede anatomical rarefaction. For example, arteriolar and capillary density are reduced in the gracilis muscle of 12- to 14-week-old SHR under innervated and denervated conditions but not after vasodilation, suggesting that the reduced vessel density is due to active closure of arterioles. However, in 16- to 18-week-old SHR, vessel density is also reduced in the vasodilated state, suggesting that some arterioles which are initially closed eventually disappear (anatomical rarefaction).[11] A complete understanding of the effect of arteriolar rarefaction upon microvascular resistance may be especially important in assessing the role of long-term autoregulatory mechanisms in controlling tissue perfusion and peripheral vascular resistance in hypertension (see below).

II. NEURAL INFLUENCES ON MICROVESSELS IN HYPERTENSION

A. Neural Control of the Microcirculation

In the microcirculation, neural control mechanisms are important in controlling vascular resistance at the arteriolar level. However, the density of innervation, the level of basal sympathetic tone, and the response of the vessels to sympathetic stimulation vary considerably between different vascular beds, and between various branching orders of microvessels within a vascular bed. In addition, metabolic and myogenic autoregulatory mechanisms often modulate the effect of changes in neurogenic input upon microvascular resistance.

Although the arterial side of the microcirculation is generally well innervated (Figure 1), the immediate precapillary arterioles are often not innervated and are primarily controlled by local autoregulatory mechanisms or humoral factors.[35,36] In skeletal muscle, the small arteries and arterioles show a fairly dense adrenergic innervation while the veins are sparsely innervated.[37] In the intestinal mesenteric circulation of the rat, adrenergic nerve fibers are found in association with the principal arteries, small arteries, and the arterioles.[38] However, the smaller precapillary arterioles and the small collecting venules are not innervated. Venules in excess of 30 μm in diameter are innervated, although the innervation is less dense than that of the corresponding arterial vessels (Figure 1).

In the brain, surface arteries and larger arterioles inside the tissue receive sympathetic and parasympathetic innervation; and pial vessels contract in response to norepinephrine and dilate in response to acetylcholine.[39] However, arterioles of the brain appear to be under very little, if any, autonomic control under resting conditions.[39] In the bat wing, acute surgical denervation dilates the larger vessels (major artery, main artery, and small artery) supplying the bed, indicating that these vessels are innervated.[40] However, the arterioles and the terminal arterioles

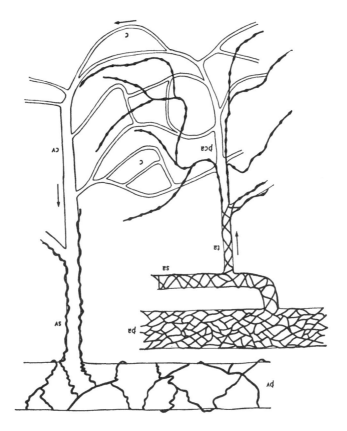

FIGURE 1. Distribution of adrenergic innervation (dense lines) in the mesenteric microcirculation of the rat. pa, principal artery; sa, small artery; ta, terminal arteriole; pca, precapillary arteriole; c, capillary; cv, collecting venule; sv, small vein; pv, principal vein. Arrows indicate the direction of blood flow. (From Furness, J. B. and Marshall, J. M., *J. Physiol. (London)*, 239, 75, 1974. With permission.)

constrict following denervation, suggesting that the smaller vessels are not innervated and are primarily controlled by local mechanisms. Finally, in rare cases (e.g., hamster cheek pouch) entire microvascular networks may be devoid of adrenergic innervation.[41,42]

It appears that both α_1 and α_2 postsynaptic receptors are present in the blood vessels of skeletal muscle[43] and the intestine.[44] In the rat, arterioles of the cremaster muscle constrict in response to carotid artery occlusion[45] and arterioles of the spinotrapezius muscle constrict in response to sympathetic stimulation.[46] In the mesenteric circulation, vessel responses to sympathetic stimulation are well correlated with the distribution of adrenergic innervation described above. For example, the principal arteries, small arteries, and arterioles of the mesenteric circulation and venules larger than 30 μm constrict in response to adrenergic nerve stimulation, whereas the smallest precapillary arterioles and the small collecting venules do not.[38] However, with the exception of the capillaries, all microvessels of the mesenteric circulation respond to norepinephrine application.[38] Small arteries and arterioles in the brain respond only modestly to autonomic stimulation.[39] However, it appears that the sympathetic innervation of cerebral vessels is of considerable importance in protecting the brain against the effects of elevated arterial pressure such as those encountered in hypertension.[47]

As noted above, arteriolar responses to sympathetic stimulation or withdrawal of sympathetic tone may be modulated by local autoregulatory mechanisms, or possibly by presynaptic compensatory mechanisms.[43] For example, in rat spinotrapezius muscle, arteriolar constriction in response to sympathetic stimulation is maintained in arterioles with diameters greater than 13 μm, while terminal arterioles (7 to 13 μm) began to relax after about 15 s.[46] In skeletal muscle, acute denervation results in a transient two- to threefold increase in blood flow which subsides fairly rapidly, suggesting that the ability of reflex sympathetic withdrawal to maintain a reduced vascular resistance is limited.[43] In the intestinal circulation, stimulation of sympathetic nerves leads to an initial constriction which subsequently decreases ("autoregulatory escape") in the arterioles, but not in the precapillary arterioles or venules. The mechanism of autoregulatory escape remains unknown but could involve release of dilator substances secondary to sympathetic stimulation or an inability of the vascular smooth muscle to remain contracted.[44] Although it is conceivable that alterations in the mechanisms which modulate the responses of microvessels to changes in the level of sympathetic efferent activity can contribute to an elevated microvascular resistance in hypertension, very little is known of the nature of these mechanisms and their interaction with the neurogenic control of microvessels in various forms of hypertension.

B. Role of Neurogenic Factors in Hypertension

Investigators in a wide variety of scientific disciplines have become interested in neural control of the circulation in hypertension.[48-52] Consequently, studies designed to assess the importance of neural influences in hypertension have not only expanded our knowledge of the role of the nervous system in the pathophysiology of this disease, but have also contributed to a better understanding of higher central nervous system (CNS) sites involved in the homeostatic control of blood pressure in normotensive humans and animals.

Evidence is accumulating in support of an early neural contribution to the elevated blood pressure in a number of forms of hypertension. The neural sites involved in the elevation of blood pressure appear to be multiple and may include aberrations both at the peripheral level (particularly neuromuscular transmission) and at the CNS level. Increased sympathetic activity may lead to a sustained increase in arterial pressure by a variety of mechanisms, including arteriolar constriction or closure, increased cardiac output, Na^+ retention and renin release, or effects upon the properties of the vascular smooth muscle cells themselves.[48]

It has long been postulated that a possible cause of essential hypertension in humans is a specific, genetic susceptibility that leads to an excessive and unusually sustained pressor response to physiological stimuli such as pain, controlled muscular exercise, cold immersion of a limb, or psychological stress.[13,53,54] Pharmacological blockade of sympathetic activity at the ganglionic level or at the neuromuscular junction usually produces larger pressure drops in the early stages of hypertension in man and in various experimental animal models of hypertension than it does in normotensive controls.[55-57] Plus, many potent antihypertensive drugs operate via inhibition of adrenergic function.[58] However, in both human hypertensives and animal models of this disease, the early increase in neural activity may become replaced once hypertension is established, as structural thickening of vessel walls encroaches upon lumen diameters[55,59-61] or anatomical rarefaction[11,12] contributes to a maintained increase in vascular resistance.

Since whole body studies cannot distinguish between an elevated sympathetic efferent-nerve activity and alterations at the level of the individual neuron, neuromuscular junction, or vascular smooth muscle cell, a number of investigators have measured levels of plasma or urinary catecholamines as an index of sympathetic nerve activity in hypertension. Such studies generally suggest that plasma catecholamines and excreted catecholamines are elevated to various degrees in hypertensive individuals relative to normotensive controls.[62-65] However, even though plasma and urinary levels of norepinephrine may closely reflect the level of sympathetic activity in a particular individual, significant variations in baseline levels exist among individuals, making it difficult to compare differences. These baseline variations are not surprising, since circulating (and excreted) levels of norepinephrine represent a variable proportion of the transmitter released at the neuromuscular junction during nerve activity.

A number of studies utilizing the genetic rat models of hypertension have indicated that an early abnormal increase in neural control of vascular smooth muscle tone occurs in hypertension. For example, studies employing neonatal sympathectomy with 6-hydroxydopamine or guanethidine have suggested that an intact nervous system is essential for the development of hypertension in the SHR,[66,67] the New Zealand genetically hypertensive rat,[68] and the Dahl salt-sensitive rat.[69,70] In addition, preganglionic and postganglionic splanchnic sympathetic nerve traffic is increased in adult SHR[71-73] and possibly in young SHR with developing hypertension.[74,75]

It is particularly important to understand the relationship between an elevated renal sympathetic efferent nerve activity and the maintenance of fluid balance in hypertension, since this relationship may provide a direct link between neurogenic hypertension and an altered renal function.[76-78] Liard[79] and Kline et al.[80] have both reported that renal denervation slows the development of hypertension in SHR, and others[75] have demonstrated a positive correlation between renal sympathetic nerve activity and mean arterial blood pressure using hybrid rats produced by backcrossing SHR and WKY controls. The reason for a delay rather than an inhibition of the elevation in pressure in the SHR following renal denervation is not known. Nonetheless, it appears as if elevated renal sympathetic efferent nerve activity in various forms of hypertension can shift the renal function curve (i.e., the rate of urine and sodium output vs. arterial blood pressure[81]) to the right on the pressure axis,[82] resulting in an alteration in the "setpoint" for the balance between the intake and output of salt and water. Alterations in this setpoint are particularly significant in forms of hypertension in which local autoregulatory mechanisms may contribute to an elevation of peripheral vascular resistance in response to tissue overperfusion resulting from volume expansion and a subsequent elevation in cardiac output (see below).

Another area of particular interest related to neural control of the circulation in hypertension concerns the possibility that trophic influences of the sympathetic nervous system can affect the properties of the blood vessels. For example, Abel and Hermsmeyer[83] have demonstrated that vascular smooth muscle cells from the caudal artery of WKY rats can assume the altered membrane characteristics of SHR rats when they are transplanted into the anterior eye chamber of SHR. However, this alteration in membrane properties will not occur if the adrenergic innervation of the iris is eliminated by superior cervical ganglionectomy.[83] If trophic influences of the sympathetic nervous system contribute to alterations in the membrane properties of vascular smooth muscle cells in arterioles of hemodynamically significant vascular beds, the reactivity of the peripheral vasculature to a wide variety of stimuli (e.g., neurotransmittters, circulating vasoactive hormones, metabolic regulators of blood flow, oxygen, etc.) could be significantly altered in hypertension. Finally, there is evidence that trophic effects of sympathetic nerves upon vascular smooth muscle can lead to an increase in vessel wall thickness,[84,85] although the significance of this effect in the microcirculation remains to be established.[12]

C. Neural Control of Microvessels in Hypertension

Present evidence supports the existence of an increased adrenergic tone in precapillary resistance vessels of spontaneously hypertensive rats in the established stage of hypertension. Neural blockade with tetrodotoxin produces a significant dilation of third-order arterioles in the cremaster muscle of 12- to 15-week-old SHR, but does not cause any change in the diameters of third-order arterioles of WKY controls or of fourth-order arterioles of either SHR or WKY.[22] The latter vessels are sparsely innervated and appear to play more of a role in controlling the distribution of blood flow within the tissue. Sympathetic influences also contribute to active closure of skeletal muscle arterioles of SHR in the established stage of hypertension. For example, Bohlen[9] reported that the increase in the percent of third-order arterioles which opened to flow following denervation of the cremaster muscle of 18- to 20-week-old SHR was significantly greater than that in age-matched WKY controls. He also observed that arterioles

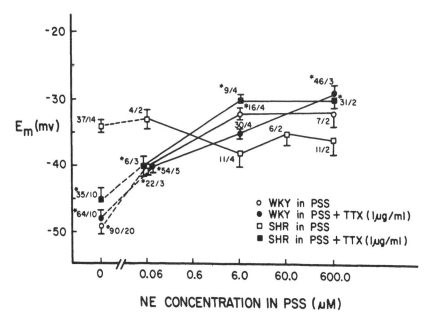

FIGURE 2.   Vascular smooth muscle transmembrane potentials (E_m) in small (200 to 500 µm) intestinal mesenteric veins of 12- to 15-week-old SHR and normotensive WKY controls before and during neural blockade with 1 µg/ml tetrodotoxin (TTX) in the physiological salt solution (PSS) superfusing the tissue. Before neural blockade, vascular smooth muscle of SHR veins is less polarized than that of WKY veins and does not depolarize further in response to norepinephrine superfusion. During neural blockade, resting E_m of SHR veins hyperpolarizes to a value which is not significantly different from that of WKY veins, and the SHR norepinephrine concentration-response curve becomes similar to that of WKY, which is unaffected by tetrodotoxin. Values are expressed as pooled mean ±SD for n impalements/a animals; asterisks represent values which are significantly different from that in SHR without neural blockade. (From Harder D. R., Contney, S. J., Willems, W. J., and Stekiel, W. J., *Am. J. Physiol.*, 240; *Heart Circ. Physiol.*, 9, H837, 1981. With permission.)

of SHR were more sensitive to iontophoretically applied norepinephrine than WKY controls, and concluded that active closure of cremasteric arterioles of SHR appears to result from hyperresponsiveness of the vessels to norepinephrine.

In contrast to observations in 12- to 15-week-old SHR with established hypertension,[22] neural blockade with tetrodotoxin does not affect the diameters of third- or fourth-order arterioles of 4- to 6-week-old or 8- to 9-week-old SHR and WKY.[109] These findings suggest that neural influences do not contribute to an active constriction of skeletal muscle arterioles of SHR in the early (4 to 6 weeks) and developing (8 to 9 weeks) stages of hypertension. However, it is possible that neurogenic contributions to active vascular smooth muscle tone in these vessels could be masked by local autoregulatory mechanisms (see above), or by an increase in the vasodilator response to β_2 adrenergic activation, which has been proposed as a compensatory mechanism to maintain blood flow regulation in the face of a reduced vascular density in SHR.[86]

Mesenteric vessels of SHR with established hypertension appear to receive a higher sympathetic efferent nervous input and exhibit an enhanced response to sympathetic stimulation than those of their WKY controls.[87] *In situ* small intestinal mesenteric arteries (100 to 400 µm) and veins (200 to 500 µm) of 12- to 15-week-old SHR exhibit a lower vascular smooth muscle transmembrane potential (E_m) (Figure 2) and an elevated active tone relative to those of normotensive WKY controls.[14-16] *In situ* vascular smooth muscle E_m is also depolarized in small mesenteric veins of SHR in the developing stage of hypertension (8 to 9 weeks old) relative to that in age-matched WKY controls, whereas small mesenteric veins of 4-week-old SHR are not depolarized relative to those of WKY.[88] Taken together, these data indicate that neurogenic constriction of capacitance vessels does not initiate hypertension in SHR, but may contribute to the elevated blood pressure after 4 to 6 weeks of age. The depolarization of small arteries and veins of SHR with established hypertension reflects adrenergic neural influences, since it can be eliminated by neural blockade with tetrodotoxin[14] (Figure 2), local chemical sympathectomy by topical application of 6-hydroxydopamine,[16] and α adrenergic blockade.[15] An elevated neurogenic vascular smooth muscle tone also appears to exist in mesenteric microvessels, since arterioles of the mesoappendix of 12- to 15-week-old SHR exhibit a significant dilation in response to neural blockade with tetrodotoxin, while those of WKY do not.[89]

Neural influences may also contribute to an elevated microvascular resistance in some forms of renal hypertension. For example, Prewitt et al.[12] reported that a greater percentage of arterioles were closed to flow in the innervated gracilis muscle of 1K-1C renal hypertensive rats than in uninephrectomized controls, suggesting that active neurogenic constriction contributes to functional rarefaction of arterioles in the hypertensive animals. In small mesenteric veins of rats with reduced renal mass hypertension, *in situ* vascular smooth muscle E_m is depolarized relative to that in noninfused controls.[90] This depolarization appears to be mediated by sympathetic nerves, since it can be eliminated by neural blockade with tetrodotoxin or local chemical sympathectomy by topical application of 6-hydroxydopamine.[90] However, small arteries of infused reduced renal-mass hypertensive animals are not depolarized relative to those of noninfused reduced renal-mass controls. The intense constriction and extremely high frequencies of arteriolar vasomotion observed in the cremaster muscle of reduced renal-mass rats infused with 145 mM NaCl for 36 h do not depend upon neurogenic influences, since they persist in the presence of neural blockade with tetrodotoxin.[6] However, this observation does not preclude the possibility that an enhanced neurogenic tone could still exist in these vessels, since local autoregulatory mechanisms (or other constrictor influences) could maintain an elevated arteriolar tone, even after neural influences are blocked. Finally, it has been postulated that neurogenic influences may also contribute to an elevated vascular resistance in DOCA-salt hypertensive animals.[91] However, little is known of the role of neural influences in controlling the microcirculation in DOCA-salt hypertension.

III. LOCAL CONTROL OF ARTERIOLES IN HYPERTENSION

A. Autoregulatory Mechanisms in the Microcirculation

Although nervous influences have an important role in regulating vascular resistance in the peripheral circulation, moment to moment regulation of blood flow in most organs is primarily mediated by local control mechanisms which are independent of the nervous system.[35,36] These local control mechanisms exist in almost all organs of the body and maintain tissue blood flow constant (i.e., autoregulate) by changing microvascular resistance in response to changes in perfusion pressure, blood flow, or metabolic requirements of the tissue. Myogenic autoregulatory mechanisms are pressure-sensitive and produce arteriolar constriction in response to an elevated transmural pressure in the vessel (or arteriolar dilation in response to a reduced transmural presssure in the vessel). Metabolic mechanisms are flow-sensitive and are believed to be mediated by changes in tissue levels of vasoactive metabolites, which occur when blood flow or tissue metabolism changes in an organ. Although many different vasoactive metabolites have been implicated in flow-dependent autoregulation in various organs, changes in oxygen availability to the tissue or alterations in tissue oxygen demand are often the primary determinants of metabolic autoregulation in a tissue. Since nearly all tissues can normally adjust their local vascular resistance in order to maintain a constant blood flow, it has been proposed that the sum of all the tissue resistances and the total blood flow through the entire circulation should be ultimately influenced by autoregulation.[21]

B. Role of Autoregulatory Mechanisms in Determining Vascular Resistance in Hypertension

The possible contribution of autoregulatory mechanisms to an elevated blood pressure in hypertension was suggested by Borst and Borst-de-Geus[92] and by Ledingham and Cohen,[93] who proposed that volume expansion with a consequent increase in cardiac output leads to overperfusion of peripheral vascular beds and a subsequent vasoconstriction to maintain normal blood flows in the tissues. Recently, two detailed reviews summarizing evidence for and against the role of autoregulatory mechanisms in contributing to the elevated total peripheral resistance in various forms of hypertension have appeared.[17,21]

A generalized vasoconstriction leading to an increase in total peripheral resistance due to local autoregulatory mechanisms could arise in cases where renal function is altered in such a way as to require increased perfusion pressures to allow the kidney to filter and excrete amounts of salt and water equivalent to the levels of daily intake.[21] This could occur with kidney damage, experimental reduction of renal mass, or renal artery constriction (due to elevated sympathetic nerve activity or other factors). Although this pattern of hemodynamic events would be expected to involve volume expansion, Coleman et al.[17] have noted that a decrease in venous compliance would also be effective in producing autoregulatory constriction as a result of tissue overperfusion resulting from an increased venous return and a subsequent elevation in cardiac output. This observation is particularly significant in view of evidence which supports the existence of an elevated venomotor tone in hypertension.[14-16]

Uncertainty about the contribution of local autoregulatory mechanisms to hypertension arises because the initial hemodynamic sequence consistent with autoregulatory-based hypertension (i.e., an elevated arterial pressure associated with volume expansion and an increased cardiac output) is not apparent in all forms of hypertension. In fact, cardiac output, blood volume, and extracellular fluid volume are often normal or reduced in hypertension.[21] Although classical autoregulatory mechanisms are clearly not involved in some forms of hypertension which are characterized by high levels of circulating vasoconstrictor agents,[17,21] it is possible that the hemodynamic changes associated with an initial volume expansion in other forms of hypertension may go undetected. Since long-term autoregulatory mechanisms possess considerable strength, only a small amount of fluid retention and a small increase in cardiac output may be required to increase vascular resistance by this mechanism. For example, Cowley[21] has noted that local autoregulatory mechanisms could theoretically sustain a 50% increase in mean arterial pressure with only a 5% increase in cardiac output.

One observation which indicates that autoregulatory mechanisms could contribute to an elevated total peripheral resistance in hypertension is that blood volume expansion is followed by a slow rise in total peripheral resistance, after which blood volume and cardiac output gradually return to nearly normal levels. This hemodynamic pattern has been observed in dogs before and after ganglionic blockade[94] and in the areflexic dog preparation, in which nervous influences are eliminated by severing connections to the brain and destroying the spinal cord with alcohol.[95]

In certain forms of hypertension (especially those with volume expansion), the initial hemodynamic alteration is often an increase in cardiac output. In these types of hypertension, total peripheral resistance is initially unaffected or slightly reduced, and then it progressively rises above the normal value and becomes maximal after a number of days. For example, in the reduced renal mass-salt loading model of hypertension,[96,97] cardiac output, arterial pressure, blood volume, and extravascular fluid volume are initially elevated while total peripheral resistance is decreased. In reduced renal-mass hypertension in the dog, skeletal muscle blood flow is initially increased, but subsequently returns to control values with an elevated regional vascular resistance, suggesting that local autoregulatory mechanisms normalize tissue blood flow in response to an initial overperfusion of the bed.[98] After 2 weeks of reduced renal-mass hypertension, there is an elevated total peripheral resistance with no significant elevation in plasma volume or extracellular fluid volume. Although autoregulation has not been directly demonstrated in this form of hypertension, all the observed changes are consistent with those predicted by autoregulatory mechanisms, and no known neurohumoral mechanisms would explain the response.[21] Hemodynamic responses, consistent with a contribution of local autoregulatory mechanisms to hypertension, have also been observed by some investigators following volume expansion by dialysis in anephric man.[99] However, this has not been a consistent finding.[100] Finally, recent evidence suggests that cardiac index in young SHR is elevated relative to WKY controls,[101] and that hindlimb blood flow is elevated early in hypertension (6 weeks) but subsequently returns to normal levels (9 weeks) because of an elevation in local vascular resistance which appears to be due to long-term autoregulatory mechanisms[102] (see below).

Another mechanism which could contribute to an elevated peripheral vascular resistance in hypertension is myogenic vasoconstriction in response to an elevated transmural pressure or wall stress in the arterioles (i.e., the Bayliss response). It is unclear whether the activity of myogenic mechanisms alone would be sufficient to explain the normal blood flow observed in most vascular beds in hypertension. However, myogenic mechanisms could contribute an additional component to the elevated vascular resistance and add to the effect of the elevated arterial pressure in hypertension. Several factors favor the contribution of myogenic mechanisms to vasoconstriction and an elevated microvascular resistance in hypertension. These include an increased intravascular pressure and wall tension at the arteriolar level,[30,103,104] alterations in the excitability of the cell membrane,[20,105] and possible depolarization of the vascular smooth muscle.[14-16,88] However, despite the possible contribution of myogenic mechanisms to the maintenance of an elevated total peripheral resistance, there have been few direct microcirculatory studies of their role in hypertension.

Recent evidence indicates that local vascular control mechanisms are indeed altered in hypertension, and that they may contribute to the elevated peripheral vascular resistance in some forms of this disease. For example, the pressure ranges for autoregulation in the cerebral[106,107] and hindlimb vascular beds[102] are shifted upward in hypertension. Alson et al.[102] reported that the autoregulatory curves of 6- and 9-week-old SHR exhibited similar slopes and open loop gains, suggesting that the acute autoregulatory response of SHR was not adversely affected by hypertension. These authors concluded that the hemodynamic events which they observed in the gracilis muscle of SHR were consistent with a structurally based long-term autoregulatory mechanism responsive to overperfusion of the tissues. Although the upward shift of the pressure range for autoregulation in hypertension may often be a response to the elevated blood pressure rather than its cause, local autoregulatory mechanisms can contribute to an elevated regional vascular resistance very soon after the onset of hypertension. For example, the increases in hindquarters[23] and mesenteric[24] vascular resistance which occur in the early stages of acute 2K-1C renal hypertension in rats appear to arise from either pressure-dependent (myogenic) or flow-dependent (metabolic) autoregulatory mechanisms.

The contribution of metabolic autoregulatory mechanisms to an elevated vascular resistance in hypertension may be magnified by an enhanced constriction of hypertensive vessels in response to increases in oxygen availability. Although the precise role of these mechanisms in controlling active vascular smooth muscle tone in hypertension remains to be determined, considerable evidence has recently been obtained which indicates that alterations in oxygen-dependent local control mechanisms may exist in various forms of hypertension, and therefore contribute to the elevated peripheral resistance in this disease. For example, Walsh and Tobia[108] reported that repeated increases in subclavian blood flow lead to an enhanced "autoregulatory" constriction in young (8-week-old) SHR in the developing stages of hypertension, but not in adult (36- to 41-week-old) SHR. In these studies, vascular resistance in young SHR was consistently greater than that of WKY when blood oxygen concentration was normal, but resistances were not different when the animals were hypoxemic. Although oxygen could merely have a permissive role in supporting active vascular smooth muscle tone in these

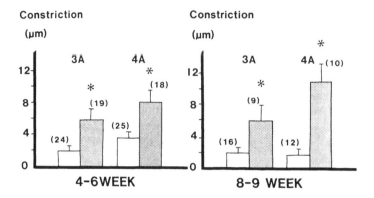

FIGURE 3. Constriction of (3A) third- and (4A) fourth-order arterioles in the cremaster muscle of SHR (stippled bars) and age-matched normotensive WKY controls (open bars) in response to elevation of the oxygen content of the superfusion solution from 0 to 5% O_2. Neurogenic tone was blocked with 0.1 mg/ml tetrodotoxin in the superfusate. Arterioles of SHR in the early (4 to 6 weeks old) and developing (8 to 9 weeks old) stages of hypertension exhibited a significantly greater constriction in response to elevation of superfusion solution PO_2 than normotensive WKY controls. (From Lombard, J. H., Hess, M. E., and Stekiel, W. J., *Am. J. Physiol.*, 250; *Heart Circ. Physiol.*, 19, H761, 1986. With permission.)

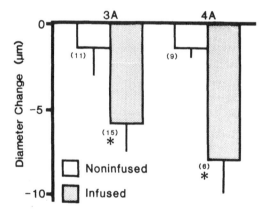

FIGURE 4. Data from preliminary studies comparing the response of neurally blocked (0.1 mg/ml tetrodotoxin in superfusate) (3A) third- and (4A) fourth-order cremasteric arterioles of reduced renal-mass rats to elevation of superfusion solution oxygen content from 0 to 5% O_2. Animals had recovered from a surgical reduction of 75% of the renal mass. Rats in the experimental group (stippled bars) received a continuous intravenous infusion of 145 mM NaCl (5 to 7 ml/h) for 36 h to produce hypertension, while those in the normotensive control group (open bars) were subjected to similar procedures without infusion. Constriction of third- and fourth-order arterioles of the hypertensive animals in response to elevation of superfusion solution PO_2 was significantly greater than that of the noninfused controls.

studies,[108] more recent observations[6,22,25,89,109] indicate that arteriolar constriction in response to an elevated PO_2 is indeed enhanced in various forms of hypertension. For example, an enhanced constriction of arterioles in response to an elevation of superfusion solution PO_2 has been observed in the very early[109] and established[22] stages of hypertension in SHR (Figure 3), in reduced renal-mass hypertension[6] (Figure 4), and in 1K-1C Goldblatt hypertension.[25] In

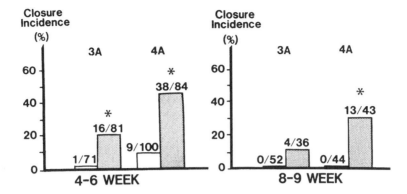

FIGURE 5. Incidence of complete closure of (3A) third- and (4A) fourth-order arterioles in the cremaster muscle of SHR (stippled bars) and normotensive WKY controls (open bars) in response to elevation of the oxygen content of the superfusion solution from 0 to 5% O_2. Neurogenic tone was blocked with 0.1 mg/ml tetrodotoxin in the superfusate. Ordinate represents the percentage of arterioles which were open during 0% O_2 superfusion but subsequently closed during 5% O_2 superfusion. Numbers above the bars represent the number of arterioles which closed during 5% O_2 superfusion/the total number of open arterioles observed during 0% O_2 superfusion. Arterioles of SHR in the early (4 to 6 weeks old) and developing (8 to 9 weeks old) stages of hypertension exhibited a significantly greater incidence of complete closure in response to elevation of superfusion solution PO_2 than those of WKY controls. (From Lombard, J. H., Hess, M. E., and Stekiel, W. J., *Am. J. Physiol.*, 250; *Heart Circ. Physiol.*, 19, H761, 1986. With permission.)

addition, small cremasteric arterioles of SHR in all stages of hypertension exhibit a significantly higher incidence of complete closure in response to elevated superfusion PO_2 than their age-matched WKY controls[22,109] (Figure 5).

The enhanced constriction of SHR arterioles[22,109] and reduced renal-mass vessels[6] in response to increased oxygen availability occurs in the presence of neural blockade with tetrodotoxin, demonstrating that it does not depend upon nervous influences. This observation suggests that the sensitivity of metabolic autoregulatory mechanisms or of the vascular smooth muscle itself to increases in oxygen availability are enhanced in SHR relative to WKY. Although it has been postulated that tissue PO_2 may be elevated in hypertension,[110] SHR exhibit a reduced number of arterioles and capillaries (and therefore an increased distance between microvascular sources of oxygen), a reduced calculated volume flow,[2] and an elevated oxygen consumption[111] relative to normotensive controls. Since all of these factors should contribute to a reduced tissue PO_2 in hypertension, it is unlikely that the enhanced response of hypertensive animals to increased oxygen availability, which was observed in the above studies,[6,22,25,89,109] reflects an initial elevation of tissue PO_2 prior to increasing the PO_2 of the superfusion solution. However, the relationship between tissue PO_2 and arteriolar diameters needs to be clarified by direct measurement in hypertensive animals and normotensive controls.

It is also important to establish whether or not the response of isolated vascular smooth muscle to changes in oxygen availability is altered in SHR and in other models of hypertension. Jackson and Duling[112] have demonstrated that arterioles of the hamster cheek pouch exhibit changes in active tone in response to alterations in oxygen availability, even when the vessels are isolated from parenchymal cell influences. Considerable evidence exists to suggest that intrinsic alterations in the function of the vascular smooth muscle cell membrane exist in hypertension,[20] and it is conceivable that these alterations could contribute to differences in the response of vascular smooth muscle cells to changes in oxygen availability in hypertension.

In addition to examining the contractile response of vascular smooth muscle to PO_2 increases in various forms of hypertension, it is important to compare the relaxation of hypertensive and normotensive vessels in response to hypoxia. Several studies suggest that decreases in oxygen availability may reduce active vascular smooth muscle tone via mechanisms which act at the level of the cell membrane, e.g., stimulation of electrogenic Na^+/K^+ transport[113] or a reduction in membrane Ca^{2+} permeability.[114,115] Although the relaxation of vascular smooth muscle in response to a wide variety of vasodilator agents has been studied in various forms of hypertension,[116] there are presently no studies of the effect of hypoxia upon isolated vessels of hypertensive and normotensive animals. Such studies could provide valuable information concerning the control of vascular function in hypertension, since whole body studies suggest that the response of the circulation to hypoxemia is altered in SHR relative to normotensive controls.[117]

As noted above, myogenic autoregulatory mechanisms could also contribute to an elevated microvascular resistance in hypertension. An enhanced activity of myogenic mechanisms may reflect an intrinsic alteration in vascular smooth muscle cell membrane properties in hypertensive individuals relative to normotensive controls. Since myogenic depolarization appears to be Ca^{2+}-dependent,[118] and vascular smooth muscle Ca^{2+} permeability may be elevated in many forms of hypertension,[105,119-121] it is likely that myogenic constrictor responses may be enhanced in hypertensive individuals relative to normotensive controls. This hypothesis is supported by the observation that middle cerebral arteries of SHR exhibit an enhanced depolarization in response to elevation of transmural pressure relative to their WKY controls.[122] However, the relationship between the electrical and mechanical response of vascular smooth muscle to elevations in transmural pressure needs to be examined in more detail, since dimensional studies of pressurized cerebral arteries in SHR and WKY[123] suggest that the myogenic autoregulatory capacity of cerebral vessels may in fact be reduced in SHR relative to WKY. In the latter study,[123] WKY vessels could constrict in response to increasing pressures, while SHR vessels maintained a constant diameter over a wide range of transmural pressures. In relating the electrical and mechanical responses of cerebral vessels to increases in transmural pressure, it is important to determine the role of several factors, including age and reduced force generation by cerebral arteries of SHR,[124] in determining the final response of the vessels to increases in transmural pressure. Moreover, the relationship between E_m, transmural pressure, and vessel diameter may differ among vascular beds. For example, in contrast to cerebral arteries, small mesenteric arteries of SHR generate more force than those of normotensive controls,[125,126] and one study[127] suggests that myogenic constrictor responses of these vessels are enhanced in SHR relative to WKY. Taken together, these studies clearly demonstrate that the relationship between E_m, vessel diameter, and transmural pressure must be further clarified in various vascular beds during the early and developing stages of different forms of hypertension.

At the present time, it is unclear whether changes in classical autoregulatory mechanisms persist indefinitely in hypertension, or whether a gradual substitution of longer-term mechanisms occurs as hypertension is sustained. Although classical short-term autoregulatory mechanisms are well suited to regulate organ blood flow during acute changes in tissue perfusion or arterial pressure, Cowley[21] has postulated that chronic conditions seem to be best met by long-term autoregulatory mechanisms which could involve alterations in the structure of the microcirculation. The hypothesis that a change from short-term autoregulatory mechanisms to chronic structural changes occurs in the course of hypertension seems to be supported by some observations which are available from human hypertensives. For example, Sullivan et al.[32] reported that capillary density and total vascular density are decreased in the conjunctiva of borderline hypertensive patients, although arteriolar diameters and numbers are not reduced. In these studies, capillary density was inversely related to the cardiac index but was not significantly related to blood pressure. Since the hypertensive patients exhibited an elevated cardiac index, a reduced peripheral vascular resistance, and an elevated forearm blood flow relative to normotensive controls, these investigators[32] hypothesized that short-term autoregulatory mechanisms may contribute to the reduced capillary density, by causing constriction and closure of the immediate precapillary arterioles. However, it is important to note that the elevated cardiac output seen in the young borderline hypertensive patients may be a response to changing metabolic needs, rather than a primary event.[17] In contrast to the lack of arteriolar narrowing and rarefaction observed in borderline hypertensives, arteriolar diameter and arteriolar density are both reduced in the conjunctiva of untreated human essential hypertensives.[33] Although it cannot be determined whether the reduction in arteriolar diameter and density in the latter study[33] was due to active constriction or structural changes, it appears that structural narrowing of vessels and anatomical rarefaction are responsible for at least part of the arteriolar constriction and reduced vessel density which develops during hypertension. This is based on the fact that autopsy specimens of the intestine taken from human hypertensives exhibit narrowing of arterioles and a decreased vascularity relative to those of normotensive controls.[34]

Although autoregulation is a powerful mechanism which could theoretically produce an increased total peripheral resistance and an elevated arterial blood pressure in some forms of hypertension, experiments to demonstrate that this mechanism is the predominant source of vasoconstriction in these types of hypertension are limited by present technology, and are therefore lacking.[17] Thus, it is impossible to say whether the time course of the resistance changes in individual organs in hypertension is compatible with the phenomenon of classic autoregulation and/or vascular restructuring or whether the ability of vascular beds to autoregulate changes with time. Nonetheless, local autoregulation of blood flow must be carefully considered for a full understanding of the hemodynamic events associated with all types of hypertension,[21] including those which do not arise as a primary result of the action of local autoregulatory mechanisms. Further investigation of the role of metabolic, myogenic, and structural mechanisms in determining microvascular resistance and tissue perfusion in various forms of hypertension should prove to be quite valuable in understanding the pathophysiology of this disease, since autoregulation of blood flow provides a mechanism (albeit poorly understood) whereby small increases in the total blood volume (or the "effective volume") could result in a chronic elevation of total peripheral resistance.[21]

REFERENCES

1. **Zweifach, B. W.,** The microcirculation in experimental hypertension, state-of-the-art review, *Hypertension,* 5 (Suppl. I), 10, 1983.
2. **Roy, J. W. and Mayrovitz, H. N.,** Microvascular blood flow in the normotensive and spontaneously hypertensive rat, *Hypertension,* 4, 264, 1982.
3. **Harper, S. L. and Bohlen, H. G.,** Microvascular adaptation in the cerebral cortex of adult spontaneously hypertensive rats, *Hypertension,* 6, 408, 1984.
4. **Joshua, I. G., Wiegman, D. L., Harris, P. D., and Miller, F. N.,** Progressive microvascular alterations with the development of renovascular hypertension, *Hypertension,* 6, 61, 1984.
5. **Abell, R. G. and Page, I. H.,** The effects of renal hypertension on the vessels of the ears of rabbits, *J. Exp. Med.,* 75, 673, 1942.
6. **Lombard, J. H., Cowley, A. W., Jr., Smits, G. J., Mazzeo, A. J., and Stekiel, W. J.,** Microcirculatory changes in rats in the early stages of reduced renal mass (RRM) hypertension, *Microvasc. Res.,* 29 (Abstr.), 236, 1985.
7. **Meininger, G. A., Harris, P. D., and Joshua, I. G.,** Distributions of microvascular pressure in skeletal muscle of one-kidney, one clip, two-kidney, one clip, and deoxycorticosterone-salt hypertensive rats, *Hypertension,* 6, 27, 1984.
8. **Hutchins, P. M. and Darnell, A. E.,** Observation of a decreased number of small arterioles in spontaneously hypertensive rats, *Circ. Res.,* 34-35 (Suppl. I), 161, 1974.
9. **Bohlen, H. G.,** Arteriolar closure mediated by hyperresponsiveness to norepinephrine in hypertensive rats, *Am. J. Physiol.,* 236; *Heart Circ. Physiol.,* 5, H157, 1979.
10. **Chen, I. I., Prewitt, R. L., and Dowell, R. F.,** Microvascular rarefaction in spontaneously hypertensive rat cremaster muscle, *Am. J. Physiol.,* 241; *Heart Circ. Physiol.,* 10, H306, 1981.

11. **Prewitt, R. L., Chen, I. I. H., and Dowell, R.,** Development of microvascular rarefaction in the spontaneously hypertensive rat, *Am. J. Physiol.,* 243; *Heart Circ. Physiol.,* 12, H243, 1982.

12. **Prewitt, R. L., Chen, I. I. H., and Dowell, R.,** Microvascular alterations in the one-kidney, one-clip renal hypertensive rat, *Am. J. Physiol. 246; Heart Circ. Physiol.,* 15, H728, 1984.

13. **Folkow, B.,** Cardiovascular structural adaptation; its role in the initiation and maintenance of primary hypertension, *Clin. Sci. Mol. Med.,* 55, 3s, 1978.

14. **Harder, D. R., Contney, S. J., Willems, W. J., and Stekiel, W. J.,** Norepinephrine effect on *in situ* venous membrane potential in spontaneously hypertensive rats, *Am. J. Physiol.,* 240; *Heart Circ. Physiol.,* 9, H837, 1981.

15. **Willems, W. J., Harder, D. R., Contney, S. J., McCubbin, J. W., and Stekiel, W. J.,** Sympathetic supraspinal control of venous membrane potential in spontaneous hypertension *in vivo, Am. J. Physiol.,* 243; *Cell Physiol.,* 12, C101, 1982.

16. **Stekiel, W. J., Contney, S. J., Lombard, J. H., and Willems, W. J.,** Effect of adrenergic denervation on small mesenteric vessel membrane potential responses to noradrenaline in spontaneously hypertensive and Wistar-Kyoto rats, in *Hypertensive Mechanisms,* Ganten, D., Ed., F. K. Schattauer, Stuttgart, p. 86.

17. **Coleman, T. G., Samar, R. E., and Murphy, W. R.,** Autoregulation versus other vasoconstrictors in hypertension. A critical review, *Hypertension,* 1, 324, 1979.

18. **Click, R. L., Gilmore, J. P., and Joyner, W. L.,** Direct demonstration of alterations in the microcirculation of the hamster during and following renal hypertension, *Circ. Res.,* 41, 461, 1977.

19. **Click, R., Gilmore, J., and Joyner, W.,** Differential response of hamster cheek pouch microvessels to vasoactive stimuli during the early development of hypertension, *Circ. Res.,* 44, 512, 1979.

20. **Harder, D. R. and Hermsmeyer, K.,** Membrane mechanisms in arterial hypertension, *Hypertension,* 5, 404, 1983.

21. **Cowley, A. W., Jr.,** The concept of autoregulation of total blood flow and its role in hypertension, *Am. J. Med.,* 68, 906, 1980.

22. **Lombard, J. H., Hess, M. E., and Stekiel, W. J.,** Neural and local control of arterioles in spontaneously hypertensive rats, *Hypertension,* 6, 530, 1984.

23. **Meininger, G. A., Lubrano, V. M., and Granger, H. J.,** Hemodynamic and microvascular responses in the hindquarters during the development of renal hypertension in rats. Evidence for the involvement of an autoregulatory component, *Circ. Res.,* 55, 609, 1984.

24. **Meininger, G. A., Routh, L. K., and Granger, H. J.,** Autoregulation and vasoconstriction in the intestine during acute renal hypertension, *Hypertension,* 7, 364, 1985.

25. **Hippensteele, J. R., Harris, P. D., and Wiegman, D. L.,** Renovascular hypertension: altered oxygen sensitivity of cremasteric arterioles in decerebrate rats, *Microvasc. Res.,* 23 (Abstr.), 258, 1982.

26. **Bohlen, H. G. and Lobach, D.,** *In vivo* study of microvascular wall characteristics and resting control in young and mature spontaneously hypertensive rats, *Blood Vessels,* 15, 322, 1978.

27. **Zweifach, B. W., Kovalcheck, S., DeLano, F., and Chen, P.,** Micropressure-flow relationships in the skeletal muscle of spontaneously hypertensive rats, *Hypertension,* 3, 601, 1981.

28. **Henrich, H., Hertel, R., and Assman, R.,** Structural differences in the mesentery microcirculation between normotensive and spontaneously hypertensive rats, *Pfluegers Arch.,* 375, 153, 1978.

29. **Bohlen, H. G.,** Intestinal microvascular adaptation during maturation of spontaneously hypertensive rats, *Hypertension,* 5, 739, 1983.

30. **Joyner, W. L., Davis, J. M., and Gilmore, J. P.,** Intravascular pressure distribution and dimensional analysis of microvessels in hamsters with renovascular hypertension, *Microvasc. Res.,* 22, 190, 1981.

31. **Wiegman, D. L., Joshua, I. G., Morff, R. J., Harris, P. D., and Miller, F. N.,** Microvascular responses to norepinephrine in renovascular and spontaneously hypertensive rats, *Am. J. Physiol.,* 236, H545, 1979.

32. **Sullivan, J. M., Prewitt, R. L., and Josephs, J. A.,** Attenuation of the microcirculation in young patients with high-output borderline hypertension, *Hypertension,* 5, 844, 1983.

33. **Harper, R. N., Moore, M. A., Marr, M. C., Watts, L. E., and Hutchins, P. M.,** Arteriolar rarefaction in the conjunctiva of human essential hypertensives, *Microvasc. Res.,* 16, 369, 1978.

34. **Short, D. S. and Thomson, A. D.,** The arteries of the small intestine in systemic hypertension, *J. Pathol. Bacteriol.,* 78, 321, 1959.

35. **Johnson, P. C.,** Principles of peripheral circulatory control, in *Peripheral Circulation,* Johnson, P. C., Ed., John Wiley & Sons, New York, 1978, chap. 4.

36. **Wiedeman, M. P., Tuma, R. F., and Mayrovitz, H. N.,** *An Introduction to Microcirculation,* Academic Press, New York, 1981.

37. **Fuxe, K. and Sedvall, G.,** The distribution of adrenergic nerve fibers to the blood vessels in skeletal muscle, *Acta Physiol. Scand.,* 64, 75, 1965.

38. **Furness, J. B. and Marshall, J. M.,** Correlation of the directly observed responses of mesenteric vessels of the rat to nerve stimulaion and noradrenaline with the distribution of adrenergic nerves, *J. Physiol. (London),* 239, 75, 1974.

39. **Lassen, N. A.,** Brain, in *Peripheral Circulation,* Johnson, P. C., Ed., John Wiley & Sons, New York, 1978, chap. 12.

40. **Wiedeman, M. P.,** Effect of denervation on diameter and reactivity of arteries in the bat wing, *Circ. Res.,* 3, 618, 1955.

41. **Joyner, W. L., Campbell, G. T., Peterson, C., and Wagoner, J.,** Adrenergic neurons: are they present in microvessels in cheek pouches of hamsters?, *Microvasc. Res.,* 26, 27, 1983.

42. **Lombard, J. H., Chenoweth, J. L., and Stekiel, W. J.,** Nonneural vascular smooth muscle tone in arterioles of the hamster cheek pouch, *Microvasc. Res.,* 29, 81, 1985.

43. **Granger, H. J., Meininger, G. A., Borders, J. L., Morff, R. J., and Goodman, A. H.,** Microcirculation of skeletal muscle, in *The Physiology and Pharmacology of the Microcirculation,* Vol. 2, Academic Press, New York, 1984, chap. 7.

44. **Greenway, C. V.,** Neural control and autoregulatory escape, in *Physiology of the Intestinal Circulation,* Shepherd, A. P. and Granger, D. N., Eds., Raven Press, New York, 1984.

45. **Hutchins, P. M., Bond, R. F., and Green, H. D.,** The response of skeletal muscle arterioles to common carotid occlusion, *Microvasc. Res.,* 7, 321, 1974.

46. **Marshall, J. M.,** The influence of the sympathetic nervous system on individual vessels of the microcirculation of skeletal muscle of the rat, *J. Physiol. (London),* 332, 169, 1982.

47. **Heistad, D. D.,** Effects of nerves on cerebral vessels in stroke, cerebral edema, and hypertension, *J. Lab. Clin. Med.,* 99, 139, 1982.

48. **Abboud, F. M.,** The sympathetic system in hypertension: state-of-the-art review, *Hypertension,* 4 (Suppl. II), 208, 1982.

49. **Brody, M. J., Haywood, J. R., and Touw, K. B.,** Neural mechanisms in hypertension, *Annu. Rev. Physiol.,* 42, 441, 1980.

50. **Abboud, F., Fozzard, H., Gilmore, J., and Reis, D., Eds.,** Neural control in hypertension, in *Disturbances in Neurogenic Control of the Circulation,* Sect. 2, Am. Physiol. Soc., Bethesda, MD, 1981, 87.

51. **Hughes, M. and Barnes, C., Eds.,** *Neural Control of the Circulation,* Academic Press, New York, 1980.

52. **Julius, S. and Ester, M., Eds.,** *The Nervous System in Arterial Hypertension,* Charles C Thomas, Springfield, IL, 1976.

53. **Boyer, J. T., Fraser, J. R., and Doyle, A. E.,** The haemodynamic effects of cold immersion, *Clin. Sci.,* 19, 539, 1960.

54. **Brod, J.,** Haemodynamic basis of acute pressor reactions and hypertension, *Br. Heart J.,* 25, 227, 1963.

55. **Doyle, A.,** Autonomic nervous system in hypertension, in *Hypertension in the Young and the Old,* Onesti, G. and Kim, K. E., Eds., Grune & Stratton, New York, 1981, 251.

56. **Korner, P. I., Shaw, J., Uther, J. B., West, M. J., McRitchie, R. J., and Richards, J. G.,** Autonomic and non-autonomic circulatory components in essential hypertension in man, *Circulation,* 48, 107, 1973.

57. **Scriabine, A., Ed.,** *Pharmacology of Antihypertensive Drugs,* Raven Press, New York, 1980.

58. **Yamori, Y.,** Neurogenic mechanisms of spontaneous hypertension, in *Regulation of Blood Pressure by the CNS,* Onesti, G. M., Fernandes, M., and Kim, K. E., Eds., Grune & Stratton, New York, 1976, 65.

59. **Folkow, B., Hallback, M., Lundgren, Y., Weiss, L., Albrecht, I., and Julius, S.,** Analysis of design and reactivity of series-coupled vascular sections in spontaneously hypertensive rats, *Acta Physiol. Scand.,* 90, 654, 1974.

60. **Hallback-Norlander, M. and Lundin, S.,** Cardiovascular reactions in young spontaneously hypertensive rats, in *Hypertension in the Young and the Old,* Onesti, G. and Kim, K. E., Eds., Grune & Stratton, New York, 1981, 107.

61. **Conway, J.,** Mechanisms sustaining hypertension, in *Hypertension in the Young and the Old,* Onesti, G. and Kim, K. E., Eds., Grune & Stratton, New York, 1981, 231.

62. **Henry, D., Luft, F., Weinberger, M., Fineberg, N., and Grim, G.,** Norepinephrine in urine and plasma following provocative maneuvers in normal and hypertensive subjects, *Hypertension,* 2, 20, 1980.

63. **Engleman, K., Portnoy, B., and Sjoerdsma, A.,** Plasma catecholamine concentrations in patients with hypertension, *Circ. Res.,* 26, 27 (Suppll. I), 141, 1970.

64. **De Quattro, V. and Chan, S.,** Raised plasma-catecholamines in some patients with primary hypertension, *Lancet,* 1, 806, 1972.

65. **Louis, W. J., Doyle, A. E., and Anavekar, S.,** Plasma norepinephrine levels in essential hypertension, *N. Engl. J. Med.,* 288, 599, 1973.

66. **Provoost, A. P. and DeJong, W.,** Differential development of renal, DOCA-salt and spontaneous hypertension in the rat after neonatal sympathectomy, *Clin. Exp. Hypertension,* 1, 177, 1978.

67. **Ikeda, H., Shino, A., and Nagaoka, A.,** Effects of chemical sympathectomy on hypertension and stroke in stroke-prone spontaneously hypertensive rats, *Eur. J. Pharmacol.,* 53, 173, 1979.

68. **Clark, D., Jones, D., Phelan, E., and Devine, C.,** Blood pressure and vascular resistance in genetically hypertensive rats treated at birth with 6-hydroxydopamine, *Circ. Res.,* 43, 293, 1978.

69. **Friedman, R., Tassinari, L. M., Heine, M., and Iwai, J.,** Differential development of salt-induced and renal hypertension in Dahl hypertension-sensitive rats after neonatal sympathectomy, *Clin. Exp. Hypertension,* 1, 779, 1979.

70. **Takeshita, A., Mark, A., and Brody, M.,** Prevention of salt-induced hypertension in the Dahl strain by 6-hydroxydopamine, *Am. J. Physiol.,* 236, H48, 1979.

71. **Okamoto, K., Nosaka, S., Yamori, Y., and Matsumoto, M.,** Participation of neural factor in the pathogenesis of hypertension in the spontaneously hypertensive rat, *Jpn. Heart J.,* 8, 168, 1967.

72. **Iriuchijima, J.,** Role of splanchnic nerves in spontaneously hypertensive rats, *Jpn. Circ. J.,* 37, 1251, 1973.

73. **Judy, W., Watanabe, A., Henry, D., Beech, H., Murphy, W., and Hockel, G.,** Sympathetic nerve activity: role in regulation of blood pressure in spontaneously hypertensive rats, *Circ. Res.,* 38 (Suppl. II), 21, 1976.

74. **Judy, W. and Farrell, S.,** Arterial baroreceptor reflex control of sympathetic nerve activity in the spontaneously hypertensive rat, *Hypertension,* 1, 605, 1979.

75. **Judy, W. V., Watanabe, A. M., Murphy, W. R., Aprison, B. S., and Yu, P.-L.,** Sympathetic nerve activity and blood pressure in normotensive backcross rats genetically related to the spontaneously hypertensive rat, *Hypertension,* 1, 598, 1979.

76. **Zanchetti, A., Stella, A., Baccelli, G., and Mancia, G.,** Neural influences on kidney function in the pathogenesis of arterial hypertension, in *Hypertension Determinants. Complications and Intervention,* Onesti, G. and Klimt, C., Eds., Grune & Stratton, New York, 1979, 99.

77. **Brody, M. J.,** New developments in our knowledge of blood pressure regulation, *Fed. Proc.,* 40, 2257, 1981.

78. **Brody, M. and Johnson, A.,** Role of anteroventral third ventricle region in fluid and electrolyte balance, arterial pressure regulation and hypertension, in *Frontiers in Neuroendocrinology,* Martini, L. and Ganong, W., Eds., Raven Press, New York, 1980, 249.

79. **Liard, J. F.,** Renal denervation delays blood pressure increase in the spontaneously hypertensive rat, *Experientia,* 33, 339, 1977.

80. **Kline, R. L., Kelton, P. M., and Mercer, P. F.,** Effect of renal denervation on the development of hypertension in spontaneously hypertensive rats, *Can. J. Physiol. Pharmacol.,* 56, 818, 1978.

81. **Guyton, A., Coleman, T., Cowley, A., Jr., Manning, R., Norman, R., and Ferguson, J.,** A systems analysis approach to understanding long range arterial blood pressure control and hypertension, *Circ. Res.,* 35, 159, 1974.

82. **Norman, R. A., Jr., Enobakhare, J. A., Declue, J. W., Douglas, B. H., and Guyton, A. C.,** Renal function curves in Goldblatt and spontaneously hypertensive rats, *Fed. Proc.,* 36 (Abstr.), 531, 1977.

83. **Abel, P. W. and Hermsmeyer, K.,** Sympathetic cross-innervation of spontaneously hypertensive rats and genetic controls suggests a trophic influence on vascular muscle membranes, *Circ. Res.,* 49, 1311, 1981.

84. **Bevan, R. D.,** Effect of sympathetic denervation on smooth muscle cell proliferation in the growing rabbit ear artery, *Circ. Res.,* 37, 14, 1975.

85. **Hart, M. N., Heistad, D., and Brody, M. J.,** Effect of chronic hypertension and sympathetic denervation on wall/lumen ratio of cerebral vessels, *Hypertension,* 2, 419, 1980.

86. **Dusseau, J. W., Smith, T. L., and Hutchins, P. M.,** Acute effects of salbutamol on arteriolar vasodilatation and blood pressure in hypertensive rats, *Microvasc. Res.,* 22, 1, 1981.

87. **Henrich, H. and Eder, M.,** Sympathetic-adrenergic regulation of the microvasculature in spontaneously hypertensive rats, *Bibl. Anat.,* 18, 187, 1979.

88. **Stekiel, W. J., Contney, S. J., and Lombard, J. H.,** Small vessel membrane potential, sympathetic input and electrogenic pump rate in SH rats, *Am. J. Physiol.,* 250 (*Cell Physiol.,* 19), C547, 1986.

89. **Lombard, J. H. and Stekiel, W. J.,** Arteriolar responses to increased O_2 availability, tetrodotoxin (TTX), and adenosine (ADO) in the mesoappendix of spontaneously hypertensive (SHR) and normotensive (WKY) rats, *Microvasc. Res.,* 27 (Abstr.), 253, 1984.

90. **Stekiel, W. J., Contney, S. J., Mazzeo, A., Cowley, A. W., Jr., and Lombard, J. H.,** Evidence for elevated sympathetic neural input to small mesenteric blood vessels in volume-induced hypertension, *Microvasc. Res.,* 29 (Abstr.), 252, 1985.

91. **Bohr, D. F.,** What makes the pressure go up? A hypothesis, *Hypertension,* 3 (Suppl. II), 160, 1981.

92. **Borst, J. G. G. and Borst-de Geus, A.,** Hypertension explained by Starling's theory of circulatory homeostasis, *Lancet,* 1, 677, 1963.

93. **Ledingham, J. M. and Cohen, R. D.,** Hypertension explained by Starling's theory of circulatory homeostasis, *Lancet,* 1, 887, 1963.

94. **Conway, J.,** Hemodynamic consequences of induced changes in blood volume, *Circ. Res.,* 18, 190, 1966.

95. **Granger, H. J. and Guyton, A. C.,** Autoregulation of the total systemic circulation following destruction of the central nervous system in the dog, *Circ. Res.,* 25, 379, 1969.

96. **Coleman, T. and Guyton, A.,** Hypertension caused by salt loading in the dog. III. Onset transients of cardiac output and other circulatory variables, *Circ. Res.,* 25, 153, 1969.

97. **Cowley, A. W. and Guyton, A. C.,** Baroreceptor reflex effects on transient and steady state hemodynamics of salt-loading hypertension in dogs, *Circ. Res.,* 36, 536, 1975.

98. **Liard, J. F.,** Regional blood flows in salt loading hypertension in the dog, *Am. J. Physiol.,* 240, H361, 1981.

99. **Coleman, T. G., Bower, J. D., Langford, H. G., and Guyton, A. C.,** Regulation of arterial pressure in the anephric state, *Circulation,* 42, 509, 1970.

100. **Onesti, G., Swartz, C., Ramirez, O., and Brest, A. N.,** Bilateral nephrectomy for control of hypertension in uremia, *Trans. Am. Soc. Artif. Internal Organs,* 14, 361, 1968.

101. **Smith, T. L. and Hutchins, P. M.,** Central hemodynamics in the developmental stage of spontaneous hypertension in the unanesthetized rat, *Hypertension*, 1, 508, 1979.
102. **Alson, R. L., Dusseau, J. W., and Hutchins, P. M.,** Arteriolar and systemic autoregulatory responses during the development of hypertension in the spontaneously hypertensive rat, *Proc. Soc. Exp. Biol. Med.*, 80, 62, 1985.
103. **Bohlen, H. G., Gore, R. W., and Hutchins, P. M.,** Comparison of microvascular pressures in normal and spontaneously hypertensive rats, *Microvasc. Res.*, 13, 125, 1977.
104. **Hertel, R., Henrich, H., and Assmann, R.,** Intravital measurement of arteriolar pressure and tangential wall stress in normotensive and spontaneously hypertensive rats (established hypertension), *Experientia*, 34 (Part 2), 865, 1978.
105. **Holloway, E., Sitrin, M., and Bohr, D.,** Calcium dependence of vascular smooth muscle from normotensive and hypertensive rats, in *Hypertension '72*, Genest, J. and Koiw, E., Eds., Springer-Verlag, Berlin, 1972, 400.
106. **Standgaard S., Olesen J., Skinhoj E., and Lassen, N. A.,** Autoregulation of brain circulation in severe arterial hypertension, *Br. Med. J.*, 1, 507, 1973.
107. **Fujishima, M. and Omae, T.,** Lower limit of autoregulation in normotensive and spontaneously hypertensive rats, *Experientia*, 32, 1019, 1976.
108. **Walsh, G. M. and Tobia, A. J.,** Vascular pressure-flow analysis in normal and hypoxemic spontaneously hypertensive rats, *Clin. Exp. Hypertension Part A, Theory and Practice*, 4, 445, 1982.
109. **Lombard, J. H., Hess, M. E., and Stekiel, W. J.,** Enhanced response of arterioles to oxygen during the development of hypertension in spontaneously hypertensive rats, *Am. J. Physiol.*, 250; *Heart Circ. Physiol.*, 19, H761, 1986.
110. **Hertel, R. and Henrich, H.,** Microvascular pressures and permeability in spontaneously hypertensive and normotensive rats, *Bibl. Anat.*, 18, 180, 1979.
111. **Tadepalli, A. S., Walsh, G. M., and Tobia, A. J.,** Normal cardiac output in the conscious young spontaneously hypertensive rat: evidence for higher oxygen utilization, *Life Sci.*, 15, 1103, 1974.
112. **Jackson, W. F. and Duling, B. R.,** The oxygen sensitivity of hamster cheek pouch arterioles. *In vitro* and *in situ* studies, *Circ. Res.*, 53, 515, 1983.
113. **Detar, R.,** Mechanism of physiological hypoxia-induced depression of vascular smooth muscle contraction, *Am. J. Physiol.*, 238; *Heart Circ. Physiol.*, 7, H761, 1980.
114. **Ebeigbe, A. B., Pickard, J. D., and Jennett, S.,** Responses of systemic vascular smooth muscle to hypoxia, *J. Exp. Physiol.*, 65, 273, 1980.
115. **Ebeigbe, A. B.,** Influence of hypoxia on contractility and calcium uptake in rabbit aorta, *Experientia*, 38, 935, 1982.
116. **Cohen, D. M., Webb, R. C., and Bohr, D. F.,** Nitroprusside-induced vascular relaxation in DOCA hypertensive rats, *Hypertension*, 4, 13, 1982.
117. **Walsh, G. M., Tsuchiya, M, Cox, A. C., Tobia, A. J., and Frohlich, E. D.,** Altered hemodynamic responses to acute hypoxemia in spontaneously hypertensive rats, *Am. J. Physiol.*, 234; *Heart Circ. Physiol.*, 3, H275, 1978.
118. **Harder, D. R.,** Pressure-dependent membrane depolarization in cat middle cerebral artery, *Circ. Res.*, 55, 197, 1984.
119. **Mulvany, M. J. and Nyborg, N.,** An increased calcium sensitivity of mesenteric resistance vessels in young and adult spontaneously hypertensive rats, *Br. J. Pharmacol.*, 71, 585, 1980.
120. **Noon, J. P., Rice, P. J., and Baldessarini, R. J.,** Calcium leakage as a cause of the high resting tension in vascular smooth muscle from the spontaneously hypertensive rat, *Proc. Natl. Acad. Sci. U.S.A.*, 75, 1605, 1978.
121. **Mulvany, M. J., Korsgaard, N., and Nyborg, N.,** Evidence that the increased calcium sensitivity of resistance vessels in spontaneously hypertensive rats is an intrinsic defect of their vascular smooth muscle, *Clin. Exp. Hypertension*, 3, 749, 1981.
122. **Harder, D. R., Smeda, J., and Lombard, J.,** Enhanced myogenic depolarization in hypertensive cerebral arterial muscle, *Circ. Res.*, 57, 319, 1985.
123. **Osol, G. and Halpern, W.,** Myogenic properties of cerebral blood vessels from normotensive and hypertensive rats, *Am. J. Physiol.*, 249; *Heart Circ. Physiol.*, 18, H914, 1985.
124. **Winquist, R. J. and Bohr, D. F.,** Structural and functional changes in cerebral arteries from spontaneously hypertensive rats, *Hypertension*, 5, 292, 1983.
125. **Whall, C. W., Jr., Myers, M. M., and Halpern, W.,** Norepinephrine sensitivity, tension development and neuronal uptake in resistance arteries from spontaneously hypertensive and normotensive rats, *Blood Vessels*, 17, 1, 1980.
126. **Mulvany, M. and Halpern, W.,** Contractile properties of small arterial resistance vessels in spontaneously hypertensive and normotensive rats, *Circ. Res.*, 41, 19, 1977.
127. **Greensmith J. E. and Duling B. R.,** Behavior of isolated, cannulated mesenteric arterioles from control (WKY) and spontaneously hypertensive rats (SHR), *Microvasc. Res.*, 23 (Abstr.), 255, 1982.

Chapter 6

NEURAL REGULATION OF BLOOD VESSELS IN NORMOTENSIVE AND HYPERTENSIVE ANIMALS

M. J. MacKay and D. W. Cheung

TABLE OF CONTENTS

I. INTRODUCTION

The contribution of the sympathetic nervous system to hypertension has long been recognized and has been a subject of intense research for several years. Many aspects concerning the role of the sympathetic nervous system in the pathogenesis of experimental hypertension have been previously reviewed.[1-5] In this chapter, we will consider the recent findings in the study of the neuroeffector interaction between the sympathetic nerves and the vascular smooth muscle cells and the changes in experimental hypertension, using mainly the spontaneously hypertensive rat (SHR) as our model.

A. The Role of the Peripheral Sympathetic Nervous System in Hypertension

Several lines of evidence suggest that an enhanced sympathetic nervous activity is associated with hypertension. Hypertensive animals and/or man have been reported to exhibit higher plasma norepinephrine levels,[6] increased firing of splanchnic[7-9] and renal[9,10] nerves, faster norepinephrine turnovers in peripheral tissues[11,12] and an enhanced release of norepinephrine from sympathetic nerve terminals.[13,14]

An indication that the peripheral sympathetic nervous system contributes to hypertension comes from studies which show that interference of this system reduces elevated blood pressure. Using the ganglionic blocking agent hexamethonium, Judy et al.[9] showed that the drop in blood pressure was greater in the SHR so that the final level was comparable to that of age-matched WKY similarly treated with hexamethonium. However, in a later study, a similar drop in blood pressure after hexamethonium in the SHR and WKY was observed.[15]

A recent assessment of the neural and nonneural contributions to blood pressure in SHR and WKY was performed using the ganglionic blocker chlorisondamine.[16] Blood pressure measurements from birth to 42 days of age showed that within 24 h, resting diastolic pressure was increased in SHR. The difference in pressures was attributed to both neural and nonneural factors. However, while the difference in the nonneural component (that remaining after chlorisondamine) remained consistent throughout development, the difference in the neurally mediated component (chorisondamine-sensitive) increased. Thus, it was concluded that an enhanced sympathetic nervous activity was associated with the development of hypertension.

Another approach to assess the contribution of the peripheral sympathetic nervous system to hypertension is sympathectomy.[17] When given repeatedly from birth by subcutaneous injection, 6-OHDA prevented the full development of hypertension in the SHR.[18-21] However, 6-OHDA also destroys central adrenergic neurones in immature rats.[22-24] Therefore, central and peripheral effects cannot be separated. Furthermore, 6-OHDA does not produce complete sympathectomy.[18] Recently, better success has been achieved by treatment of young SHR with nerve growth factor antiserum alone or in combination with guanethidine.[25,26] These studies thus implicate the importance of an intact peripheral sympathetic nervous system for the full development of hypertension in the SHR.

II. NEUROEFFECTOR MECHANISMS

The major determinants in the neuroeffector interaction are (1) the density of innervation and the width of the synaptic cleft; (2) the presynatpic mechanisms involved in the release and reuptake of the transmitter; and (3) the response at the postsynaptic membrane. Many aspects in the sympathetic regulation of vascular activity have been reviewed in recent years.[27-30] In this chapter, our emphasis will be on the new developments in the study of neuroeffector interaction in blood vessels and the changes in the SHR.

A. Innervation

Components of the blood vessel wall are concentrically arranged. Surrounding the vascular smooth muscle in the tunica media are the postganglionic sympathetic nerve endings which form a network of slender processes, the neural plexus. The plexus consists of nonmyelinated axons, 0.25 to 5 μm in diameter, surrounded by a Schwann cell sheath. At regular intervals of about 3 to 10 μm, each axon exhibits swellings or varicosities of 1.5 to 2 μm in diameter, which are devoid of Schwann cells where they face the vascular smooth muscle cells. The varicosities contain small granular vesicles, the major sites of transmitter synthesis, storage, release, and uptake. In most arteries, sympathetic nerves do not penetrate into the tunica media.[31,32] The density of innervation varies between different blood vessels and between species. Even within the same artery, the density of innervation may vary. Thus, in the rabbit ear artery[33] and the rat tail artery,[34] the innervation of the proximal region is about twice as dense as that in the distal region.

Transmitter released from the vesicles must diffuse across a gap in order to reach receptors on the vascular smooth muscle cell. In general, clefts 20 to a few hundred nm are considered narrow, while those several hundred nm to a few μm are considered wide.[35] The narrowest clefts are found in arterioles, small arteries, and some veins,[36] and the widest in cerebral arteries.[37] However, the cleft width may be dependent on the functional state of the artery itself, being narrow in a dilated artery and wider when the artery is constricted. Functional significance has been attributed to cleft width since, as compared to tissues with wide clefts, those with narrow clefts exhibit: (1) a larger difference in transmitter concentration inside and outside the cleft;[39] (2) a more easily demonstrated negative-feedback release mechanism;[39] (3) a larger proportion of transmitter taken back into varicosities;[27] (4) a lower threshold for neurogenic responses and larger responses to a given frequency of nerve stimulation;[27] and (5) more rapid neurogenic responses.[40]

In the SHR, the density of innervation in blood vessels is increased. The number of nerve axons innervating the tail artery,[34] the jejunal artery,[41] and the mesenteric arterioles[41] are significantly increased in the SHR. The intensity of catecholamine fluorescence is also larger in the SHR.[34,41] These findings are in good agreement with the observed increase in catecholamine content in the blood vessels of SHR.[34] In the jejunal arteries, there appears to be no change in the distance between the smooth muscle cell and the nerve axon in the SHR.[41]

B. Presynaptic Mechanisms

1. Norepinepherine (NE) Release in Hypertension

Studies to compare sympathetic nervous activity and NE release in SHR and WKY have often been performed by using plasma catecholamine and/or dopamine β-hydroxylase levels as indices of nerve activity. In general, this approach has shown an increase in sympathetic activity in young SHR.[43-47] Results obtained from adult SHR however, are more controversial, with some investigators reporting an increase,[45] and others reporting no change[48,49] in plasma NE or dopamine β-hydroxylase levels. Because plasma catecholamine levels reflect the net overflow of transmitter from adrenergic nerve terminals, and not the amount actually reaching postsynaptic receptors, more refined methods of comparing sympathetic nervous activity have been developed which allow NE release, uptake, and plasma clearance to be assessed independently. Experiments involving the measurement of either ³H-NE release or NE content before and after stimulation while preventing reuptake have shown a greater release in SHR, especially in young animals. An increased release was reported in response to nerve stimulation in the perfused kidney,[13,50-52] perfused mesentery,[53-56] isolated portal vein,[57,58] and isolated tail artery.[14,59] Thus, for young SHR, conclusions were similar to those made when measuring plasma catecholamine levels. In contrast, an attenuated release was reported for adult SHRs,[56,60] prompting the suggestion that the rise in blood pressure in adults is compensated by a decreased transmitter release.

2. Presynaptic Regulation of Release in Hypertension

It is now generally accepted that the release of noradrenaline from adrenergic nerves can be modulated by endogenous substances acting on presynaptic receptors. Activation of angiotensin and β-adrenergic receptors enhances release,[61-65] while activation of α_2-adrenoceptors and possibly purinoceptors attentuates release.[66-69] Results from several laboratories suggest that angiotensin receptor-mediated facilitation of release and contraction is enhanced in both young and old SHR.[53,58] In the isolated mesenteric vascular bed, β-adrenoceptor agonists were found to produce a greater increase in perfusion pressure in response to nerve stimulation in SHR as compared to WKY, suggesting an enhanced β-receptor mediated facilitation of release.[70] However, there are also reports of a similar presynaptic β_2-adrenoceptor function in isolated vessels of SHR and WKY.[53]

In addition to altered facilitation, there is some evidence that autoinhibition of noradrenaline release is altered in SHR. In the tail artery[59] and portal vein[58] of 28-week-old animals, yohimbine was found to enhance the release of noradrenaline in response to nerve stimulation to a lesser extent in SHR than in WKY. This would suggest a decreased presynaptic α_2-adrenoceptor-mediated inhibition in the adult SHR. However, similar responses to presynaptic α_2-blockade were found in the tail artery, portal vein and perfused mesentery of 6-, 10-, and 18-week-old SHR as compared to age-matched WKY.[53,54,58,69,71] In 5- and 15- to 18-week-old SHR, a decreased purine-mediated inhibition was observed in the perfused mesentery.[72,73]

3. Neuronal Reuptake

A major role of the nerves in the disposition of the released transmitter is reuptake into the nerve terminals. In the SHR, enhanced uptake of noradrenaline was observed in the tail artery[74,75] and the mesenteric artery.[76,77] The increased neuronal uptake may be related to the higher density of innervation. Alterations in the presynaptic mechanisms regulating noradrenaline release in hypertension have been reviewed by Westfall and Meldrum recently.[78]

C. Postsynaptic Mechanisms

Changes in the vascular smooth muscle properties have been implicated in the pathogenesis and maintenance of hypertension.[79-81] Therefore, it is very important to consider these postsynaptic changes when comparing the neural responses in normotensive and hypertensive animals.

1. Postsynaptic Reactivity in Hypertension

Accumulating evidence suggests that postsynaptic reactivity to NE and other vasopressor agents may be altered in hypertension.[50,82-88] In many vessels, differences in reactivity between SHR and WKY may only be unmasked when the neural influence is removed, as with denervation procedures and blockade of neuronal uptake with cocaine.[34,76,89,90] It has been proposed that the altered reactivity observed in SHR is due to changes in the vascular smooth muscle membrane. An increase in membrane permeability to K^+, Na^+, and Ca^{2+} [91-93] and an altered ionic transport mechanism for Na^+ and Ca^{2+} [93,94] have been reported. Since membrane permeability and active electrogenic transport are the main determinants of membrane potential in vascular smooth muscle, the altered vascular function in hypertension may be related to the resetting of the membrane potential to a more depolarized level,[93] thereby increasing the tone and reactivity to vasoactive agents.[95]

Results from this laboratory support the proposal that membrane properties are altered in hypertension. Intracellular recordings showed that the resting membrane potential of the tail artery is significantly decreased with the development of hypertension.[96] The electrical responses to perivascular nerve stimulation observed in normotensive Wistar rats (the excitatory junction potential [e.j.p.] and slow depolarization[97]) were also observed in both SHR and WKY. However, given similar stimulation parameters, both responses were smaller in amplitude and faster in time course in SHR (Table 1). The time constant for the decay of the e.j.p. was also much faster in SHR (281.1 ± 16.8 ms) than in WKY (400.6 ± 23.6 ms). Since the time constant of the e.j.p. is related to the time constant of the membrane,[98,99] these findings suggest a decreased membrane resistance in the SHR, which supports the theory that the SHR membrane is more

Table 1
NERVE-EVOKED RESPONSES OF TAIL ARTERIES FROM SHR AND WKY

	WKY	SHR
Blood pressure (mmHg)	118.6 ± 1	183.7 ± 2^a
Membrane potential (mV)	-65.9 ± 1.3	-56.2 ± 2.2^a
s.e.j.p.		
Cells(%)	41	66
Frequency/min/cell	0.45	1.62^a
e.j.p.		
Amplitude[b] (mV)	9.3 ± 0.4	6.6 ± 1.2^a
Time constant (ms)	400.6 ± 23.6	281.1 ± 16.8^a
Time to peak (ms)	103.8 ± 6.8	86.4 ± 5.0^a
Duration at half-peak amplitude (ms)	386.2 ± 20.2	228.4 ± 14.4^a
Slow depolarization		
Amplitude[c] (MV)	6.0 ± 0.8	4.6 ± 1.3^a
Duration at half-peak amplitude(s)	22.6 ± 4.8	16.8 ± 2.2^a

Note: Each value is expressed as mean ± s.e. of at least five experiments.

[a]   Denotes statistical significance with $p < 0.05$.
[b]   Single stimulus of 60V and 0.1 ms duration.
[c]   Single stimulus of 80V and 0.1 ms duration.

leaky to ions. A decreased membrane resistance in SHR would account for the depolarization and altered electrical responses observed. It would also account for the the smaller ouabain-sensitive electrogenic component of the membrane potential in the SHR.[96] Interestingly, long-term treatment with captopril, which prevents the development of hypertension and decreases the enhanced membrane permeability to ions in the SHR,[100] also prevents membrane depolarization in SHR tail arteries.[96] That membrane depolarization in SHR is indeed related to a decreased membrane resistance was evidenced by the good correlation found between the resting membrane potential and the e.j.p. time constant ($r = 0.80$, $p < 0.01$) (Figure 1).

Another determinant in the postsynaptic response is the type and density of the receptors activated by the neurotransmitters. It is now well established that noradrenaline released from nerve endings activates two subtypes of α-adrenoceptors on the vascular smooth muscle membrane to elicit vasoconstriction. There appears to be no change in the density or sensitivity of the α_1 receptors in the tail artery[101] and the mesenteric artery[102] of the SHR. However, an increase in density of α_2 receptors was observed in these arteries in the SHR.[102,103] In the tail artery of the SHR, there was also an increase in the vasoconstrictor responses to α_2 receptor activation.[103,104]

In addition to the α-adrenoceptors, other receptors and transmitters may participate in the neuroeffector interaction. There is good evidence to suggest that both vasoactive intestinal peptide and neuropeptide Y are neurotransmitters in certain vessels, although their role in the hypertension process has yet to be determined. The type of receptor receiving most attention recently is the "γ receptor".[105,106] Electrophysiological recordings show that a synaptic potential, the e.j.p., that is resistant to blockade by α-adrenoceptor antagonists, is elicited in the vascular smooth muscle cell with stimulation of the perivascular nerves. Studies by Hirst and Neild[107,108] suggest that the e.j.p. is mediated by a new type of adrenoceptor — the γ-receptor. However, Sneddon and Burnstock[109] suggest that the e.j.p. is mediated by a purinoceptor with ATP as the transmitter. Their evidence was based on desensitization studies with an ATP analogue α,β-

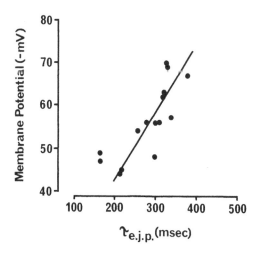

FIGURE 1.   Relationship between resting membrane potential and e.j.p. time constant in the SHR. There was a positive correlation (r = 0.80, *p* <0.01) between the resting membrane potential and the time constant of decay of the e.j.p. in the SHR.

methylene-ATP.[110,111] The α,β-methylene-ATP sensitive response seems to have a greater role in the tail artery of the SHR.[112] It will be interesting to know whether the density and the affinity of the receptor responsible for the e.j.p. is altered in the SHR.

III. NEUROMUSCULAR TRANSMISSION

The synaptic responses involved in the neuroeffector interaction in blood vessels are now being studied by electrophysiological techniques. Nerve stimulation elicits a fast, transient depolarization of the vascular smooth muscle membrane, the e.j.p. E.j.p.s have been recorded in response to nerve stimulation *in vivo* and/or *in vitro* in a number of vascular preparations including the guinea pig mesenteric artery,[113-115] guinea pig ear artery,[116] guinea pig main pulmonary artery,[117] rabbit ear artery,[118-120] rabbit saphenous artery,[99] rat tail artery,[97] dog middle cerebral artery,[121] dog mesenteric artery,[122] rat saphenous vein,[123] dog mesenteric vein,[124] and guinea pig mesenteric vein.[125] Although the e.j.p. itself (when subthreshold) is not associated with contraction, in some vessels an action potential can be elicited from the e.j.p. when a threshold level of depolarization is reached. A fast, phasic contraction is associated with the action potential.[120,126] Contractions triggered by e.j.p.s are mediated by electro-mechanical coupling since (1) a threshold level of depolarization is required to produce contraction, and (2) the depolarization preceeds contraction, reflecting a causal relationship.[120,126] In support of this, it has been found that agents affecting voltage-regulated Ca^{2+} channels such as Bay K 8644 (a Ca^{2+} channel agonist) and nifedipine (a Ca^{2+} channel antagonist) potentiate and inhibit e.j.p.-mediated responses, respectively.[120]

Although e.j.p.-mediated contractions have been observed to predominate in some vascular preparations, (e.g., rabbit ear artery[120]), it has become evident that in others the e.j.p.s are so small that they contribute little to contractions evoked by nerve stimulation (e.g., rat saphenous vein[123]). Recently, a second component of the cellular electrical response to nerve stimulation — a slow depolarization — has been identified.[97] In contrast to the fast, phasic contraction mediated by the e.j.p. and action potential, the contraction associated with the slow depolarization is slow and sustained.[123,126] Contractions predominantly mediated by slow depolarization have been reported in a number of veins.[123-125] In the rat tail artery[97] and rabbit ear artery,[119] slow depolarization is mediated by α_1-adrenoceptors and is selectively blocked by prazosin. In the rabbit saphenous vein,[143] rat saphenous vein,[123] and dog mesenteric vein,[125] the slow depolarization and contraction are mediated by α_2-adrenoceptors. It has been suggested that while α_2-mediated responses proceed by electro-mechanical coupling mechanisms only,[123] α_1-mediated responses may be mediated by both pharmaco- and electro-mechanical coupling.[126]

Unlike the slow depolarization and its associated contraction, which is mediated by α-adrenoceptors, the nature of the e.j.p. and fast phasic contraction is of great controversy since they are not sensitive to α-blockade. Phentolamine-resistant e.j.p.s have been observed in a number of preparations[97,118,119] and could account for neurally mediated contractile components remaining after α-adrenoceptor blockade.[119,126]

Although insensitive to α-blockade, e.j.p.s have been shown to be of neural origin since they are effectively blocked by agents such as TTX and guanethidine[97,118] and surgical denervation.[127] Similarly, chemical denervation with reserpine, 6-OHDA, and a combination treatment of guanethidine and nerve growth factor antiserum effectively blocks the e.j.p. response.[97]

Three main hypotheses regarding the phentolamine-resistant component of the vascular neural response have been proposed: (1) intrasynaptic noradrenaline concentrations are so high that exogenously applied α-blockers are ineffective;[128] (2) adrenoceptors other than α_1 or α_2 mediate the response;[106-108,129] or (3) the neurotransmitter is one other than NE.[109-111]

The first hypothesis was based on the premise that NE concentrations were lower outside the synapse in the plexus region (perisynaptic) than immediately within the synapse (intrasynaptic). This was especially true for vessels such as the rat portal vein with a narrow junctional cleft width. Presumably, the narrow cleft prevents the diffusion of NE from the junction, thus enabling it to reach the postsynaptic membrane in high concentrations. Furthermore, the narrow cleft hinders the accessability of blocking agents to the postsynaptic receptors acted upon by the released transmitter. These mechanisms, taken together, were thought to be responsible for the phentolamine-resistant component of the neural response.[128,130]

That adrenoceptors other than α_1 or α_2 subtypes mediate the phentolamine-resistant response led to the γ-adrenoceptor hypothesis. According to this hypothesis, α_1- and α_2-adrenoceptors are both located extra-junctionally, while γ-adrenoceptors are located at the neuromuscular junction close to the sites of noradrenaline release. The γ-adrenoceptors, unlike the α_1- and α_2-adrenoceptors, are not blocked by α-adrenergic antagonists.[106,107] Evidence leading to this proposal came mainly from studies involving the ionophoretic application of NE in guinea pig arterioles. When NE was applied to some regions of the arteriole, a phentolamine-sensitive localized contraction was produced which was not associated with membrane potential change. In other regions, NE caused a depolarization similar to the e.j.p. produced by nerve stimulation. The depolarizations persisted in the presence of phentolamine, and if large enough, they could elicit an action potential and contraction of the entire arteriole. By matching the location of the nerves with the responses from the ionophoretic pipette at different locations on the arteriole, it was found that the e.j.p.-like depolarizing responses could only be evoked in regions close to sympathetic nerve terminals.[108] Because pharmacological evidence for the existance of γ-adrenoceptors is lacking (i.e., specific γ-adrenoceptor agonists and/or antagonists have not been found), the validity of the γ-adrenoceptor hypothesis remains to be proven.

The possibility that the phentolamine-resistant vascular response to nerve stimulation may be mediated by a transmitter other than noradrenaline was prompted by initial studies in the guinea pig vas deferens. In this tissue, nerve stimulation produces a biphasic contraction, a fast twitch associated with e.j.p.s that sum and facilitate to elicit action potentials, and a slow contraction not associated with the e.j.p. Both the e.j.p. and fast twitch could be mimicked by local application of ATP and were unaffected by α-blockers. The slow contraction was mimicked by NE and was sensitive to α-blockade.[131,132] Selective blockade of the first component (e.j.p. and associated twitch) could be accomplished by the P_2-purinoceptor photoaffinity antagonist ANAPP$_3$[132] or by desensitization with the P_2-purinoceptor agonist α,β-

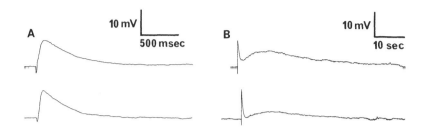

FIGURE 2. (A) Time course of e.j.p. in WKY (top) and SHR (bottom). In comparing e.j.p.s of similar size, the time course (i.e., the time to peak and the rate of decay) was faster in the SHR. (B) Time course and amplitude of slow depolarization in WKY (top) and SHR (bottom). A single stimulus of 80 V and 0.1 ms elicited an e.j.p. and slow depolarization in both WKY and SHR. However, the slow depolarization was smaller in amplitude and faster in time course in the SHR.

methylene ATP.[131] Thus, in the guinea pig vas deferens, it appears likely that ATP mediates the first component of the neural response, while NE mediates the second component.

In vascular smooth muscle, experiments with NE and ATP agonists and antagonists have yielded results similar to those found in the guinea pig vas deferens. In the rabbit ear artery, e.j.p.-like responses were elicited by local application of ATP.[133,134] In the rat tail artery,[109] guinea pig mesenteric artery, and rabbit mesenteric artery,[135] α,β-methylene ATP inhibited e.j.p.s evoked by nerve stimulation. Thus, in vascular smooth muscle, both NE and ATP may be involved in the neuromuscular transmission process.

A. Neuromuscular Transmission in SHR

We have recently compared the synaptic events underlying neuromuscular transmission in the tail artery of the WKY and SHR (10 to 12 weeks old). The resting membrane potential of cells from WKY tail arteries averaged –65.9 ± 1.3 mV (n = 11 animals, 4 to 5 cells each), while in the SHR the resting membrane potential was significantly depolarized to –56.2 ± 2.2 mV (n = 15 animals, 4 to 5 cells each). In the absence of stimulation, small spontaneous depolarizations-spontaneous excitatory junction potentials (s.e.j.p.s) were observed in 41% of the cells sampled in the WKY (n = 6 animals, 5 to 7 cells each) and 66% of the cells sampled in the SHR (n = 6 animals, 5 to 7 cells each). The mean s.e.j.p. frequencies in unstimulated cells for a recording period of 2 min/cell was 0.45 s.e.j.p.s/min/cell for WKY, and 1.62 s.e.j.p.s/min/cell for SHR (Table 1). In a previous study on the tail artery of normotensive Wistar rats, we concluded that cells with high s.e.j.p. frequencies are very close to narrow neuromuscular junctions.[136] Thus, the higher number of cells showing s.e.j.p.s in the SHR indicates that there are a greater number of close neuromuscular contacts, which is in agreement with morphological studies showing denser innervation in the vasculature of the SHR.[34]

In the Wistar rat tail artery, stimulation of perivascular nerves elicits two types of electrical responses, a fast depolarization — the e.j.p. and a second slow depolarization.[97,126] These two electrical components were also found in the SHR and WKY (Figure 2). However, given similar stimulation parameters, the electrical responses, viz., the e.j.p. and the slow depolarization of the SHR were smaller in amplitude and faster in time course as compared to WKY. At a single stimulating pulse of 60 V, the average e.j.p. amplitude was 9.28 ± 0.41 mV for WKY (n = 6 animals, 2 to 3 cells each) and 6.64 ± 1.22 mV for SHR (n = 9 animals, 2 to 3 cells each). Similarly, a single pulse of 80 V produced an average slow depolarization amplitude of 5.98 ± 0.78 mV for WKY (n = 5 animals, 2 cells each) and 4.65 ± 1.35 mV for SHR (n = 9 animals, 2 cells each) (Table 1).

Within a preparation, e.j.p. amplitudes were more variable between cells given similar stimulation parameters in the SHR (Figure 3). Larger amplitudes were observed in cells with

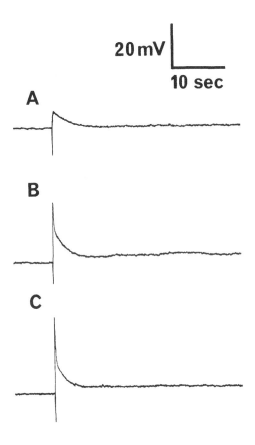

20 mV

10 sec

A

B

C

FIGURE 3. Variation in amplitude of e.j.p.s in the SHR. Within the same preparation, single stimulus pulses of 60 V and 0.1 ms duration elicited e.j.p.s of variable amplitude. A, B, and C show three cells in close proximity to each other.

greater s.e.j.p. frequencies, as previously reported.[136] When comparing e.j.p.s of similar amplitudes (5 to 10 mV), the time course was significantly faster in the SHR (Figure 2, Table 1), with the time to peak averaging 103.8 ± 6.8 ms for WKY (n = 10 animals, 3 to 5 cells each) and 86.4 ± 5.0 ms for the SHR (n = 11 animals, 3 to 5 cells each). Similarly, the average duration at half peak amplitude was 386.2 ± 20.2 ms for WKY, and only 228.4 ± 14.4 ms for SHR. As seen in other arteries,[98,99] the decay of the e.j.p. in both WKY and SHR was exponential, with a time constant (τ) of 400.6 ± 23.6 ms for WKY (n = 11 animals, 2 to 3 cells each) and 281.1 ± 16.8 ms for SHR (n = 15 animals, 2 to 3 cells each) (Table 1). In the SHR, a significant correlation (r = 0.80; $p < 0.01$) was found between the e.j.p. time constant and the membrane potential, this being that the more depolarized the membrane, the faster the time constant (Figure 1).

With increasing stimulation intensity, action potentials can be elicited from e.j.p.s in the Wistar tail artery.[97,126] In the WKY, there was a distinct transition from an e.j.p. to an action potential at a threshold potential of about –47 mV. However, in the SHR no such obvious transition from e.j.p. to action potential could be observed (Figure 4).

As with the e.j.p., the time course of the slow depolarization was faster in the SHR than in the WKY (Figure 2; Table 1). The duration at half amplitude averaged 22.6 ± 4.82 s in the WKY (n = 4 animals, 1 to 2 cells each) and only 16.83 ± 2.23 s in the SHR (n = 9 animals, 1 to 2 cells each).

One possible explanation for the smaller and faster responses in the SHR is that less

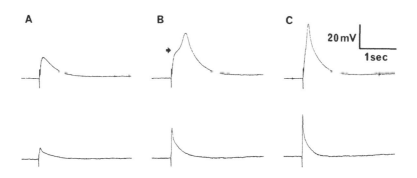

FIGURE 4.   Transition of e.j.p. to action potential in WKY (top) and SHR (bottom). (A) Electrical stimulation elicited by an e.j.p. (B) Increasing stimulus intensity elicited an action potential when the e.j.p. reached a threshold potential of about –47 mV (arrow) in the WKY. However, no obvious transition from e.j.p. to action potential could be distinguished in the SHR. (C) With higher stimulus strength, the amplitude of the action potential is increased.

transmitter was released from the nerve terminals per stimulus. Conversely, increased neuronal reuptake of noradrenaline has been demonstrated in many vasculatures of the SHR,[74-77] and it may also account for the diminished response.

Another factor in determining the amplitude and time course of the electrical responses is the membrane properties of the smooth muscle cells. In a previous study, we reported a depolarization of the resting membrane potential in the tail artery with the development of hypertension in the SHR.[96] In the present study, we found that the time course for the e.j.p. and the time constant for the decay of the e.j.p. was much faster in the SHR than WKY. Since the time constant of the e.j.p. is related to the time constant of the membrane,[98,99] this finding implicates that the membrane resistance itself was lowered in the SHR. A lower membrane resistance in the muscle cells of the SHR is in good agreement with the conclusion that the membrane is more leaky to ions[92,93] and it can account for the observed changes in electrical responses. A cell with low membrane resistance would have a faster time course and smaller amplitude for the e.j.p. and slow depolarization.

A decrease in membrane resistance, together with more close neuromuscular contacts, would also explain the variability in the e.j.p. amplitude in the SHR. Since e.j.p. originates from cells at close neuromuscular contacts, these cells would show large amplitude e.j.p.s.[136] However, electrotonic spread of the potential to neighboring cells in the SHR would be greatly attenuated because of the low membrane resistance, i.e., a smaller space constant. Therefore, there is a rapid decrement of the e.j.p. away from the neuromuscular junctions, giving rise to the great variability in amplitude of the e.j.p. in the SHR.

IV. VASCULAR RESPONSES TO NERVE STIMULATION

It is obvious from the above discussions that the final effector response to nerve stimulation is the result of interaction between many different factors. These factors must be taken into consideration in studying neuroeffector interaction, especially when comparing SHR and WKY. For example, the increase in perfusion pressure of isolated kidneys to nerve stimulation was significantly larger in 6-week-old SHR than WKY.[13] This difference was due to a greater release of endogenous NE from the SHR, since the reactivity of the postsynaptic membrane to exogenous NE, angiotensin II, and barium was not altered. However, similar studies with adult animals (4 to 6 months old) showed that the perfusion pressure increase with nerve stimulation in the SHR was not different from the WKY.[60] This is surprising in view of the fact that the postsynaptic reactivity to vasoactive agents was significantly increased in the adult SHR.

Similar results were obtained with the tail artery of adult rats.[75,89,90] These observations have led to the suggestion that the sympathetic nerve terminals of SHR can modulate the junctional concentration of neurotransmitters so that the final response, even with the changes in hypertension, approximates that of normotensive rats.[60,89] Thus, the apparently normal response to nerve stimulation in the tail artery of the SHR is due to an enhanced uptake of NE by the nerve terminals.[89,90] An enhanced response to nerve stimulation and exogenous NE in the SHR could be unmasked upon blockade of neuronal uptake with cocaine.[90] In the isolated perfused kidney of the SHR, the normal response to nerve stimulation was probably due to a reduced exocytotic release of noradrenaline.[60]

Another important change in the neural responses of the SHR is the greater role of the α_2 receptors. In the tail artery, idazoxan at low concentrations antagonized the responses to perivascular nerve stimulation in the SHR only.[104] Since contraction mediated by α_2 receptors is due to influx of extracellular calcium through voltage-dependent channels,[123,137,138] the neural responses in the tail artery of the SHR, but not those of the WKY, were also very sensitive to blockade by calcium antagonists.[139]

A recent study showed that the purinoceptors also play a more significant role in the neural responses in the tail artery of the SHR. Using α,β-methylene ATP to desensitize the ATP or e.j.p. component of the response, Vidal et al.[112] showed that vasoconstrictor response to nerve stimulation was inhibited in the SHR but not in the WKY. A greater role of the e.j.p. component and the α_2 receptors in the tail artery of the SHR may be related to its lower membrane potential.[96] Since contraction mediated by both the e.j.p. and the α_2 adrenoceptors is dependent on membrane depolarization,[120,123,126] vasoconstriction could be more readily initiated in the SHR, where the resting membrane potential is already depolarized to a level very close to the threshold for contraction.

V. FUTURE TRENDS

There has been tremendous progress in recent years in the understanding of the neuroeffector interaction in blood vessels. Two findings are of particular importance to future research. First, there are at least two excitatory components in the neural response, an α-adrenoceptor component and an e.j.p. component. (The neurotransmitter and receptor type responsible for the e.j.p. have yet to be firmly established.) Second, both the α_1 and α_2 receptors participate in the neural regulation process. In the SHR, a more important role for both the e.j.p. and the α_2 receptors have been implicated, but only in the tail artery. It is therefore important to test how common these findings are in other vessels and whether similar changes apply to human essential hypertension. Since vasoconstriction induced by both the e.j.p. and α_2 receptors are mediated by voltage operated calcium channels, it will also be important to study the role of calcium antagonists in neural regulation in hypertension. Another area of importance to future research is the effect of low sodium diets. Reduced sodium intake results in an attenuation of transmitter release from sympathetic nerve terminals.[140-142] There is evidence that the SHR is more sensitive to dietary sodium than the age-matched WKY.[140]

REFERENCES

1. **Abboud, F. M.,** The sympathetic nervous system in hypertension, *Clin. Exp. Hypertension, Theory Practice,* A6, 43, 1984.
2. **Abboud, F. M.,** The sympathetic nervous system in hypertension — state-of-the-art review, *Hypertension,* 4 (Suppl. II), 208, 1982.
3. **Brody, M. J., O'Neill, T. P., and Porter, J. P.,** Role of central catecholaminergic systems in pathogenesis and treatment of hypertension, *J. Cariovasc. Pharmacol.,* 6, S727, 1984.
4. **Brody, M. J., Barron, K. W., Berecek, K. H., Faber, J. E., and Lappe, R. W.,** Neurogenic mechanisms of experimental hypertension, in *Hypertension,* Genest, J., Kuchel, O., Hamet, P., and Cantin, M., Eds., McGraw-Hill, New York, 1983, chap. 9.

5. **Kuchel, O.,** The autonomic nervous system and blood pressure regulation in human hypertension, in *Hypertension,* Genest, J., Kuchel, O., Hamet, P., and Cantin, M., Eds., McGraw-Hill, New York, 1983, chap. 10.

6. **Goldstein, D. S.,** Plasma norepinephrine in essential hypertension, *Hypertension,* 3, 48, 1981.

7. **Okamoto, K., Nosaka, S., and Yamori, Y.,** Participation of neural factor in the pathogenesis of hypertension in the spontaneously hypertensive rat, *Jpn. Heart J.,* 8, 168, 1967.

8. **Iriuchijima, J.,** Sympathetic discharge rate in SHR, in *The Nervous System in Arterial Hypertension,* Julius, J. and Esler, M. D., Eds., Charles C Thomas, Springfield, IL, 1975, 51.

9. **Judy, W. V., Watanabe, A. M., Henry, D. P., Besch, H. R., Murphy, W. R., and Hockel, G. M.,** Sympathetic nerve activity, role in regulation of blood pressure in the spontaneously hypertensive rat, *Circ. Res.,* 38(6) (Suppl. II), 21, 1976.

10. **Lundin, S., Ricksten, S.-E., and Thoren, P.,** Renal sympathetic activity in spontaneously hypertensive rats and normotensive controls, as studied by three different methods, *Acta Physiol. Scand.,* 120, 265, 1984.

11. **DeChamplain, J., Krakoff, L. R., and Axelrod, J.,** Catecholamine metabolism in experimental hypertension in the rat, *Circ. Res.,* 20, 136, 1967.

12. **Yamori, Y.,** Interaction of neural and non-neuronal factors in the pathogenesis of spontaneous hypertension, in *The Nervous System in Arterial Hypertension,* Julius, J. and Esler, M. D., Eds., Charles C Thomas, Springfield, IL, 1975, 17.

13. **Collis, M. G., DeMey, C., and Vanhoutte, P. M.,** Renal vascular reactivity in the young spontaneously hypertensive rat, *Hypertension,* 2, 45, 1980.

14. **Zsoter, T. T., Wolchinsky, C., Lawrin, M., and Sirko, S.,** Norepinephrine release in arteries of spontaneously hypertensive rats, *Clin. Exp. Hypertension, Theory Practice,* A4(3), 431, 1982.

15. **Touw, K. B., Haywood, J. R., Shaffer, R. A., and Brody, M. J.,** Contribution of the sympathetic nervous system to vascular resistance in conscious young and adult spontaneously hypertensive rats, *Hypertension,* 2, 408, 1980.

16. **Smith, P. G., Poston, C. W., and Mills, E.,** Ontogeny of neural and non-neural contributions to arterial blood pressure in spontaneously hypertensive rats, *Hypertension,* 6, 54, 1984.

17. **Provoost, A. P.,** Sympathectomy and the development of hypertension in rats, in *Handbook of Hypertension,* Vol. 4, DeJong, W., Ed., Elsvier, Amsterdam, 1984, chap. 25.

18. **Finch, L., Cohen, M., and Horst, W. D.,** Effects of 6-hydroxydopamine at birth on the development of hypertension in the rat, *Life Sci.,* 13, 1403, 1973.

19. **Yamori, Y., Yamabe, H., DeJong, W., Lovenberg, W., and Sjoerdsma, A.,** Effect of tissue norepinephrine depletion by 6-hydroxydopamine on blood pressure in spontaneously hypertensive rats, *Eur. J. Pharmacol.,* 17, 135, 1972.

20. **Provoost, A. P., Bohus, B., and DeJong, W.,** Neonatal chemical sympathectomy: functional control of denervation of the vascular system and tissue noradrenaline level in the rat after 6-hydroxydopamine, *Naunyn Schmiedebergs Arch. Pharmacol.,* 284, 353, 1974.

21. **Mulvany, M. J., Korsgaard, N., Nyborg, N., and Nilsson, H.,** Chemical denervation does not effect the medial hypertrophy and increased calcium sensitivity of mesenteric resistance vessels from spontaneously hypertensive rats, *Clin. Sci.,* 61, 62S, 1981.

22. **Clark, D. W. J., Laverty, R., and Phelan, E. L.,** Long-lasting peripheral and central effects of 6-hydroxydopamine in rats, *Br. J. Pharmacol.,* 44, 233, 1972.

23. **Lew, G. M., and Quay, W. B.,** Noradrenaline contents of hypothalamus and adrenal gland increased by postnatal administration of 6-hydroxydopamine, *Res. Commun. Chem. Pathol. Pharmacol.,* 2, 807, 1971.

24. **Jacks, B. R., DeChamplain, J., and Corbeau, J. P.,** Effects of 6-hydroxydopamine on putative transmitter substances in the central nervous system, *Eur. J . Pharmacol.,* 18, 353, 1972.

25. **Folkow, B., Hallback, M., Lundgren, Y., and Weiss, L.,** The effects of immunosympathectomy on blood pressure and vascular reactivity in normal and spontaneously hypertensive rats, *Acta Physiol. Scand.,* 84, 512, 1972.

26. **Johnson, E. M. and Macia, R.,** Unique resistance to guanethidine-induced chemical sympathectomy of spontaneously hypertensive rats, *Circ. Res.,* 45, 243, 1979.

27. **Bevan, J. A., Bevan, R. D., and Duckles, S. P.,** Adrenergic regulation of vascular smooth muscle, in *Handbook of Physiology, Vascular Smooth Muscle,* Section 2, Vol. 2, Bohr, D. F., Somylo, A. P., and Sparks, H. V., Eds., American Physiological Society, Baltimore, MD, 1980, chap. 18.

28. **Vanhoutte, P. M., Verbeuren, T. J., and Webb, R. C.,** Local modulation of adrenergic neuroeffector interaction in the blood vessel wall, *Physiol. Rev.,* 61, 151, 1981.

29. **Osswald, W. and Guimaraes, S.,** Adrenergic mechanisms in blood vessels; morphological and pharmacological aspects, *Rev. Physiol. Biochem. Pharmacol.,* 96, 53, 1983.

30. **Shephard, J. T. and Vanhoutte, P. M.,** Local modulation of adrenergic neurotransmission in blood vessels, *J. Cardiovasc. Pharmacol.,* 7 (Suppl. 3), S167, 1985.

31. **Burnstock, G. and Costa, E.,** *Adrenergic Neurons,* John Wiley & Sons, New York, 1975, 255.

32. **Bevan, J. A.,** Some bases of differences in vascular response to sympathetic activity. Variations on a theme, *Circ. Res.,* 45, 161, 1979.

33. **Griffith, S. G., Crowe, R., Lincoln, J., Haven, A. J., and Burnstock, G.,** Regional differences in the density of perivascular nerves and varicosities, noradrenaline content and responses to nerve stimulation in the rabbit ear artery, *Blood Vessels,* 19, 41, 1982.

34. **Cassis, L. A., Stitzel, R. E., and Head, R. J.,** Hypernoradrenergic innervation of the caudal artery of the spontaneously hypertensive rat: an influence upon neuroeffector mechanisms, *J. Pharmacol. Exp. Ther.,* 234(3), 792, 1985.

35. **Rowan, R. A. and Bevan, J. A.,** Distribution of adrenergic synaptic cleft width in vascular and nonvascular smooth muscle, in *Vascular Neuroeffector Mechanisms,* Bevan, J. A., Fujiwara, M., Maxwell, R. A., Mohri, K., Shibata, S., and Toda, N., Eds., Raven Press, New York, 1983, 75.

36. **Moffatt, D. B.,** The fine structure of the blood vessels of the renal medulla with particular reference to the control of the medullary circulation, *J. Ultrastruct. Res.,* 19, 532, 1967.

37. **Lee, T. J. F., Chiueh, C. C., and Adams, M.,** Synaptic transmission of vasoconstrictor nerves in rabbit basilar artery, *Eur. J. Pharmacol.,* 61, 55, 1980.

38. **Govyrin, V. A.,** Mechanism of vascular tone regulation based on instability of neuromuscular cleft widths in blood vessels, *Proc. Int. Union Physiol. Science,* 16, 149, 1986.

39. **Bevan, J. A.,** Some functional consequences of variation in adrenergic synaptic cleft width and in nerve density and distribution, *Fed. Proc.,* 36, 2439, 1977.

40. **Gero, J. and Gerova, M.,** In vivo studies of sympathetic control of vessels of different function, in *Physiology and Pharmacology of Vascular Neuroeffector Systems,* Bevan, J. A., Furchgott, R. F., Maxwell, R. A., and Somylo, A. P., Eds., S. Karger, Basel, 1971, 86.

41. **Scott, T. M. and Pang, S. C.,** The correlation between the development of sympathetic innervation and the development of medial hypertrophy in jejunal arteries in normotensive and spontaneously hypertensive rats, *J. Autonom. Nerv. Syst.,* 8, 25, 1983.

42. **Lee, R. M. K., Coughlin, M. D., and Cheung, D. W.,** Relationship between sympathetic innervation, vascular changes and hypertension in the SHR, *J. Hypertension,* 1986, in press.

43. **Nagaoka, A. and Lovenberg, W.,** Plasma norepinephrine and dopamine-beta-hydroxylase in genetic hypertensive rats, *Life Sci.,* 19, 29, 1976.

44. **Nagatsu, T., Kato, T., Numata, Y., Ikuta, K., Umezawa, H. et al.,** Serum dopamine beta-hydroxylase activity in developing hypertensive rats, *Nature (London),* 251, 630, 1974.

45. **Pak, C. H.,** Plasma adrenaline and noradrenaline concentration of the spontaneously hypertensive rat, *Jpn. Heart J.,* 22, 987, 1981.

46. **Affara, S., Denoroy, L., Renaud, B., Vincent, M., and Sassard, J.,** Serum dopamine-beta-hydroxylase activity in a new strain of spontaneously hypertensive rat, *Experientia,* 36, 1207, 1980.

47. **Palermo, A., Constantini, C., Mara, G., and Libretti, A.,** Role of the sympathetic nervous system in spontaneous hypertension: changes in central adrenoceptors and plasma catecholamine levels, *Clin. Sci.,* 61(7), 195s, 1981.

48. **Picotti, G. B., Carruba, M. O., Ravazzani, G., Bondiolotti, G. P., and DaPrada, M.,** Plasma catecholamine concentrations in normotensive rats of different strains and in spontaneously hypertensive rats under basal conditions and during cold exposure, *Life Sci.,* 31, 2137, 1982.

49. **McCarty, R., Chiueh, C. C., and Kopin, I. J.,** Spontaneously hypertensive rats: adrenergic hyperresponsivity to anticipation of electric shock, *Behav. Biol.,* 22, 405, 1978.

50. **Collis, M. G. and Vanhoutte, P. M.,** Vascular reactivity of isolated perfused kidneys from male and female spontaneously hypertensive rats, *Circ. Res.,* 41(6), 759, 1977.

51. **Ekas, R. D., Steenberg, M. L., and Lokhandwala, M. F.,** Increased presynaptic alpha-adrenoceptor mediated regulation of noradrenaline release in the isolated perfused kidney of spontaneously hypertensive rats, *Clin. Sci.,* 63, 309S(8), 1982.

52. **Ekas, R. D., Steenberg, M. L., Woods, M. D., and Lokhandwala, M. F.,** Presynaptic alpha- and beta-adrenoceptor stimulation and norepinephrine release in the spontaneously hypertensive rat, *Hypertension,* 5, 198, 1983.

53. **Eikenberg, D. C., Ekas, R. D., and Lokhandwala, M. F.,** Presynaptic modulation of norepinephrine release by alpha-adrenoceptors and angiotensin II receptors in spontaneously hypertensive rats, in *Central Nervous System Mechanisms in Hypertension,* Buckley, P. and Ferraro, C. M., Eds., Raven Press, New York, 1981, 215.

54. **Ekas, R. D. and Lokhandwala, M. F.,** Sympathetic nerve function and vascular reactivity in spontaneously hypertensive rats, *Am. J. Phyiosl.,* 241, R379, 1981.

55. **Tsuda, K., Kuchii, M., Kusuyama, Y., Hano, T., Nishio, I., and Masuyama, Y.,** Neurotransmitter release and vascular reactivity in spontaneously hypertensive rats, *Jpn. Circ. J.,* 48, 1263, 1984.

56. **Masuyama, Y., Tsuda, K., Kusuyama, Y., Hano, T., Kuchii, M., and Nishio, I.,** Neurotransmitter release, vascular responsiveness and their calcium-mediated regulation in perfused mesenteric preparation of spontaneously hypertensive rats and DOCA-salt hypertension, *J. Hypertension,* 2 (Suppl. 3), 99, 1984.

57. **Westfall, T. C., Peach, M. J., and Tittermary, V.,** Enhancement of the electrically induced release of norepinephrine from the rat portal vein: mediation by beta-2-adrenoceptors, *Eur. J. Pharmacol.*, 58, 67, 1979.

58. **Westfall, T. C., Meldrum, M. J., Badino, L., and Earnhardt, J. T.,** Noradrenergic transmission in the isolated portal vein of the spontaneously hypertensive rat, *Hypertension*, 6, 267, 1984.

59. **Galloway, M. P. and Westfall, T. C.,** The release of endogenous norepinephrine from the coccygeal artery of spontaneously hypertensive and Wistar-Kyoto rats, *Circ. Res.*, 51, 225, 1982.

60. **Vanhoutte, P. M., Browning, D., Coen, E., Verbeuren, T. J., Zonnekeyn, L., and Collis, M. G.,** Decreased release of norepinephrine in the isolated kidney of the adult spontaneously hypertensive rat, *Hypertension*, 4, 251, 1982.

61. **Zimmerman, B. G. and Whitmore, L.,** Effect of angiotensin and phenoxybenzamine on the release of norepinephrine in vessels during sympathetic nerve stimulation, *Int. J. Neuropharmacol.*, 6, 27, 1967.

62. **Zimmerman, B. G.,** Actions of angiotensin in adrenergic nerve endings, *Fed. Proc.*, 37, 199, 1978.

63. **Adler-Grascinsky, E. and Langer, S. Z.,** Possible role of a beta-adrenoceptor in the regulation of noradrenaline release by nerve stimulation through a positive feed-back mechanism, *Br. J. Pharmacol.*, 53, 43, 1975.

64. **Dahlof, C.,** Studies on beta-adrenoceptor mediated facilitation of sympathetic neurotransmission, *Acta Physiol. Scand.*, 500, 1, 1981.

65. **Stjarne, L. and Brundin, J.,** Beta-2-adrenoceptors facilitating noradrenaline secretion from human vasoconstrictor nerves, *Acta Physiol. Scand.*, 97, 88, 1976.

66. **Starke, K.,** Regulation of noradrenaline release by presynaptic receptor systems, *Rev. Physiol. Biochem. Pharmacol.*, 77, 1, 1977.

67. **Westfall, T. C.,** Local regulation of adrenergic neurotransmission, *Physiol. Rev.*, 57, 659, 1977.

68. **Vizi, E. S.,** Presynaptic modulation of neurochemical transmission, *Prog. Neurobiol.*, 12, 181, 1979.

69. **Su, C., Bevan, J. A., and Burnstock, G.,** ³[H]-Adenosine triphosphate release during stimulation of enteric nerves, *Science*, 173, 337, 1971.

70. **Kawasaki, I., Clin, W. H., Jr., and Su, C.,** Enhanced presynaptic beta-adrenoceptor mediated modulation of vascular adrenergic neurotransmission in spontaneously hypertensive rats, *J. Pharmacol. Exp. Ther.*, 223, 721, 1982.

71. **Su, C., Kamikawa, Y., Kubo, T., and Cline, W. H., Jr.,** Inhibitory modulation of vascular adrenergic neurotransmission in the SHR, in *Proceedings of the Springfield Blood Vessel Symposium*, Su, C., Ed., Southern Illinois University Press, Springfield, IL, 1982, 33.

72. **Kamikawa, Y., Cline, W. H., Jr., and Su, C.,** Diminished purinergic modulating of the vascular adrenergic neurotransmission in the spontaneously hypertensive rat, *Eur. J. Pharmacol.*, 66, 347, 1980.

73. **Kubo, T. and Su, C.,** Effects of adenosine on ³H-norepinephrine release from perfused mesenteric arteries of SHR and renal hypertensive rats, *Eur. J. Pharmacol.*, 87, 349, 1983.

74. **Zsoter, T. T. and Wolchinsky, C.,** Norepinephrine uptake in arteries of spontaneously hypertensive rats, *Clin. Invest. Med.*, 6(3), 191, 1983.

75. **Webb, R. C., Vanhoutte, P. M., and Bohr, D. F.,** Inactivation of released norepinephrine in rat tail artery by neuronal uptake, *J. Cardiovasc. Pharmacol.*, 2, 121, 1980.

76. **Whall, C. W., Myers, M. M., Jr., and Halpern, W.,** Norepinephrine sensitivity, tension development and neuronal uptake in resistance arteries from spontaneously hypertensive and normotensive rats, *Blood Vessels*, 17, 1, 1980.

77. **Rho, J. H., Newman, B., and Alexander, N.,** Altered in vitro uptake of norepinephrine by cardiovascular tissues of spontaneously hypertensive rats. 1. Mesenteric artery, *Hypertension*, 3, 704, 1981.

78. **Westfall, T. C. and Meldrum, M. J.,** Alterations in the release of norepinephrine at the vascular neuroeffector junction in hypertension, *Annu. Rev. Pharmacol. Toxicol.*, 25, 621, 1985.

79. **Webb, R. C. and Bohr, D. F.,** Recent advances in the pathogenesis of hypertension: consideration of structural, functional, and metabolic vascular abnormalities resulting in elevated arterial resistance, *Am. Heart J.*, 102, 251, 1981.

80. **Mulvany, M. J.,** Do resistance vessel abnormalities contribute to the elevated blood pressure spontaneously hypertensive rats?, *Blood Vessels*, 20, 1, 1983.

81. **Mulvany, M. J.,** Pathophysiology of vascular smooth muscle in hypertension, *J. Hypertension*, 2 (Suppl. 3), 413, 1984.

82. **Haeusler, G. and Finch, L.,** Vascular reactivity to 5-hydroxytryptamine and hypertension in the rat, *Naunyn Schmiedebergs Arch. Pharmacol.*, 272, 101, 1972.

83. **Bohr, D. F.,** The role of altered vascular reactivity in hypertension, *Hosp. Pract.*, 9, 107, 1974.

84. **Lais, L. and Brody, M.,** Mechanisms of vascular hyperresponsiveness in the spontaneously hypertensive rat, *Circ. Res.*, 36/37(1), 216, 1975.

85. **Mulvany, M. J., Hansen, P. K., and Aalkjaer, C.,** Direct evidence that the greater contractility of resistance vessels in spontaneously hypertensive rats is associated with a narrower lumen, a thicker media and a greater number of smooth muscle cell layers, *Circ. Res.*, 43, 854, 1978.

86. **Bohlen, H. G.,** Arteriolar closure mediated by hyperresponsiveness to norepinephrine in hypertensive rats, *Am. J. Physiol.,* 236, H157, 1979.

87. **Kubo, T.,** Increased pressor responses to pressor agents in spontaneously hypertensive rats, *Can. J. Physiol. Pharmacol.,* 57, 59, 1979.

88. **Whall, C. W., Havlik, R. J., Halpern, W., and Bohr, D. F.,** Potassium depolarization of adrenergic varicosities in resistance arteries from SHR and WKY rats, *Blood Vessels,* 20, 23, 1983.

89. **Webb, R. C., Vanhoutte, P. M., and Bohr, D. F.,** Adrenergic neurotransmission in vascular smooth muscle from spontaneously hypertensive rats, *Hypertension,* 3, 93, 1981.

90. **Webb, R. C. and Vanhoutte, P. M.,** Cocaine and contractile responses of vascular smooth muscle from spontaneously hypertensive rats, *Arch. Int. Pharmacodyn.,* 253, 241, 1981.

91. **Friedman, S. M.,** An ion-exchange approach to the problem of intracellular sodium in the hypertensive process, *Circ. Res.,* 34 (Suppl. 1), 123, 1974.

92. **Noon, J. P., Rice, P. J., and Baldessarini, R. J.,** Calcium leakage as a cause of the high resting tension in vascular smooth muscle from the spontaneously hypertensive rat, *Proc. Natl. Acad. Sci.,* 75, 1605, 1978.

93. **Jones, A. W.,** Reactivity of ion fluxes in rat aorta during hypertension and circulatory control, *Fed. Proc.,* 33, 133, 1974.

94. **Kwan, C. Y., Belbeck, L., and Daniel, E. E.,** Abnormal biochemistry of vascular smooth muscle plasma membrane as an important factor in the initiation and maintenance of hypertension in rats, *Blood Vessels,* 16, 259, 1979.

95. **Casteels, R., Kitamura, L., Kuriyama, H., and Suzuki, H.,** Excitation-contraction coupling in the smooth cells in the rabbit main pulmonary artery, *J. Physiol.,* 271, 63, 1977.

96. **Cheung, D. W.,** Membrane potential of vascular smooth muscle and hypertension in spontaneously hypertensive rats, *Can. J. Physiol. Pharmacol.,* 62, 957, 1984.

97. **Cheung, D. W.,** Two components in the cellular response of rat tail arteries to nerve stimulation, *J. Physiol.,* 328, 461, 1982.

98. **Hirst, G. D. S. and Neild, T. O.,** Some properties of spontaneous excitatory junction potentials recorded from arterioles of guinea pigs, *J. Physiol.,* 303, 43, 1980.

99. **Holman, M. E. and Surprenant, A. M.,** Some properties of the excitatory junction potentials recorded from saphenous arteries of rabbits, *J. Physiol.,* 287, 237, 1979.

100. **Ito, K., Koike, H., Miyamoto, M., and Urakawa, N.,** Long-term blockade of angiotensin converting enzyme alters passive ion transport of vascular smooth muscle, *Life Sci.,* 26, 1023, 1980.

101. **Aqel, M. B., Sharma, R. V., and Bhalla, R. C.,** Increased Ca sensitivity of alpha-1-adrenoceptor-stimulated contraction in SHR caudal artery, *J. Physiol.,* 250, C275, 1986.

102. **Agarwal, D. K. and Daniel, E. E.,** Increased density of ^{3}H-yohimbine binding sites in spontaneously hypertensive rat mesentery artery, *J. Hypertension,* 2 (Suppl. 3), 107, 1984.

103. **Weiss, R. J., Webb, R. C., and Smith, C. B.,** Comparison of alpha-2 adrenoceptors on arterial smooth muscle and brain homogenates from spontaneously hypertensive and Wistar-Kyoto normotensive rats, *J. Hypertension,* 2, 249, 1984.

104. **Medgett, I. C., Hicks, P. E., and Langer, S. Z.,** Smooth muscle alpha-2 adrenoceptors mediate vasoconstrictor responses to exogenous norepinephrine and to sympathetic stimulation to a greater extent in spontaneously hypertensive than in Wistar Kyoto rat tail arteries, *J. Pharmacol. Exp. Ther.,* 231, 159, 1984.

105. **Neild, T. O. and Zelcer, E.,** Noradrenergic neuromuscular transmission with special reference to arterial smooth muscle, *Prog. Neurobiol.,* 19, 141, 1982.

106. **Hirst, G. D. S., De Gleria, S., and van Helden, D. F.,** Neuromuscular transmission in arterioles, *Experientia,* 41, 874, 1985.

107. **Hirst, G. D. S. and Neild, T. O.,** Evidence for two populations of exictatory receptors for noradrenaline on arteriolar smooth muscle, *Nature (London),* 283, 767, 1980.

108. **Hirst, G. D. S. and Neild, T. O.,** Localization of specialized noradrenaline receptors at neuromuscular junctions on arterioles of the guinea-pig, *J. Physiol.,* 313, 343, 1981.

109. **Sneddon, P. and Burnstock, G.,** ATP as a co-transmitter in rat tail artery, *Eur. J. Pharmacol.,* 106, 149, 1985.

110. **Burnstock, G.,** The changing face of autonomic neurotransmission, *Acta Physiol. Scand.,* 126, 67, 1986.

111. **Burnstock, G. and Kennedy, C.,** A dual function of adenosine 5'-triphosphate in the regulation of vascular tone, *Circ. Res.,* 58, 319, 1986.

112. **Vidal, M., Hicks, P. E., and Langer, S. Z.,** Differential effects of alpha-beta-methylene ATP on responses to nerve stimulation in SHR and WKY tail arteries, *Naunyn Schmiedebergs Arch. Pharmacol.,* 332, 384, 1986.

113. **Speden, R. N.,** Electrical activity of single smooth muscle cells of the mesenteric artery produced by splanchnic nerve stimulation in the guinea-pig, *Nature (London),* 202, 193, 1964.

114. **Kuriyama, H. and Suzuki, H.,** Adrenergic transmission in the guinea-pig mesenteric artery and their cholinergic modulations, *J. Physiol.,* 317, 383, 1981.

115. **Kuriyama, H. and Makita, Y.,** Modulation of noradrenaline transmission in the guinea-pig mesenteric artery: an electrophysiological study, *J. Physiol.,* 335, 609, 1983.

116. **Kajiwara, M., Kitamura, K., and Kuriyama, H.,** Neuromuscular transmission and smooth muscle membrane properties in the guinea-pig ear artery, *J. Physiol.,* 315, 283, 1981.
117. **Suzuki, H.,** An electrophysiological study of excitatory neuromuscular transmission in the guinea-pig main pulmonary artery, *J. Physiol.,* 336, 47, 1983
118. **Holman, M. E. and Surprenant, A. M.,** An electrophyiological analysis of the effects of noradrenaline and alpha-receptor antagonists on neuromuscular transmission in mammalian muscular arteries, *Br. J. Pharmacol.,* 71, 651, 1980.
119. **Suzuki, H. and Kou, K.,** Electrical components contributing to the nerve-mediated contractions in the smooth muscles of the rabbit ear artery, *Jpn. J. Physiol.,* 33, 743, 1983.
120. **Cheung, D. W. and Mackay, M. J.,** The effects of BAY K 8644 and nifedipine on the neural responses of the rabbit ear artery, *Br. J. Pharmacol.,* 88, 363, 1986.
121. **Suzuki, H. and Fujiwara, S.,** Neurogenic electrical responses of single smooth muscle cells of the dog middle cerebral artery, *Circ. Res.,* 51, 751, 1982.
122. **Kou, K., Kuriyama, H., and Suzuki, H.,** Effects of 3,4-dihydro-8-(2-hydroxy-3-isopropylaminopropoxy)-3-nitroxy-2H-1-benzopyran (K-351) on smooth muscle cells and neuromuscular transmission in the canine mesenteric artery, *Br. J. Pharmacol.,* 77, 679, 1982.
123. **Cheung, D. W.,** An electrophysiological study of alpha-adrenoceptor mediated excitation — contraction coupling in the smooth muscle cells of the rat saphenous vein, *Br. J. Pharmacol.,* 84, 265, 1985.
124. **Suzuki, H.,** Adrenergic transmission in the dog mesenteric vein and its modulation by alpha-adrenoceptor antagonists, *Br. J. Pharmacol.,* 81, 479, 1984.
125. **Suzuki, H.,** Effects of endogenous and exogenous noradrenaline on the smooth muscle of guinea-pig mesenteric vein, *J. Physiol.,* 321, 495, 1981.
126. **Cheung, D. W.,** Neural regulation of electrical and mechanical activities in the rat tail artery, *Pfluegers Arch.,* 400, 335, 1984.
127. **Hirst, G. D. S.,** Neuromuscular transmission in arterioles of guinea-pig submucosa, *J. Physiol.,* 273, 263, 1977.
128. **Bevan, J. A. and Su, C.,** Distribution theory of resistance of neurogenic vasoconstriction to alpha receptor blockade in the rabbit, *Circ. Res.,* 28, 179, 1971.
129. **Hirst, G. D. S., Neild, T. O., and Silverberg, G. D.,** Noradrenaline receptors on the rat basilar artery, *J. Physiol.,* 328, 351, 1982.
130. **Bevan, J. A. and Su, C.,** Variation of intra- and perisynaptic adrenergic transmitter concentrations with width of synaptic cleft in vascular tissue, *J. Pharmacol. Exp. Ther.,* 190, 30, 1974.
131. **Meldrum, L. A. and Burnstock, G.,** Evidence that ATP acts as a co-transmitter with noradrenaline in sympathetic nerves supplying the guinea-pig vas deferens, *Eur. J. Pharmacol.,* 92, 161, 1983.
132. **Sneddon, P. and Westfall, D. P.,** Pharmcological evidence that adenosine triphosphate and noradrenaline are co-transmitters in the guinea-pig vas deferens, *J. Physiol.,* 347, 561, 1984.
133. **Suzuki, H.,** Electrical responses of smooth muscle cells of the rabbit ear artery to adenosine triphosphate, *J. Physiol.,* 359, 401, 1985.
134. **Suzuki, H., Mishima, S., and Miyahara, H.,** Effects of reserpine on electrical responses evoked by perivascular nerve stimulation in the rabbit ear artery, *Biomed. Res.,* 5(3), 259, 1984.
135. **Ishakawa, S.,** Actions of ATP and alpha-beta-methylene ATP on neuromuscular transmission and smooth muscle membrane of the rabbit and guinea-pig mesenteric arteries, *Br. J. Pharmacol.,* 86, 777, 1985.
136. **Cheung, D. W.,** Spontaneous and evoked excitatory junction potentials in rat tail arteries, *J. Physiol.,* 328, 449, 1982.
137. **Cheung, D. W.,** The effect of BAY K 8644 on contraction mediated by alpha-adrenoceptors in the rat saphenous vein, *Br. J. Pharmacol.,* 85, 317, 1985.
138. **Godfraind, T., Miller, R. C., and Lima, J. S.,** Selective alpha-1- and alpha-2-adrenoceptor agonist-induced contractions and 45Ca fluxes in the rat isolated aorta, *Br. J. Pharmacol.,* 77, 597, 1982.
139. **Hicks, P. E., Tiernery, C., and Langer, S. Z.,** Preferential antagonism by diltiazem of alpha-2-adrenoceptor mediated vasoconstrictor responses in perfused tail arteries of spontaneously hypertensive rats, *Naunyn Schmiedebergs Arch. Pharmacol.,* 328, 388, 1985.
140. **Meldrum, M. J., Xue, C., Badino, L., and Westfall, T. C.,** Effect of sodium depletion on the release of 3H-norepinephrine from central and peripheral tissue of Wistar-Kyoto and spontaneously hypertensive rats, *J. Cardiovasc. Pharmacol.,* 7, 59, 1985.
141. **Nilsson, H., Ely, D., Friberg, P., and Folkow, B.,** Effects of low and high Na diets on cardiovascular dynamics in normotensive and hypertensive rats: neuroeffector characteristics of the resistance vessels, *J. Hypertension,* 2 (Suppl. 3), 433, 1984.
142. **Gradin, K., Dahlof, C., and Persson, B.,** A low dietary sodium intake reduces neuronal noradrenaline release and the blood pressure in spontaneously hypertensive rats, *Naunyn Schmiedebergs Arch. Pharmacol.,* 332, 364, 1986.
143. **Cheung, D. W.,** unpublished observations.

Chapter 7

ELECTROPHYSIOLOGICAL MECHANISMS OF FORCE DEVELOPMENT BY VASCULAR SMOOTH MUSCLE MEMBRANE IN HYPERTENSION

William J. Stekiel

TABLE OF CONTENTS

I. GENERAL INTRODUCTION

A. Rationale for Measurement of Vascular Muscle (VSM) Transmembrane Potentials in Hypertension

The overall rationale for study of the role of changes in VSM transmembrane electrical potential E_m in the development of cardiovascular hypertension is based on two fundamental hypotheses. The first can be expressed in terms of hemodynamic factors. An increase in total peripheral resistance (TPR)[1-6] coupled with an inappropriately low venous capacitance[3,5] are necessary to sustain the elevated blood pressure in most forms of experimental as well as human primary (i.e., essential) hypertension. Based on the variety of aberrations that have been postulated to occur in the mechanisms controlling TPR in hypertension,[2,19] it is clear that the mechanisms underlying its initiation and early etiology either in animal models or man remain to be established. However, it is now well established that a sustained increase does occur in the active contractile force (i.e., tone) of VSM in the media of blood vessels that contribute significantly to the increase in TPR and to the inappropriately small venous capacitance observed during the developing and the established phases of hypertension.[4-7]

The second fundamental hypothesis underlying the rationale for measurement of E_m of VSM in hypertension is that this parameter can be used to quantitatively assess aberrations in both extrinsic (i.e., neural and humoral) and intrinsic (i.e., VSM membrane and intracellular) mechanisms that control VSM tone. A necessary corollary to this second hypothesis is the existence of electromechanical coupling in VSM. This is defined for both arterial and venous VSM of resistance and capacitance vessels, respectively, as the negative correlation that exists between the absolute magnitude of E_m and VSM tone, once a threshold depolarization is reached.[8-14] Thus, at the level of the VSM membrane, interrelated mechanisms exist for regulation of both the transmembrane potential and active tension.

B. Central Role of an Elevated Total Peripheral Resistance and a Decreased Venous Capacitance in Hypertension

Research efforts over the past 3 decades on basic cardiovascular regulatory mechanisms, coupled with the introduction of a large number of genetically controlled animal models of hypertension, have generated an enormous amount of additional data describing many new detailed mechanisms and loci that are involved in the pathogenesis of hypertension. An ever increasing myriad of neural, humoral, and VSM cellular mechanisms has been postulated to modulate the two hemodynamic factors — cardiac output (CO) and TPR —that regulate blood pressure (BP) according to the hemodynamic counterpart of Ohm's Law (viz., $BP = CO \times TPR$). Unfortunately, even a clear picture of the sequential temporal changes that occur in these basic hemodynamic variables during the development of hypertension still remains to be established.[1,2,6,7,19] Added to this need is a better understanding of the modulation of the two right-hand variables in this equation by changes in vascular and extravascular volumes and vascular capacity during the development of hypertension.

Figure 1 depicts a scheme particularly emphasizing the many interacting regulatory mechanisms that control the CO factor in the above equation.[18] This figure helps clarify the rationale for study of E_m changes in venous VSM in hypertension since it clearly indicates that blood volume and venous capacity contribute to the regulation of systemic arterial pressure through their effect on venous return and, hence, on cardiac output.[3] This relationship and the importance of changes in it for regulation of arterial blood pressure, particularly in volume-expanded hypertension, have been well described by Guyton[20] and his colleagues. Particularly relevant to the relationship between blood volume, venous capacity, and CO is the quantitative concept of mean circulatory filling pressure.[21] This is the steady-state pressure that would exist throughout the entire circulatory system if the heart were stopped suddenly and the existing intravascular fluid volume were allowed to redistribute itself passively to fill the existing vascular capacity.

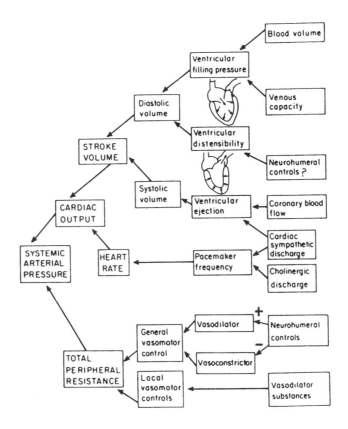

FIGURE 1. Factors determining systemic arterial pressure. (From Rushmer, R. F., *Cardiovascular Dynamics*, 4th ed., W. B. Saunders, Philadelphia, 1976, 206. With permission.)

Experimentally, this pressure level is usually determined during a short temporary arrest of the heart by rapidly transferring blood from the arterial to the venous side of the circulation without loss until the pressures in these respective compartments reach a common value.[22] This pressure concept is particularly useful in relating changes in the blood volume/vascular capacity ratio of an actively regulated distensible vascular system to venous return and CO under steady-state conditions.[20,21] The gradient for venous return (and for CO under steady state) is represented by the difference between mean circulatory filling pressure and right atrial pressure. This difference, in turn, is directly proportional to the volume/capacity ratio. Since active regulation of the denominator of the ratio is a direct function of tone in venous VSM, it is clear that measurement of venous E_m can be used to indirectly assess the magnitude of capacitance vessel tone and its effect on venous return, CO, and BP. This will be true as long as these vessels exhibit electromechanical coupling.

Figure 2, in turn, specifically illustrates some of the potentially abnormal mechanisms and sites of peripheral vascular control that could be responsible for the increased TPR that occurs during the development and maintenance of hypertension.[7] These specific mechanisms are included on the basis of studies made primarily in the Okamoto-Aoki rat model of genetically controlled spontaneous hypertension (SHR).[5-7] Though various strains of spontaneously hypertensive rats are now available for study,[16,36] the SHR continues to be the most widely studied animal model of primary hypertension. This has been true since its development over 20 years ago.[15]

To date, in addition to countless articles in individual journals, several symposia have been devoted to mechanisms underlying the genesis and maintenance of hypertension in the SHR and

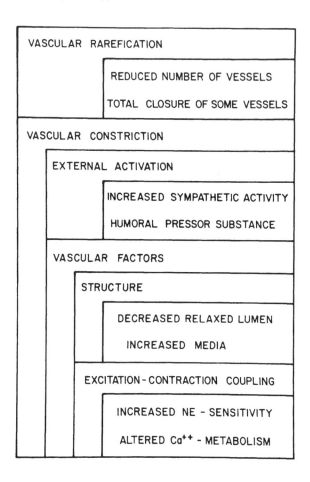

FIGURE 2. Potentially abnormal mechanisms and sites of peripheral vascular control that could be responsible for the increased TPR and decreased venous compliance in hypertension. (From Mulvany, M. J., *Blood Vessels,* 20, 1, 1983. With permission.)

other genetically derived rat models of spontaneous hypertension. In the fourth of these symposia proceedings and in the latest comprehensive treatise in hypertension, Yamori[16,36] has tabulated a very useful set of pathogenetic similarities and differences among various strains of spontaneously hypertensive rats. In addition, Trippodo and Frohlich have summarized[5] a substantial body of evidence to establish SHR as a reasonably accurate model of human essential hypertension, despite the fact that the model is not perfect.[17] In general, most hemodynamic studies indicate that the elevation in BP during the established phase of hypertension is sustained by an elevation in TPR primarily on the arterial side of the circulation. CO is usually normal or only slightly elevated. This is true both for the spontaneously hypertensive animal model (i.e., SHR),[23-25] the reduced renal mass volume expanded hypertensive animal model,[20,26,27] and the experimental renal hypertensive animal model.[28,29] It is also true for established human essential hypertension.[1,3,5,30,31,33-35] Though less appreciated, an equally important hemodynamic change in sustained hypertension is a decrease in venous compliance. Such a decrease, which has been observed in animals and in man, involves both functional and structural changes in the vascular wall that remain to be clarified.[32,33] In contrast, no consistent hemodynamic pattern of change is evident during the developmental stage of hypertension. For example, CO has been shown to undergo a transient elevation while TPR is normal during early development of hypertension in the unanesthetized SHR.[23] A similar hemodynamic pattern occurs in the volume expanded reduced renal mass dog and rat models, except that TPR undergoes a transient reduction below normal at the beginning of the CO elevation.[26,27,37] In the DOCA-treated young pig the early rise in BP can be caused either by a rise in CO or TPR, but in either case it is accompanied by an increase in water intake.[6] CO is elevated in one- to two thirds of patients with developing (i.e., borderline) hypertension, whereas it may be normal or even below normal in the remainder.[30,31,34]

Thus, during the development of hypertension, somewhat unpredictable variations occur in the time patterns of change of the two operational variables controlling BP in different animal models as well as humans. This emphasizes the need for further longitudinal studies of changes in the VSM cell membrane mechanisms that control these operational variables (as diagrammed in Figures 1 and 2). Inclusion of E_m measurements in VSM from both resistance and capacitance vessels during the development of hypertension is important since such measurements can delineate changes in both external as well as internal mechanisms controlling active tone in VSM.

II. IONIC AND MEMBRANE REGULATION OF THE VASCULAR SMOOTH MUSCLE TRANSMEMBRANE POTENTIAL

A. General Characteristics and Measurement of E_m in VSM

As in other excitable cells, the E_m across the VSM membrane is a steady-state potential difference dependent upon a constant supply of metabolic energy to maintain the gradients for permeable ions. Due to the small diameters of mammalian VSM cells (2 to 5 μm),[38,39] direct measurement of their E_m with glass capillary microelectrodes is technically difficult, particularly *in situ*. Consequently, the first successful direct measurements using such microelectrodes with ultrafine tips (0.1 μm diameter) were reported by Funaki[40] almost 10 years after Ling and Gerard[41] refined the original glass capillary microelectrode impalement technique introduced by Graham and Gerard.[42] Since this time, a large number of VSM E_m measurements have been reported using this technique both in a variety of mammalian blood vessels and under a variety of experimental conditions. Most measurements have been made in *in vitro* preparations.

Several important conclusions can be derived from these measurements. First, VSM cells exhibit a wide range of mean resting values of E_m (e.g., −30 to −70 mV). They also exhibit a wide range of E_m responses to various exogenous agonists and perivascular electrical stimulation. Second, VSM in most *in vitro* small blood vessel preparations exhibits steady resting E_m (i.e., no spontaneous action potentials) and graded, rather than phasic, electrical and mechanical responses to agonists.[43-45] We have also observed only graded E_m responses to K+ and NE in *in situ* as well as *in vitro* small mesenteric arteries and veins of SHR and WKY rats.[46-48] Third, a heterogeneity exists in the mechanisms by which VSM membrane receptors[49] and ion channels[50-52] exert control over both electrical and mechanical responses to various stimuli.[53] However, such heterogeneity has not precluded development of an empirical quantitative relationship between E_m, ion activity gradients, and VSM membrane conductance for specific ions, similar to that developed for other excitable tissues.

B. Diffusion Potential Component of E_m in VSM

Under steady-state conditions, the E_m across VSM cells can be divided into two regulatory components, namely a passive diffusion potential and an electrogenic potential.[12,43,54,55] Both are a function of the coupled active transport of Na+ out of and K+ into the VSM cell via the membrane Na/K exchange pump. Figure 3 illustrates a simple schematic relating these components and the factors that in turn regulate their magnitudes.

Steady state is defined as the condition where the sum of net ionic currents across the membrane is zero. The diffusion potential component of E_m derived from this steady-state

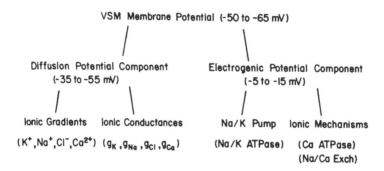

FIGURE 3. Simple schematic illustrating the two major components of the VSM membrane potential and the factors that regulate their magnitudes. (From Hermsmeyer, K., in *New Trends in Arterial Hypertension*, Worcel, M. et al., Eds., Elservier/North Holland, Amsterdam, 1981. With permission.)

current relationship can be expressed in terms of the conductances and equilibrium (or Nernst) potentials for the permeable ions not in electrochemical equilibrium across the VSM membrane. In its most simple form the diffusion potential can be expressed as the electrical analog or chord conductance equation,[12,56] namely:

$$E_{diff} = \frac{g_K}{\Sigma_g} E_K + \frac{g_{Na}}{\Sigma_g} E_{Na} + \frac{g_{Ca}}{\Sigma_g} E_{Ca} + \frac{g_{Cl}}{\Sigma_g} E_{Cl} \tag{1}$$

Each g_{ion} term in this equation represents the electrical conductance (measured in siemens) for the current carried through a membrane ionic channel that is relatively specific for the designated permeable ion. The specific conductance for an ion is directly proportional to its membrane permeability (P_{ion}), its concentration, and the existing E_m. Fractional conductance for each permeable ion is designated by the ratio of specific ion conductance to the total ionic conductance

$$\frac{(g_{ion})}{\Sigma_g}$$

Each E_{ion} term represents the equilibrium potential for the designated ion (i.e., the membrane potential at which net passive flux for the ion is zero). It is expressed by its Nernst equation:[57]

$$E_{ion} = \frac{-RT}{F} \ln \frac{[ion]_i}{[ion]_o} \tag{2}$$

where

$$\frac{[ion]_i}{[ion]_o}$$

is the ratio of intracellular to extracellular activation for the ion. The magnitude of Ediff under the steady-state condition can also be expressed in terms of the intra- and extracellular products of permeability and activity for each permeable ion not in electrochemical equilibrium across the membrane. Expressed in this form, the E_{diff} relation is known as the Goldman, Hodgkins,

Katz (G.H.K.) equation.[43,56,57] The equilibrium potential for each ion that is in electrochemical equilibrium across the membrane is equal to the E_m at steady state. These ions are not included in either E_{diff} equation since they do not contribute net current across the membrane and hence do not contribute to the diffusion potential. By definition they also are not actively transported across the membrane.

The membrane resistance (r_m), which is equal to the reciprocal of total ionic conductance (Σ_g), can be estimated as the fraction of input resistance (r_{in}) in the microelectrode circuit remaining after subtraction of the microelectrode resistance. In practice r_m is calculated from the slope of the plot of step voltage changes in response to small step changes in externally injected input current.[58] A bridge circuit is used to balance out microelectrode resistance prior to cell impalement.[59] The limitations of this single electrode method for determination of r_m are primarily a function of error associated with point sources of current injection[60] and resistance coupling between neighboring VSM cells in VSM preparations containing large numbers of tightly coupled cells.[12,61]

Agents that inhibit transmembrane fluxes of specific ions can be used to estimate the relative contribution of specific ionic conductances and their related permeabilities to the steady-state E_m. For example, barium (Ba^{2+}) and tetraethylammonium (TEA) have been shown to elevate r_m by selective reduction of g_K. Thus, in isolated guinea pig mesenteric artery and in VSM cells cultured from rat aorta, addition of Ba^{2+} or TEA to the physiological salt solution (PSS) causes a specific decrease in outward K^+ current. This leads to VSM membrane depolarization, induction of spontaneous action potentials, and/or generation of action potentials upon electrical stimulation of a normally unexcitable membrane.[13,58,62] However, the VSM membrane mechanisms by which many of these agents inhibit specific ion fluxes are not well understood and involve more than simple blockade of a specific ion channel. For example, amiloride, a K^+ sparing diuretic, causes hyperpolarization of isolated, resting guinea pig superior mesenteric artery but does not cause elevation of r_{in}. Evidence from studies with other tissues suggests that this agent may inhibit Na^+ influx across the cell membrane not merely by simple blockade of membrane Na channels, but by competitive inhibition with Na^+ for a membrane transport site involved in facilitated diffusion.[63]

Continued application of the recently developed gigaseal voltage clamp technique[64-67] to isolated whole VSM cells and to patches of VSM cell membrane should provide additional quantitative information about the properties and voltage control of ionic channels that regulate specific ionic conductances. These techniques have already been used to identify two types of Ca^{2+} channel in the membrane of VSM cells isolated from rat mesenteric and rabbit ear artery, viz., a rapidly inactivated transient "T" type and a slowly inactivated "L" type.[50,51] These channels are characterized by differences in their voltage activation thresholds and in the kinetics of opening and closing.

As expressed in the chord equation (Equation 1), the contribution made to the E_m by each permeable ion whose passive chemical and electrical gradient forces are not balanced across the cell membrane is a function of the product of the ion's relative conductance and its equilibrium potential. Similar to skeletal muscle, g_K for the VSM cell membrane at rest is significantly higher than for all other permeable ions. However, unlike the resting E_m of vertebrate skeletal muscle,[68] mean *in vitro* magnitude of E_m VSM in various vessels ranges significantly below that of E_K (which is approximately -90 mV). In addition, beyond approximately twice normal K^+_o (i.e., 10 mM), the negative slope of E_m vs. log K^+_o for VSM in most arteries ranges between 30 mV and 48 mV/decade.[13,43,58,70] An exception is the middle cerebral artery of the cat where the slope is 58 mV/decade.[69] Hence, for most arteries studied thus far, this slope is significantly smaller than the 60 mV per 10-fold change in K^+_o that would be observed if the VSM membrane behaved like a K^+ electrode. This indicates that even at rest the P_{Na} of most VSM cells is a significantly greater fraction of P_K (ranging from 0.1 to 0.2) than for the skeletal muscle cell membrane (ranging from 0.01 to 0.05). Based on measurements of a relatively high input resistance for arterial VSM, this higher P_{Na}/P_K ratio has been attributed to a low P_K in VSM relative to skeletal muscle.[13,58] Hence, a significant factor that contributes to the lesser electronegativity of the VSM cell interior compared to that of skeletal muscle is the inward diffusion of Na^+ down its electrochemical gradient.[43,71]

The relative contribution made by anions such as Cl^- to the resting E_m is less clear than that of K^+ and Na^+. For rat aorta, portal vein, and rabbit main pulmonary artery, E_{Cl} is only one half the measured membrane potential.[71] Also, Kreye et al.[72] have obtained evidence for an active Cl^- transport into VSM cells of rabbit aorta and main pulmonary artery based on use of furosamide. Furosamide is a known inhibitor of active Cl^- transport in several nonmuscular tissues. These investigators demonstrated that incubation with 1 mM furosamide led to an inhibition of $^{36}Cl^-$ efflux which, in the steady state, is equal to active influx. This inhibition was accompanied by a decrease in Cl^-_i, a slow hyperpolarization, and a rise in the calculated equilibrium potential for Cl^- until it became equal to the E_m. Such observations indicate that the Cl_o/Cl_i ratio normally is not determined by a passive Donnan equilibrium and that Cl^- contributes to the resting E_m across these VSM membranes.[73]

In contrast to these studies supporting an active role for Cl^- in the regulation of the resting E_m in VSM, anion replacement studies do not. For example, replacement of Cl^- by sulfate in PSS suffusing isolated rabbit common carotid artery[74] and by glutamate or nitrate in isolated guinea pig superior mesenteric artery[58] did not lead to a significant change in the E_m of either vessel. From such observations it was concluded that E_{Cl} is close to the resting E_m and that Cl^- is passively distributed in VSM cells. Otherwise if Cl were actively transported into the cell, E_{Cl} would be less negative than E_m and removal of Cl^-_o would lead to a hyperpolarization. Further, in their study, Harder and Sperelakis[58] utilized directly measured E_m and the G.H.K. equation to calculate the P_{Na}/P_K ratio before and after suppression of the Na/K electrogenic VSM membrane pump with ouabain. This ratio was found to be equally high in normal PSS and in Cl^- deficient solutions. From this observation they concluded that the low resting E_m of VSM results from the distributions and permeabilities of K^+ and Na^+ with little contribution from the Cl^- anion. The discrepancy between this conclusion and the strong evidence for a non-Donnan distribution (i.e., active influx) of Cl^- across the VSM cell membrane emphasizes the heterogeneity in the membrane properties of these cells and the lack of a simple relation between E_m and anions in general.[73]

Even less well understood, but of physiological importance, are the VSM membrane mechanisms relating the vasoactive and electrical effects of circulating endogenous agents such as norepinephrine (NE) to their effects on anion permeability (including P_{Cl}). For example, it has been shown that the vasoconstrictor effect of NE is coupled to an increased P_{Cl} and hence Cl^- efflux in rat portal vein,[75] rabbit ear artery,[76] and common carotid artery.[74] However, the membrane mechanisms by which anion substitution can alter resting VSM tone and sensitivity to endogenous vasoconstrictor and vasodilator agents in different blood vessels are not clear. For example, cerebral vessels are highly sensitive to substitution of other anions for Cl^-_o.[77] However, the vasoconstrictor effect of such Cl^-_o substitution in cerebral vessels is minimal if the anion is $H_2PO_4^-$.[78] This is of general interest in the study of the regulation of blood pressure and flow since a vasodilator effect of phosphate ions has been assumed to be the mediator of functional hyperemia in working skeletal muscle.[79] The general topic of the relation between anion substitution and the regulation of electrical and mechanical activity of VSM is beyond the scope of this review, but is well summarized in the literature.[43,71,73]

C. Electrogenic Potential Component of E_m in VSM

The second regulatory component that can contribute significantly to the E_m and the regulation of active tone in VSM is the electrogenic potential (E_p) generated by a membrane bound Na^+/K^+ exchange pump.[80,81] This component has received considerable attention in studies designed to explain the elevation in TPR in experimental and human primary hypertension.[82-85] The enzyme correlate of this ion pump is an ATPase within the VSM membrane that is regulated primarily by the intracellular Na^+ concentration and the external K^+ concentration.[86] Such a pump is necessary to maintain the steady-state activity gradients of these ions across the VSM membrane and hence the diffusion potential. In addition, since the Na/K exchange coupling ratio for this pump is approximately three Na^+ out of the VSM cell for each two K^+ in, a net positive outward ionic current (I_p) is generated.[82-87] Passage of this I_p across the membrane resistance (r_m) produces the ($i \times r_m = E_p$) potential drop defined as the electrogenic potential component of the total E_m. The magnitude of this contribution is a function of the relative magnitude of passive and active fluxes of Na^+ and K^+. A quantitative relationship for total E_m incorporating the electrogenic transport of Na^+ and K^+ was first formulated by Mullins and Noda.[88] The following equation (which assumes a passive equilibrium for Cl^-) is a generalization of this relationship as developed by Sjoden and Ortiz[89] and utilized by Hermsmeyer[90] to explain the effect of NE on E_p in SHR caudal artery:

$$E_m = \frac{RT}{F} \ln \frac{ar\,[K^+]_o + b\,[Na^+]_o}{ar\,[K^+]_i + b\,[Na^+]_i} \tag{3}$$

where: E_m = total membrane potential, R and F = the gas constant and Faraday constant, T = temperature, $[K^+]$ and $[Na^+]$ = respective K^+ and Na^+ activities outside (o) and inside (i) the VSM cell, a = variable ratio of

$$\frac{\text{passive/active } Na^+ \text{ flux}}{\text{passive/active } K^+ \text{ flux}}$$

r = the coupling ratio for Na^+/K^+ transport (ex. 1.5), and b = ratio of P_{Na}/P_K.

Under resting (steady-state) conditions, "a" equals unity, since the ion concentration gradients across the membrane are maintained constant. Also, if the coupling ratio is unity, the Na^+/K^+ exchange pump is by definition an exchange-diffusion (i.e., nonelectrogenic) pump and Equation 3 would reduce to the steady-state diffusion potential expressed in the form of the G.H.K. equation.[56,57] It is apparent that under steady-state conditions the relative contribution of an E_p to the total E_m is a function of the coupling ratio and permeability ratio for Na^+ and K^+. Further, at a constant coupling ratio (i.e., 1.5) under steady-state conditions, the magnitude of E_p is directly proportional to the magnitude of the passive "leak" current for Na^+ into the cell relative to the passive "leak" current for K^+ out of the cell. Thus for example, for squid axon, where K^+_o and K^+_i are 10 and 400 mM, respectively, and Na^+_o and Na^+_i are 440 and 50 mM, respectively, with r = 1.5 and b = 0.03, the theoretical E_m = –88 mV. This value is 6 mV or approximately 7% greater than the resting E_m that would exist if the pump were nonelectrogenic (i.e., r = 1).[91] On the other hand, the relative contribution of E_p to total E_m is significantly greater for VSM cells where b is an order of magnitude greater than 0.03. Thus, using the data from Jones[71,85] for VSM in normal rat aorta where b is approximately 0.2, the total E_m with r = 1.5 is –50 mV, whereas with r = 1.0, it would be –39 mV. Hence, the E_p is 11 mV and represents approximately 20% of the resting E_m. It is clear that Na/K pump blockade would produce a significant depolarization and increase in VSM active contractile force in this vessel via electromechanical coupling. (See Section II.D.) Also, agonists such as NE, that generate active tension via electromechanical coupling involving increased P_{Na}, P_K, P_{Cl}, P_{Ca}, and thus ion fluxes, will significantly reduce net i_p and r_m, and hence E_p. This is reflected by a reduction of the (a $\times$ r) product in Equation 3.

Several important properties of the Na/K pump serve as a basis for analytical techniques to verify its existence and to quantify its electrogenic activity. First, early in studies of the role of the pump in smooth muscle, it was shown that rubidium (Rb) can substitute for K^+_o in the regulation of the enzymatic correlates of the pump (viz., the membrane bound Na^+/K^+ ATPase).[92] Second, as in other smooth muscle cells, cardiac glycosides (for example, ouabain) act on the external surface of the VSM membrane to specifically inhibit the pump and membrane-bound ATPase.[93] Third, further studies have also demonstrated specific, high affinity binding of ^{3}H-ouabain to plasma membranes of a variety of cells, including VSM. Such binding is antagonized by external K^+ which has been shown to produce allosteric change on the external surface of the Na^+/K^+ membrane pump.[94]

These properties have provided a variety of techniques to assess the transport capacity of the Na/K pump in smooth muscle and blood cells in both normal and hypertensive animals and man. For example, ouabain-sensitive ^{86}Rb uptake by an isolated blood vessel segment can be used to assess its pump capacity following VSM intracellular loading with Na^+. Initial elevation of $[Na^+]_i$ can be accomplished by a timed period of preincubation of the vascular tissue in normal PSS under conditions where pump activity is inhibited (for example, low temperature, ouabain, K^+-free PSS). VSM membrane pump receptor site density and affinity have been assessed in blood vessel segments,[96] single VSM cells,[97] and red blood cells[98] from normo- and hypertensive animals and man using Scatchard plot analysis of ^{3}H-ouabain binding.

Direct measurement of VSM transmembrane E_m with microelectrodes in *in vitro* blood vessel segments, under conditions of Na/K pump stimulation or inhibition, can be used to assess its electrogenic contribution to total E_m. Since electrogenicity in VSM is a function of both $[Na^+]_i$ and $[K^+]_o$,[12,55,80,81,99] its maximum contribution to total E_m can be estimated from the transient negative increase in E_m that occurs in response to elevated $[K^+]_o$ following pump inhibition and consequent intracellular Na^+ loading. Most commonly such inhibition has been produced by preincubation of isolated vessel segments in 0 mM K^+ for a fixed time period.[12,55,70] This technique has been used extensively to demonstrate electrogenicity in a wide variety of both visceral and vascular smooth muscle cells.[12,55,70,71,81,99] For example, Hermsmeyer[70] measured a 12-mV hyperpolarization in SHR and 5 mV in WKY *in vitro* caudal artery segments upon resuffusion with PSS containing 30 mM K^+ after 1 h incubation in 0 mM K^+. Such hyperpolarizing responses were pump dependent since they were totally blocked by 1 mM ouabain or by cooling the PSS suffusate from normal 37° to 16°C. As additional evidence for such electrogenic activity, the 12 and 5 mV hyperpolarizations were shown to be 7 and 2 mV more negative, respectively, than the calculated E_K for the SHR and WKY vessel. Much emphasis has been placed on this negative overshoot of E_m beyond the calculated E_K as evidence for electrogenicity.[12,70,81] However, such overshoot is difficult to quantitate due to lack of accurate techniques to measure the true activity of K^+_i (and hence to calculate E_K) during the transient change of K^+_o from 0 to 15 or 30 mM.

The contribution made by electrogenic pumping to the E_m in VSM under resting conditions can be estimated indirectly as the difference between total E_m, measured directly with microelectrodes, and the diffusion potential, calculated from the G.H.K. equation. Due not only to the assumptions and errors in calculating ion permeabilities and measuring their intra- and extracellular activities, but also to the heterogeneity of VSM in different vessels, the E_p determined in this manner vary widely (e.g., from −3 mV for rat portal vein to −20 mV for guinea pig taenia coli).[43,71,75,81]

E_p can also be determined from the E_m difference measured with microelectrodes before and after pump inhibition (e.g., with ouabain, low K^+_o, low temperature). However, this method of measuring Ep can also be subject to error if concomitant changes in E_{diff} occur. For example, pump inhibition can lead to a decrease in E_m due to: (1) gradual loss in $[K^+]_i$; (2) accumulation of K^+ outside the VSM cell membrane; (3) changes in P_{Na} and P_K secondary to depolarization itself.[80,81] On the other hand, opposition to depolarization can occur as a result of: (1) elevation of the Cl⁻ gradient, secondary to altered movement of positive ions; (2) elevation of E_{diff} if pump inhibition is produced by reducing K^+_o. However, it is generally accepted that E_p can be estimated reasonably well from E_m measurements if made within the first several minutes following pump blockade (i.e., before significant changes in ion gradients and permeabilities can occur).[55,80,81] Measured in this way, most reported values of E_p for arterial VSM preparations range between 5 and 10 mV with an Na^+/K^+ coupling ratio of 1.5 to 2.0.[71,81] However, in a recent study using $10^{-3}M$ ouabain blockade, we measured an E_p of 8 ± 1.5 mV in isolated small mesenteric arteries of WKY rats, but only 3 ± 1 mV in the corresponding isolated small mesenteric veins.[100]

In a detailed study using rabbit carotid artery, Heidlage and Jones[87] showed that half saturation of Na^+ efflux occurred at $K^+_o = 2$ mM and full saturation at 10 mM. Hence, it is important to emphasize that at normal K^+_o (approximately 5 mM for mammalian VSM) a significant physiological reserve exists for regulation of E_p and coupled VSM active tension via relatively small changes in K^+_o or any other factor that can modulate Na/K pump activity. For example, an elevated Na/K pump activity (and E_p) stimulated by an increase in K^+_o from contracting skeletal muscle has been invoked as a cause of skeletal muscle bed vasodilation in exercise.[101] On the other hand, beginning with the early studies of Overbeck,[102] a controversial hypothesis implicating Na/K pump inhibition (and an implied reduction in E_p) has been advanced to explain the elevated TPR in low renin forms of volume-expanded hypertension[95] and in selected humans with essential hypertension and/or end stage renal disease.[98] Simply stated, this hypothesis invokes a circulating Na/K pump inhibitor derived from the hypothalamus and possessing digitalis or ouabain-like properties to explain the elevated VSM tone observed in this type of hypertension.[93,95] Thus, it is clear from this description of the components of the total E_m that the electromechanically coupled active tone generated by elevated excitatory neural input and/or endogenous agonists can include VSM membrane depolarization attributable to a reduction of both the electrogenic and diffusion potential component of the total E_m.

D. Electromechanical vs. Pharmacomechanical Coupling in VSM

As discussed above, a key hypothesis relating E_m changes in VSM of the small resistance and capacitance vessels with the development and maintenance of hypertension is that transmembrane E_m changes are coupled to changes in VSM active tone over a range of E_m values that exist *in vivo*. In addition, it is now well established that the intracellular free calcium ion (i.e., the activator Ca^{2+}) serves as an indispensible link between changes in VSM membrane permeabilities for specific ions and the generation of active tension. It has also been well established that such tension is directly proportional to the myoplasmic Ca^{2+} activity between 10^{-7} and 10^{-5} M. Within this range Ca^{2+} activity regulates actin-myosin bridge formation via coupling with calmodulin and activation of myosin light chain kinase.[43,103-106] Beginning with the demonstration by Su et al.[107] that changes in VSM tension are not necessarily accompanied by changes in E_m and with the introduction of the concept of pharmacomechanical coupling by Somlyo and colleagues,[108-110] debate has persisted to the present day concerning the physiological role of E_m in regulating VSM tone *in vivo*.

As defined by Somlyo and Somlyo[108] pharmacomechanical coupling is a process through which drugs can cause contraction or relaxation of smooth muscle without a necessary change in the resting E_m or in action potential frequency (for VSM that exhibits action potentials either spontaneously or in response to neural or chemical stimuli). To date, the question of the relative importance of pharmacomechanical vs. electromechanical coupling in VSM has been investigated primarily *in vitro* with isolated lengths of relatively large diameter blood vessels. Classically, direct electrical (or perivascular neural) stimulation or elevated (80 to 120 mM) extracellular potassium (K^+_o) has been used to demonstrate electromechanical coupling whereas a variety of agonists (e.g., NE, serotonin, acetylcholine (ACh)) has been used primarily to demonstrate pharmacomechanical coupling.[108-111] As outlined by Johansson and Somlyo[43] and reviewed in detail elsewhere,[110,112,113] several general observations in different smooth muscle preparations form the basis for pharmacomechanical coupling in polarized smooth muscle:

1. The same blocking and potentiating agents are effective in polarized and in depolarized smooth muscle
2. Depolarization by drugs may be less, but the maximum contraction may be greater than the respective effects of high K^+ solutions
3. The differences in the maximum contractile effects of different drugs are maintained after depolarization
4. Drug-induced contractions may be sustained in smooth muscles that respond to depolarization by high potassium with a transient phasic contracture
5. Relaxing agents can relax polarized smooth muscles without evidence of hyperpolarization or inhibition of spike electrogenesis.

Even though these observations demonstrate the existence of pharmacomechanical coupling in smooth muscle, a major question remains concerning the *in vivo* physiological importance of this type of coupling and whether endogenous vasoconstrictors and vasodilators can exert their effects by pure nonelectrical mechanisms even in normally polarized cells.

Most of the published data supporting such electrically uncoupled changes in VSM tone in response to agonists such as NE have been obtained from relatively large conduit blood vessels not participating directly in the control of peripheral vascular resistance or capacitance (e.g., rat aorta,[114] rabbit ear artery,[76] rabbit main pulmonary artery,[107,115] guinea pig coronary artery[116]). Data from our own lab indicate that denervated *in situ* and *in vitro* preparations of small mesenteric resistance and capacitance vessels obtained from adult SHR and WKY rats are depolarized in a graded manner when suffused with physiological salt solution (PSS) containing increasing concentrations of either K^+ (0 to 100 mM) or NE (10^{-8} to $10^{-6}M$). We have also found that the slopes and positions of the concentration-E_m response curves of respective vessels from SHR and WKY are equal (Figure 4).[46,47]

In addition, we have also observed a tight electromechanical coupling when isolated small mesenteric arteries of SHR and WKY were mounted *in vitro* in a Mulvany-Halpern type myograph[117] and their VSM was activated with the above concentration range of NE or KCl. These vessels do not exhibit action potentials either spontaneously or in response to NE unless the increase in VSM membrane K^+ conductance (g_K) that occurs with activation is blocked or at least attenuated with an agent such as TEA (see Section II.B). The electromechanical coupling ratio (i.e., the percent of maximum active stress per millivolt depolarization between 0 and 80% of the maximum stress capable of being generated by NE) was similar for small (150 to 200 μm internal diameter) mesenteric arteries from WKY and SHR (3 ± 0.7% vs. 4 ± 1% per mV, respectively, n = 6).[244] We have also observed similar coupling ratios in these vessels when K^+ is used as an agonist. Hermsmeyer and Trapani and co-workers have observed similar coupling ratios in response to K^+ in isolated rat caudal artery[9] and in response to NE in isolated rabbit ear artery.[10] Electromechanical coupling in response to NE stimulation has also been observed *in vitro* in small mesenteric arteries from WKY by Mulvany and co-workers,[118] though beginning at a high threshold concentration of NE. In contrast, Bolton et al.[119] observed minimal electromechanical coupling in response to NE in helical strips of small mesenteric arteries of the guinea pig. From their studies, the latter investigators concluded that diffuse application of NE to VSM can activate both a potential-dependent and -independent mechanism of VSM contraction.

The membrane mechanisms underlying electromechanical coupling are complicated as demonstrated by the heterogeneity of responses to the same agonist in VSM from different vessel sources. An explanation of this variability is dependent upon a better understanding of: (1) the intramembrane transduction mechanisms that selectively regulate the opening of specific types of ion channels following agonist-receptor combination; (2) the long-term *in vivo* influence of neural, humoral, and local membrane factors that regulate the surface density of ion-specific membrane channels in VSM of blood vessels; and (3) the acute regulatory effect of

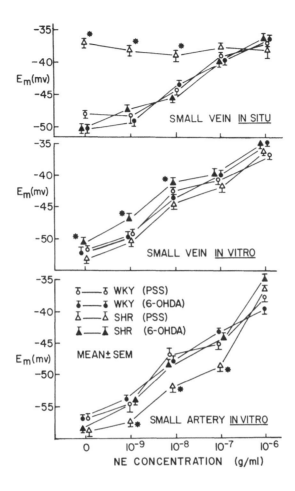

FIGURE 4. Small mesenteric vessel membrane potential (E_m) responses to NE in the presence and absence of adrenergic nerve terminals (denervation with 6-hydroxydopamine). Minimum of 50 impalements in 6 rats for each mean point. *, Significant difference from corresponding animal type at $p \leq 0.05$. (From Stekiel, W. J. et al., in *Hypertensive Mechanisms, The SHR as a Model to Study Human Hypertension*, Rascher, W. et al., Eds., F. K. Schattauer, Stuttgart, 1982, 252. With permission.)

humoral agents and ions on the duration and frequency of opening of ion-specific membrane channels. For NE there is good evidence that its combination with VSM membrane receptors increases conductance not only for the Ca^{2+} necessary for sustaining excitation-contraction coupling, but also for K^+, Na^+, and Cl^-.[75,115,120-122]

As described earlier, the relative contribution of specific ion gradients to the absolute magnitude of the E_m is a function of their respective ion conductances. From simultaneous measurements of E_m and active tension in rabbit main pulmonary artery in response to α–adrenoceptor stimulation with NE, Haeusler[123] has observed that active tension is initiated and coupled to decreases in E_m magnitude beginning at –60 mV. Such coupling was maintained to –45 mV where active contraction was 50 to 60% of maximum. This occurred over a NE concentration range of 10^{-8} to $10^{-6} M$. Above $10^{-6} M$ NE, no further depolarization was observed (Figure 5), in spite of substantial further development of contraction.[123] We have observed a break in the *in vitro* electromechanical coupling curve at a similar NE concentration in WKY and SHR small mesenteric artery.[244] Similar results were obtained with methoxamine (a specific

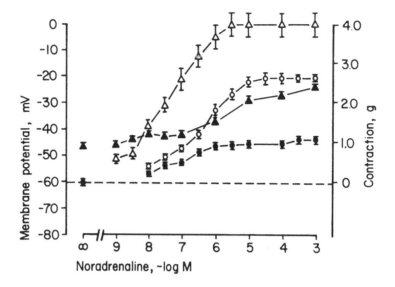

FIGURE 5. Dose-response curves for the contractile effect (open circles) and depolarizing effect (closed circles) of NE on strips of rabbit main pulmonary artery. The dose-response curves of NE in the presence of $10^{-2}M$ tetraethylammonium are also indicated by open triangles (contractile effect) and closed triangles (depolarizing effect). Shown are mean values (±SEM) in 10 vascular strips (contraction) and of at least 15 intracellular measurements of E_m for each NE concentration. (From Haeusler, G., *Blood Vessels*, 15, 46, 1978. With permission.)

α_1-agonist).[124] Since membrane resistance (r_m) continues to decrease over the entire concentration range of methoxamine[124] and since NE increases the membrane conductance (g) for Na$^+$, Cl$^-$ K$^+$, and Ca^{2+} in the rabbit main pulmonary artery,[120] Haeusler[124] has postulated that at low concentrations of NE and other α_1-receptor agonists, VSM cells are depolarized mainly by an increase in g_{Na}. A concomitant rise occurs in Ca$^{2+}_i$ upon increasing NE concentration as a result of transmembrane influx and/or release of Ca^{2+} from plasma membrane and sarcoplasmic reticular stores.[49,123-127] This rise in Ca$^{2+}_i$ is postulated to raise g_K leading to a further reduction in r_m and attenuation of further depolarization, despite the continuing elevation of active tone.[123,124] Direct control of g_K by Ca$^{2+}_i$ has been demonstrated in a variety of electrically excitable tissues including nerve,[128] cardiac,[129] visceral,[130] and vascular[13] smooth muscle. This postulated mechanism of electromechanical uncoupling at high concentrations of NE is further supported by the reestablishment of coupling at high NE concentrations if the concomitant rise in g_K is blocked with TEA (Figure 5).[124]

As mentioned earlier, in isolated large vessels active tension responses to agonists that are also neurotransmitters (e.g., NE and ACh) have been reported to occur in the absence of VSM membrane depolarization. However, general agreement about such pharmacomechanical coupling is lacking among various investigators, even when studied in the same isolated vessel preparation. Thus, in isolated rabbit ear artery, Droogmans et al.[76] reported contraction without depolarization up to $10^{-6}M$ NE, whereas Trapani et al.[10] demonstrated a tight active tension vs. voltage coupling between 10^{-8} and $10^{-5}M$ NE. A similar discrepancy exists for isolated rabbit main pulmonary artery. Coupled depolarization and active contraction to NE have been observed by Haeusler[8,123] (up to $10^{-6}M$) and by Somlyo et al. (up to $3 \times 10^{-6}M$).[131] In contrast, contraction to NE in one early study was observed in the absence of depolarization,[107] and in another, contraction was not coupled to membrane depolarization up to $10^{-7}M$ NE.[115] One clear exception to electromechanical coupling, as defined above for normally polarized cells, is the observation by Kitamura and Kuriyama[116] that guinea pig coronary artery responds to ACh (10^{-8}

to $10^{-6} M$) with a gradual increase in contractile force that is accompanied by a gradual membrane hyperpolarization rather than a depolarization. These investigators attribute the hyperpolarization of VSM in this vessel to a selective increase in g_K which is at least in part attributable to an increase in g_{Ca}. The concomitant contractile response to ACh is also attributed to the elevation of g_{Ca}. A hyperpolarizing action of ACh was also observed in rabbit superior mesenteric artery,[132] whereas it produced a depolarization in other arterial vessels such as sheep carotid[133] and rabbit pulmonary artery.[134] In each of these VSM preparations ACh produced a contraction, though in the superior mesenteric artery of the mature rabbit, ACh was also shown to suppress the contraction due to NE or K^+ via its action on the endothelium.[135]

This variability of electrical and mechanical responses of the VSM cell to ACh as a function of blood vessel source and size illustrates the overall complexity of the membrane and intracellular mechanisms underlying VSM electrical and mechanical responses to agonists. This complexity is reflected by many newly described membrane and intracellular mechanisms by which agonists act to regulate excitation-contraction coupling. For example, it is now known that agonists regulate active tone not only by combination with specific VSM membrane receptors,[49,122-124] but also with specific receptors on the adjacent endothelial cell membrane to produce an endothelium-derived vasodilator factor (or EDRF).[135,136]

Relative to the mechanism of excitation-contraction coupling and its possible aberrations in the development and maintenance in hypertension, a major question concerns the mechanisms by which activator Ca^{2+} concentration is regulated by transmembrane influx and release from intracellular stores. The controversy concerning mechanisms for regulation of transmembrane influx of Ca^{2+} is directly related to the controversy concerning the physiological importance of pharmacomechanical vs. electromechanical coupling in VSM. This relationship is the result of the distinction that has been made between receptor-operated Ca^{2+} channels (ROCs) and membrane potential-operated Ca^{2+} channels (POCs).[49,122-127] Opening of the former by agonist occupation of specific membrane receptors has been proposed to increase Ca^{2+} influx across VSM membranes in some blood vessels independently of changes in membrane potential.[125-127]

Four observations have been cited[127] in support of the hypothesis that receptor occupation and membrane depolarization can open separate ROCs and POCs, respectively: (1) additivity of $^{45}Ca^{2+}$ influx stimulated by high K^+ (80 mM) and by NE in rabbit aorta[137] and in rabbit mesenteric resistance vessels;[127] (2) selective blockade by Ca^{2+} antagonists (e.g., D-600, diltiazem, nisoldipine) of K^+-induced Ca^{2+} influx and contraction via the POC in VSM of large conduit arteries (e.g., rabbit aorta); (3) selective blockade by these Ca^2 antagonists of the NE-induced Ca^{2+} influx and contraction via the ROC in resistance vessels (e.g., rabbit small mesenteric artery); (4) differential activation of the two types of Ca^{2+} channels as evidenced by the ability of NE, but not K^+, to increase Ca^{2+} influx and active tone in the absence of depolarization in the rabbit aorta. However, such electromechanical uncoupling has not been observed in the rabbit mesenteric resistance vessel where both NE and K^+ stimulate a coupled Ca^{2+} influx and depolarization of the VSM. According to Cauvin and van Breemen,[127] this does not indicate that NE opens POCs in this vessel since they found that NE was capable of stimulating virtually the same contraction and Ca^{2+} influx in 80 mM K^+ depolarized VSM as in normally polarized VSM, but without any further depolarization. Thus, they suggest that the depolarization observed with NE in the rabbit mesenteric resistance vessels is secondary to the opening of ROCs that mediate entry of Ca^{2+} (and possibly Na^+). The observed lack of depolarization of rabbit aorta VSM by NE is suggested to result from a rectifying increase in outward g_K (as observed in rabbit ear artery by Droogmans et al.[76]) that balances an increase in g_{Na} and g_{Ca}. In effect, then, the net flux of charge across the membrane induced by NE may be insufficient to produce a measurable depolarization. This is similar to the explanation proposed by Haeusler for the uncoupling of tension and depolarization at high NE concentrations in rabbit main pulmonary artery.[122,123] It must be noted, however, that both electromechanical and pharmacomechanical coupling have been observed in isolated rabbit ear artery in response to NE.[10,76] Thus, the possibility of an increase in all ion permeabilities by an equal factor[76] is open to question.

Current pharmacological evidence for existence of separate ROCs and POCs in the VSM membrane is indirect and the generalization of this concept of separate Ca^{2+} channels for all VSM under normal physiological conditions has been challenged by Hermsmeyer[111] on several counts. For example, the assumption that KCl specifically depolarizes the VSM surface membrane to open POCs is an implicit assumption that remains to be proven directly. Similarly, stimulation of VSM by NE, particularly in small blood vessels, normally involves electromechanical coupling. As discussed above, this is true both *in situ* and *in vitro*.[8,9,12,13,46-48] The evidence for separate ROCs based on an observed additional Ca^{2+} influx and contractile response to NE in VSM completely depolarized in high K^+ concentrations (e.g., 100 mM) is open to question for several reasons. First, there is little possibility for any further changes in E_m to occur during such an abnormally depolarized state. Second, the intracellular distribution of Ca^{2+} may be significantly altered in VSM subjected to sustained depolarization.[43] Third, in small mesenteric blood vessels the additional Ca^{2+} influx into K^+ depolarized VSM in response to NE is significantly less than that into normally polarized VSM.[127]

On the other hand, application of the recently developed gigaseal voltage clamp technique[64,65] to whole VSM cells and to patches of cell membrane has provided direct evidence for ROCs. Thus, in a recent study applying the patch clamp technique to isolated VSM cells from rabbit ear artery, Benham and Tsien[51] have demonstrated ROCs for Ca^{2+} that can be activated by ATP when cell membrane E_m were held at very negative levels where voltage-gated channels were not activated. However, upon application of the whole cell voltage clamp technique to isolated VSM cells from rat azygous veins, Hermsmeyer[111] was unable to demonstrate any effect of NE on the amplitude and duration of opening of slow channels. Such channels are known to regulate Ca influx in other cells.[66,67] The whole cell and membrane patch clamp technique has also been used to obtain data that questions the pharmacological evidence for separate nonvoltage-dependent membrane Ca^{2+} channels in VSM cells. The latter evidence is based on the assumption that the dihydropyridine class of Ca^{2+} antagonists selectively blocks voltage-dependent Ca^{2+} channels. However, it was recently shown in patch-clamped isolated VSM cells from rat mesenteric artery and rabbit ear artery that only the Ca^{2+} current passing through the slowly inactivated "L" type Ca^{2+} channels is affected by dihydropyridine agonists and antagonists, being respectively enhanced by the former and blocked by the latter.[51,52] Hence, it cannot be assumed that agonist induced Ca^{2+} influx and mechanical responses of VSM remaining in the presence of dihydropyridines is necessarily mediated by nonvoltage-dependent Ca channels.

In summary, a contraction without depolarization has been demonstrated mostly in VSM of larger blood vessels. However, there is little convincing evidence to suggest that such pharmacomechanical coupling occurs *in vivo* in the absence of VSM membrane depolarization in the small resistance and capacitance vessels directly involved in the regulation of blood pressure. The conflicting evidence presented here for pharmacomechanical vs. electromechanical coupling and for the existence of NE sensitive ROCs emphasizes the poorly understood heterogeneity of VSM membrane properties at varying locations in the cardiovascular system. Accurate generalizations about these properties and functions must await clarification of the physiological function of the multitude of VSM membrane channels that contribute to this heterogeneity.[50,52]

III. MECHANICAL AND ELECTRICAL ALTERATIONS OF VSM IN HYPERTENSION

A. Altered Vascular Structure in Hypertension

Interest in the possible contribution of altered vascular wall structure to the generation of an elevated TPR in the pathogenesis of hypertension has continued ever since the early demonstration by Tobian and Binion[138] of increased water and Na^+ contents in postmortem specimens of renal arteries from hypertensive patients. Increased vascular wall water and ion contents were demonstrated in many early studies that focused primarily on renal and steroid animal models of hypertension. In these early studies a vessel wall swelling with consequent reduction in lumen diameter was postulated to result from such increases and to contribute to the elevated TPR in both animal models and human essential hypertension.[141] However, later studies demonstrated that ion accumulation (e.g., Na^+) and waterlogging of the vascular wall occur early in the development of renal and DOCA-salt hypertension but not in the SHR.[85,139,140]

Later, Folkow and co-workers (and other investigators) demonstrated an increased baseline flow resistance upon complete relaxation of VSM and an increased vascular reactivity to neural and humoral stimuli in several perfused regional vascular beds. These included hindlimb, myocardium, and kidney in both animal models and humans with essential hypertension. Reactivity was defined in terms of the rate of increase and maximum calculated resistance generated by increasing concentrations of agonist in the blood perfusing a vascular bed at constant flow. Both baseline flow resistance and vascular reactivity increases can be interpreted as evidence for an increased adventitial and medial hypertrophy that occur in resistance vessels as a structural adaptation in response to the elevated intraluminal pressure and consequent increase in passive wall tension. The importance of these concepts is well described in Folkow's two comprehensive reviews.[2,142] In the case of the SHR, a genetic predisposition is also suggested as a cause for the hypertrophy.[2] Demonstration of an early amino acid incorporation into SHR myocardium and resistance vessels lends further support for such structural adaptation.[143] In addition, Lee has described initiation of a VSM hyperplasia in 128 μm diameter muscular small artery and 50 μm diameter arteriolar mesenteric blood vessels isolated from 3- to 4-week-old SHR. Such young animals were determined to be in a prehypertensive state.[144] At least one stimulus for such early hyperplasia in these mesenteric resistance vessels appears to be a trophic effect attributable to an equally early overactive sympathetic efferent neural input.[145] Comparative morphometric measurements made by Lee et al.[146] and by Mulvany et al.[147] on small mesenteric vessels from SHR in the later developing and in the more established phase of hypertension demonstrate a correlation between increasing blood pressure, media thickness, and vascular wall media to lumen diameter ratio. Also, the data of both investigators support the hypothesis of an increased geometric gain in hypertension. This hypothesis postulates that the increased media thickness resulting primarily from VSM cell hyperplasia in the SHR mesenteric resistance vessels, gives rise to a significantly greater reduction in their lumen diameter upon neural or humoral stimulation. Such a structurally mediated gain elevation contributes significantly to the elevated vascular resistance observed in the mesenteric bed of SHR with established hypertension.[2,142]

However, the data of Lee et al.[144-146] do not indicate that the elevated media thickness to lumen diameter ratio includes a diameter reduction in relaxed small arteries from SHR with established hypertension. Hence, their data negate encroachment of the thickened wall upon the lumen as an explanation for the increased baseline resistance observed in perfused vascular beds of both animal models and humans with hypertension.[2,142] Lee's data also do not agree with the smaller calculated lumen diameter reported by Mulvany and co-workers[4,7,147,148] for relaxed SHR small mesenteric resistance vessels of similar size and age. This difference has been attributed by Lee and co-workers[146] to differences in the level of relaxation of the vessels during the time of fixation. Since these two groups of investigators used different perfusion fluids and mechanical techniques (i.e., wire mounting vs. *in situ* perfusion) for relaxation during preparation of the vessels for fixation, it is difficult to compare their results.

When normalized to media thickness, *in vitro* small mesenteric and cerebral resistance vessel segments from SHR with established hypertension have been reported to exhibit no change[147] or a decreased[148] active stress response to a 10 μM NE + 125 mM KCl stimulus compared to WKY. This suggests a possible reduction in active force generation on a per muscle cell basis particularly in the mesenteric resistance vessels where both a hyperplasia and hypertrophy have been observed.[147,149] However, based on morphometric measurements, Mulvany and co-workers[7,147,150] have calculated that the maximum force generating capacity of the individual smooth muscle cells of SHR and WKY mesenteric vessels is the same both in absolute terms and per cell cross-sectional area. Relative to this possibility, it is of interest that the amounts of actin and myosin, when normalized to DNA content, were unchanged as measured in small mesenteric arteries, but are decreased by 25 and 49%, respectively, in the small posterior cerebral arteries from 25-week-old SHR and WKY.[151] These results are in agreement with our observed lack of difference in the depolarization produced by 10 μM NE or by 100 mM K in VSM of *in vitro* segments of small mesenteric arteries from SHR and WKY with established hypertension.[47,48] In summary, strong evidence exists in support of a genetically facilitated, pressure-induced, adaptive cardiovascular structural alteration in both resistance and capacitance blood vessels that contributes to the maintenance of established hypertension once it is initiated. The evidence particularly favors an elevated geometric gain attributable to hypertrophy of the vascular wall. Evidence for a reduced lumen in nonstimulated (i.e., relaxed) blood vessels in hypertensive subjects is conflicting.

B. Altered Mechanical Sensitivity of VSM in Hypertension

In addition to vascular structural changes, a variety of quantitative and qualitative changes in the mechanisms regulating contractile responses of isolated blood vessels have also been reported for both pre- and established hypertensive animals. Thus, functional alterations of active tone at the level of the VSM cell also can contribute to hypertension both in animal models and humans. Two unanswered questions include the nature and extent of alteration of: (1) *extrinsic* neural and humoral mechanisms regulating VSM tone and (2) *intrinsic* membrane coupled excitation-contraction (e-c) steps that regulate activator Ca^{2+} (and hence tone) in VSM prior to and during development of hypertension. As pointed out by Mulvany,[148] abnormalities of vascular e-c properties in hypertension are rather small and difficult to demonstrate. Further, their causal relationship to hypertension has not been clearly demonstrated. For example, the effectiveness of antihypertensive drugs acting as excitatory VSM receptor antagonists clearly illustrates that reductions in VSM sensitivity (e.g., expressed as an elevated EC_{50} for the agonists) can cause changes in blood pressure. However, it is difficult to establish that an increased VSM cell sensitivity per se to endogenous neural or humoral stimuli (usually determined in an *in vitro* vessel preparation) is necessarily a primary *in situ* mechanism for elevation of the TPR in any specific form of hypertension. An increasing number of factors continue to be recognized as primary modulators of intrinsic sensitivity of VSM even in *in vitro* isolated vessel preparations. Lack of control continues to contribute significantly to the extreme variability of vascular responses to neural and humoral stimuli observed in hypertension when these responses are measured in vessels of different size and location. Lack of control also continues to hinder accurate assessment and clear explanation of changes in VSM sensitivity that may precede and/or accompany development of hypertension in both animal models and in man.[153,154] Included in these factors are

1. Primary cause of hypertension
2. Time of measurement in the course of hypertension
3. The anatomical location of the involved vascular beds and vessels within them
4. Technique used to evaluate changes in sensitivity (e.g., use of perfused vascular beds vs. isolated vessel segments; pressurized, perfused vessels vs. wire-mounted vessels or isolated vessel strips; level of initial perfusion pressure, flow or passive tension, etc.)
5. Magnitude of presynaptic neuronal uptake of agonist (for example, NE)
6. Functional status of the vascular endothelium

Despite lack of awareness and/or control of some of these factors in many studies, a large amount of evidence has been accrued favoring an elevated intrinsic VSM sensitivity to

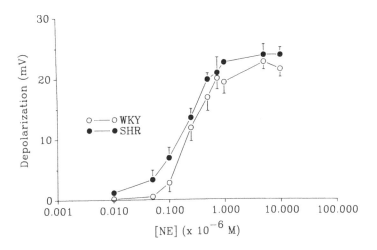

FIGURE 6. NE dose-electrical response curves for SHR and WKY small mesenteric artery segments wire-mounted in a Mulvany-Halpern type myograph. Mean E_m values for each point were calculated from means of approximately 5 impalements per vessel from each of 8 rats. ED_{50} values for NE were not significantly different between SHR and WKY.

exogenously applied neurotransmitters and circulating humoral agents. Such elevated sensitivity has been demonstrated in both isolated vessels and intact perfused vascular beds of animals with various forms of hypertension. For an in-depth review, see References 2, 7, 142, 153, and 154. However, because of the poorly understood modulating factors listed above, there is also little agreement as to the causes of this elevated intrinsic VSM sensitivity. Further, the existence of a structurally independent elevation in sensitivity has not been clearly established even for a specific agonist and vessel type isolated from a well studied animal model of hypertension. For example, NE sensitivity of isolated rat caudal artery with presynaptic nerve terminal NE uptake eliminated has been reported increased,[70,155] unchanged,[156,157] and decreased[158] in the SHR model with established hypertension. Also, contrary to results obtained by others,[159,160] we[47,48] (Figures 6 and 7) and our colleague, Dr. Nancy Rusch[245] have not been able to detect an elevated electrical or mechanical sensitivity to NE (i.e., decreased EC_{50}) when measured in PSS suffused, denervated, small segments of mesenteric resistance arteries isolated from SHR with established hypertension. The reason for this lack of agreement is unclear but may be related to differences in passive VSM lengths at which the sensitivity measurements were made. Coskinas and Price[161] have shown recently that NE sensitivity is a function of passive VSM cell length and preload. Thus, they found no differences in NE sensitivity of SHR and WKY aortic rings maintained at equal VSM cell lengths.

However, differences have been reported in VSM cell membrane properties that could underlie elevated agonist sensitivity in SHR resistance and capacitance vessels. In a recent study, Bevan and Nyborg[162] demonstrated a significant increase in both the pD_2 and pK_a for NE in isolated small mesenteric arteries from SHR. From this they concluded that sensitivity to this agonist is elevated due to a greater affinity of the NE recognition site on the α_1 adrenoreceptors. In an earlier important series of measurements, Mulvany and co-workers[7,163-165] showed that at low Ca^{2+}_o concentrations, NE-dependent Ca^{2+} sensitivity (determined by a cumulative increase in Ca^{2+}_o in the presence of 10 μM NE) is significantly greater in isolated small mesenteric resistance vessels from SHR (ED_{50} for $Ca^{2+} = 0.1$ mM) compared to WKY ($ED_{50} = 0.2$ mM). This difference was significant over a Ca^{2+}_o range of 0.05 to 0.2 mM in both 4-week and 4-month SHR and was not affected by antihypertensive therapy or chronic sympathectomy.[163,164] Increase in NE-activated Ca^{2+}_o sensitivity in SHR vessels was also observed in small branches of the femoral

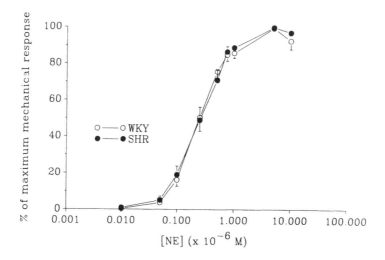

FIGURE 7. NE dose-mechanical response curves for SHR and WKY small mesenteric artery segments wire-mounted in a Mulvany-Halpern type myograph. Mean E_m values for each point were calculated using 8 vessels, 1 from each of 8 rats. ED_{50} values for NE were not significantly different between SHR and WKY.

artery[164] and portal vein,[166] but not in tail artery.[158] It was also not observed in small mesenteric arteries of WKY rats made hypertensive by the two kidney, one clip Goldblatt procedure.[164,167] Maintenance of an elevated NE-dependent Ca^{2+} sensitivity in chemically sympathectomized SHR and SHR made normotensive by antihypertensive therapy supports the hypothesis that an inherent (i.e., genetically induced) increase in P_{Ca} exists in the VSM membrane of certain SHR vessels. It is of interest that this difference in Ca^{2+}_o sensitivity can be eliminated by exposing the vessels to the Ca antagonist felodipine in concentrations which inhibit potential-dependent but not receptor-dependent responses.[167] Thus, it is possible that NE, by means of its depolarizing action via increases in P_{Na} and P_K (see Section II.B), opens POCs in the SHR VSM membrane which are more permeable to Ca^{2+} and/or have a higher surface density.[167] The functional importance of this elevated Ca sensitivity of VSM in SHR vessels relative to its possible contribution to the elevated TPR remains to be established since no differences were observed in the SHR and WKY resistance vessel contractile responses to NE at Ca^{2+} concentrations normally present *in vivo* (i.e., 1.6 mM).[163,167]

In their studies of altered structural and functional properties of VSM in hypertension, Mulvany and co-workers[117,163] did not observe any difference in K+ sensitivity between SHR and WKY isolated small mesenteric vessels. This is in agreement with our own unpublished observations. However, an elevated K+ sensitivity has been reported recently for isolated femoral artery from SHR with early developing and established hypertension (i.e., at 6, 13, and 30 weeks of age)[168] and for large mesenteric artery from SHR with established hypertension (10 weeks of age).[169] The femoral artery of 6-week SHR was also reported to be more sensitive to the Ca^{2+} agonist Bay K 8644 suggesting that the POCs for Ca^{2+} may be partially activated before and after the development of elevated blood pressure. In their study, MacKay and Cheung[169] showed that the isolated large mesenteric artery of SHR is more sensitive to the phorbol ester, phorbol 12,13-dibutyrate (PDBu) as well as to K+ and Bay K 8644. This phorbol ester has been shown to produce contractions that are at least partially dependent upon a Ca^{2+} influx[170] which can be inhibited by the Ca^{2+} entry blocker nifedipine.[169] Based on these observations and on an *in vitro* measured 10 mV reduction in E_m of the mesenteric artery from SHR, MacKay and Cheung[169] suggest that the elevated K+ and Bay K 8644 sensitivity may be due to an elevated VSM membrane excitability. The increased reactivity of SHR VSM to PDBu may be due to changes in membrane regulated e-c coupling and recruitment of new POCs for Ca^{2+}. However, the functional importance of this elevated K$^+$ sensitivity of VSM in SHR vessels relative to its possible contribution to the elevated TPR also remains to be established since significant differences were observed only at K^+_o concentrations well beyond the normal *in vivo* physiological range existing in either SHR or WKY.[16,36]

In addition to the many studies suggesting that an enhanced VSM sensitivity to neural and humoral input contributes significantly to the elevated TPR in hypertension, other studies using a variety of vascular preparations report evidence favoring a decreased ability of VSM from hypertensive animals to undergo active relaxation. However, as in studies of sensitivity to vasoconstrictors, the heterogeneity of response is a function of vessel preparation, type of hypertension, and the "test" vasodilator agonist employed. Thus, once again, the evidence is conflicting. For example, aortic strip preparations from SHR have been shown to undergo decreased, no change, and increased ability to relax actively in response to such vasodilators as isoproterenol, acetylcholine, nitroprusside, nitroglycerin, and papaverine (see review by Webb[153] for extensive references). However, at the membrane and subcellular level there is good evidence in support of an impaired ATP-dependent sequestration of activator Ca^{2+} by intracellular and plasma membrane vesicle preparations isolated from VSM of small and large arteries of both SHR and DOCA-salt hypertensive rats.[171-174] According to Kwan and Daniel,[175] there is no convincing evidence that the Ca^{2+} sequestration by endoplasmic reticulum is functionally altered in VSM in hypertension. Further, it is the active outward transport of Ca^{2+} (rather than membrane binding of Ca^{2+}) that is reduced in plasma membrane vesicles prepared from hypertensive rats compared to normotensive controls.[175] In addition, this reduction in ATP-dependent Ca^{2+} transport is coupled with an increase in membrane alkaline phosphatase activity. Both of these changes precede the blood pressure elevation in SHR and are reversed in DOCA-salt hypertensive rats that exhibit a return of blood pressure toward normal upon DOCA withdrawal. Thus, the reduced efficacy of an ATP-dependent Ca^{2+} extrusion mechanism and an increased alkaline phosphatase activity suggest a causal role for an intrinsic defect in the Ca^{2+} transport function of the VSM cell membrane in the generation of genetic, renal, and DOCA-salt induced models of hypertension. However, little is known about the real biochemical and/ or the methodological factors that may play a role in reducing Ca^{2+} extrusion in VSM of hypertensive animal models (e.g., increased g$_{Ca}$ of the VSM membrane; decreased efficiency of a VSM membrane Ca^{2+} pump; increased proportion of right-side-out vs. inside-out plasma membrane vesicles). As emphasized by Kwan and Daniel,[175] valid techniques for assessment of permeability, orientation, and intactness of isolated membrane vesicles have not been established for smooth muscle membranes.

One new factor recently discussed undoubtedly has contributed to the conflicting evidence in support of an altered intrinsic VSM cell tone and sensitivity to excitatory and inhibitory vasoconstrictor stimuli in *in situ* and *in vitro* vessel preparations from hypertensive subjects. This is the extent of vascular endothelial cell integrity and function. Unfortunately, many of the studies designed to evaluate the role of altered VSM sensitivity in hypertension were performed prior to the pioneering work of Furchgott and co-workers demonstrating the critical role of the endothelium in modulating VSM tone. Using strips of rabbit thoracic aorta, Furchgott and Zawadzki[176] demonstrated that low concentrations of ACh can combine with muscarinic receptors on endothelial cells to release an endothelial cell-derived relaxing factor (EDRF).[177] This as-yet unidentified substance actively dilates most arteries and some veins that are under either spontaneous or agonist-induced tone.[135] The early work of Furchgott and colleagues has been confirmed in many more recent studies which have also demonstrated that the vasodilatory action of a variety of both physiological and pharmacological agents is mediated via an EDRF. (e.g., ADP; ATP; thrombin; bradykinin; trypsin; peptides such as VIP, substance P, and Ca^{2+} gene-related peptide; histamine, hydralazine, the Ca^{2+} ionophore, A23187, and mellitin).[135,178,180,181]

EDRF-mediated relaxation occurs through activation of a guanylate cyclase which converts guanosine triphosphate into a 3′,5′-cyclic GMP (cGMP). This, in turn, activates a cGMP-dependent protein kinase which phosphorylates specific proteins of the contractile apparatus and of the Ca^{2+} regulatory system leading to relaxation. Thus, the relaxing action of EDRF and of the nitric oxide released from the endothelium-independent vasodilator, nitroprusside, are mediated through the common soluble guanylate cyclase pathway.[135,177-181] Similar EDRF-mediated vasodilation also has been demonstrated in small resistance arteries that directly support the elevated TPR in hypertension.[182,183] Changes in EDRF-mediated relaxation are of particular relevance to the study of altered VSM sensitivity in hypertension since such relaxation can attenuate the direct vasoconstrictor action of neurotransmitters and endogenous humoral vasoconstrictor agents.[181] For example, combination of NE or serotonin with respective α_2 and S_1 membrane receptors on endothelial cell membranes of canine and porcine coronary arteries can lead to EDRF-mediated attenuation of the contractile response of these agonists via respective α_1 and S_2 receptors on the VSM membrane.[181,184]

More recent studies have demonstrated that endothelial cells not only release an EDRF, but one or more EDCFs (i.e., endothelium derived vasoconstrictor substances) which can contribute to endothelium-mediated excitatory responses.[180,185] Known stimuli for such EDCF release include arachidonic acid (particularly in systemic and pulmonary veins),[180,186] vascular wall stretch (canine basilar and feline middle cerebral artery),[187,188] ACh and serotonin (aorta of SHR),[189] and acute anoxia/hypoxia (systemic, cerebral, coronary, and pulmonary arteries and veins).[180] The EDCF released in response to hypoxia differs from that released in response to arachidonic acid, stretch, or ACh since endothelium-dependent hypoxic contractions are not prevented by inhibitors of cyclooxygenase.[180,186]

Currently, little is known about the physiological importance *in situ* of the EDRF and EDCF mechanisms for regulation of peripheral resistance in normotensive subjects relative to other vasoactive mechanisms. Need for further study of this question is obvious since even less is known about the role observed changes in these mechanisms may play in the development and/or maintenance of hypertension. It is now clear that the release and VSM action of EDRF differ with vessel type, location, and stimulus.[135,191] However, some tentative conclusions about altered endothelium-mediated vascular responses in hypertension can be drawn from studies reported to date. First, the maximal response to endothelium-dependent vasodilators in endothelium-intact, actively contracted, large conduit arteries, resistance arteries, and arterioles from hypertensive animals is significantly decreased relative to the response of endothelium-intact normotensive controls. This has been observed in a variety of experimental hypertensive rat models (e.g., genetic, renal, DOCA-salt, Dahl S, and aortic coarctation).[182,186,190-198] Second, though some of these studies report a small decrease in the endothelium-independent vasodilator sensitivity of the artery preparations from hypertensive animals relative to controls, most report no difference in the concentration of the endothelium-independent vasodilator (e.g., nitroprusside) required to produce maximum (i.e., 100%) relaxation.[189,192-195,197,198] Third, antihypertensive therapy can prevent or restore the depressed endothelium-mediated vasodilation in hypertensive rats to levels exhibited by normotensive controls in parallel with arterial pressure reduction. Such reversal has been observed in isolated aorta preparations from DOCA-salt and 1K,1C renovascular hypertensive rats[193] and Dahl S rats.[197]

The overall conclusion from these reversal studies is that the loss of endothelium-dependent vasodilation is a result, rather than a cause, of blood pressure elevation in hypertension. Currently, the mechanism(s) responsible for the attenuation of EDRF-mediated relaxation in vessels from hypertensive animals is/are not clear. Based on measurements made on both large and small arteries from both genetic and renal hypertensive rats, it has been suggested that synthesis and/or release of EDRF by endothelial cells is impaired.[192,193,195-197] This could result from changes in replication rate, vessel lumen surface density, or surface morphology of the endothelial cell.[193,199] However, using a bioassay technique, Van de Voorde and Leusen[194] have demonstrated that depression of endothelium-dependent relaxation is not due to a diminished

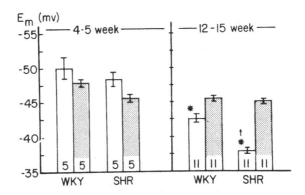

FIGURE 8. *In situ* VSM transmembrane potentials (E$_m$) of small mesenteric arteries topically suffused with physiological salt solution in 4- to 5-week-old and 12- to 15-week-old SHR and WKY. Open columns: innervated arteries; shaded columns: arteries sympathetically denervated locally by pretreatment with 6-hydroxydopamine. Column heights represent mean E$_m$ ± SE in mV. Number of animal preparations listed at base of each column. * Mean E$_m$ in 12- to 15-week-old SHR and WKY significantly less than in respective 4 to 5 wk old animals. † Mean E$_m$ in SHR vessel significantly less than in WKY vessel at same age. (From Stekiel, W. J. et al., *Am. J. Physiol.*, 250, C547, 1986. With permission.)

release of EDRF from aorta of renal and DOCA-salt hypertensive rats. They suggest that the most probable cause for depression of endothelium-mediated relaxation in vessels from hypertensive animals is a defect in the coupling mechanism between EDRF and the VSM cell. Their suggestion is based on the observed short half-life of EDRF (approximately 6 s)[180,181] and the possibility of an increase in diffusion pathway for EDRF due to the demonstrated thickening of the subendothelial layer.[198] A third plausible mechanism that may participate in the decreased arterial relaxation by endothelium-dependent vasodilators in hypertensive animals is a "push-pull" mechanism involving simultaneous release of EDRF and EDCF. Release of a prostaglandin-like EDCF by ACh has been demonstrated in relaxed rings of aorta from SHR but not WKY rats.[189]

This brief description of research on altered endothelial cell control of VSM tone in hypertensive animal models brings attention to an additional complex factor that must be clarified before a satisfactory understanding of the mechanisms of elevated peripheral vascular tone in hypertension can be achieved.

C. Altered Electrical Responses in Hypertension

As discussed in Section II.D, a tight electromechanical coupling has been demonstrated *in vitro* in VSM of blood vessels from both hypertensive and normotensive animals.[9,10,12,48] Thus, longitudinal *in situ* and *in vitro* measurements of E$_m$ changes in individual VSM cells provide an additional parameter to help quantify alterations in extrinsic and intrinsic control of VSM tone that occur with age and contribute to the elevated TPR in hypertension.

Our own *in situ* measurements of E$_m$ in small mesenteric arteries and veins in SHR and WKY as a function of age and sympathetic neural input demonstrate the value of such electrical data.[100] These vessels do not routinely exhibit spontaneous action potentials *in situ* or *in vitro* when suffused with normal PSS. They also respond to humoral stimuli (e.g., NE, AVP, K$^+$) with graded rather than phasic depolarization.[9,10,12,13,46-48,100] Figures 8 and 9, respectively, illustrate mean E$_m$ measured *in situ* in small (150- to 250-μm O.D.) mesenteric arteries and in small (200- to 400-μm O.D.) mesenteric veins in anesthetized SHR and WKY at 4 to 5 weeks of age (initial

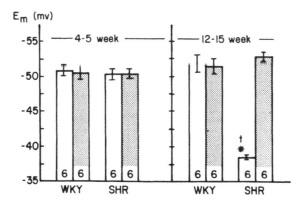

FIGURE 9   *In situ* VSM E$_m$ values of small mesenteric veins in 4-to 5- and 12- to 15-week-old SHR and WKY. Column designation and symbols for significant differences are the same as for Figure 8. (From Stekiel, W. J. et al., *Am. J. Physiol.,* 250, C547, 1986. With permission.)

stage of hypertension) and 12 to 15 weeks of age (established stage of hypertension). The nonshaded columns in Figure 8 illustrate that VSM in *in situ* innervated small mesenteric arteries in SHR with established, but not with initial, hypertension were significantly less polarized (smaller absolute magnitude of E$_m$) than respective WKY control arteries. Figure 9 illustrates that the same was true for the small mesenteric veins in the SHR with established hypertension. The shaded columns in Figures 8 and 9 illustrate that local *in situ* sympathetic neural denervation with 6-hydroxydopamine leads to a significantly greater hyperpolarization of VSM in both small mesenteric arteries and veins of SHR relative to WKY, but only during the established phase of hypertension. These observations suggest that an elevated sympathetic input to both resistance and capacitance vessels is a major cause of the elevated VSM tone underlying the increased TPR in SHR with established hypertension. This follows from the observation that after denervation, the mean E$_m$ values in the SHR vessels were no longer different from mean E$_m$ of respective WKY control vessels. The increased sympathetic neural tone in VSM of the small mesenteric veins in adult SHR suggests a consequent reduction in venous capacitance. As discussed in Section I.B, this would be necessary as hypertension develops in order to maintain an optimal cardiac filling of a hypertrophied left ventricle[2] and to maintain normal cardiac output in the face of elevated TPR.[5,23] We have recently demonstrated similar *in situ* E$_m$ responses in small branches of the femoral artery and vein supplying the anterior gracilis muscle in SHR and WKY with established hypertension.[200,244]

These results are in agreement with a significant body of other evidence in support of an elevated sympathetic neural input to peripheral vascular beds during the early established phase of SHR hypertension.[16,36] For example, the study of Thorén and Ricksten,[201] using a single nerve fiber recording technique to avoid the errors inherent in whole nerve recording, is particularly relevant. These investigators demonstrated a significant elevation in spontaneous renal sympathetic efferent single nerve fiber activity in anesthetized, adult SHR (3.3 ± 0.45 Hz) relative to WKY controls (1.6 ± 0.23 Hz). Additionally, Nilsson and Folkow[202] have observed a hyperresponsiveness of isolated segments of small mesenteric artery from adult SHR to perivascular neural stimulation. They have attributed this elevated response to an increased release of NE neurotransmitter per neural impulse due either or both to a greater release capacity of the individual nerve terminals or a denser sympathetic innervation in adult SHR vessels.[202,203] The latter possibility is of particular interest since increases in neuronal activity can increase the density of neuroeffector junctions per VSM cell.[204] Further, the elevated heart rate and cardiac output, but not TPR, observed in young SHR suggest that sympathetic neural control may be

Table 1
**IN SITU VS. IN VITRO COMPARISON OF MEAN E$_m$ LEVELS IN VSM OF
12- TO 15-WEEK-OLD SHR AND WKY**

Vessel and conditions	WKY		SHR	
	N	Mean E$_m$, mV	N	Mean E$_m$, mV
Small mesenteric artery				
In situ				
Innervated	11	−43 ± 0.9	11	−38 ± 0.5
6-OHDA denervated	11	−45 ± 0.3	11	−45 ± 0.2[a]
In vitro				
Innervated	31	−56 ± 0.3[b]	22	−57 ± 0.3[b]
6-OHDA denervated	31	−56 ± 0.3[b]	22	−57 ± 0.4[b]
Small mesenteric vein				
In situ				
Innervated	6	−52 ± 1.0	6	−38 ± 0.3
6-OHDA denervated	6	−52 ± 1.3	6	−53 ± 0.8[a]
In vitro				
Innervated	33	−52 ± 0.3	34	−53 ± 0.3
6-OHDA denervated	34	−53 ± 0.3	24	−52 ± 0.3

Note: Values are means ± SE. Mean E$_m$ was calculated using N vessel preparations with 1 per animal and average of 5 to 10 impalements per vessel for each value. VSM, vascular smooth muscle cells; 6-OHDA, 6-hydroxydopamine.

[a] Significant hyperpolarization upon denervation in situ in SHR vessels only.

[b] Denervated as well as innervated arteries of SHR and WKY significantly more polarized in vitro than *in situ*.

From Stekiel, W. J., Contney, S. J., and Lombard, J. H., *Am. J. Physiol.,* 250 (*Cell Physiol.,* 19), C547, 1986. With permission.

significantly elevated selectively to the heart but not to the small mesenteric vessels in either SHR or WKY at 4 to 5 weeks of age.[23,100] Such selectivity would explain why the magnitude of E$_m$ *in situ* is not reduced and hyperpolarization is not observed in response to 6-OHDA denervation in small mesenteric arteries and veins of the young SHR (Figures 8 and 9).[100]

Multiple reports of an increased vascular tissue content and release of NE, as well as an increased activity of NE synthesizing enzyme provide additional evidence in favor of a gradually elevated sympathetic neural control of peripheral vascular beds in SHR. Such elevations have been demonstrated during developing (6 weeks of age) and early established hypertension in both mesenteric and caudal arteries of SHR, SHRSP (stroke prone SHR), and M-SHRSP[205-210] (a new SHR rat strain with an augmented rate of development of hypertension). However, it must be noted that hyperreactivity of the sympathetic nervous system and an elevated NE content of blood vessels may not be directly correlated in all models of hypertension. Thus, in DOCA-salt hypertension, where there is indirect evidence for an elevated neurogenic component for control of TPR and cardiac output,[6,211] the circulating level of NE is increased and the content of mesenteric and renal artery and cardiac tissues, but not vena cava, aorta, and mesenteric vein, is reported to be reduced. Such reduction has been attributed to an enhanced efflux of NE from sympathetic neural storage sites in these tissues. Such enhanced efflux in turn, is attributed to a sodium-stimulated increase in neurogenic activity and a reduction in the capacity of these sites to store NE.[211,212]

An *in situ* vs. *in vitro* comparison of E$_m$ in VSM of SHR and WKY small mesenteric vessels is also of interest (Table 1).[100] In both the SHR and WKY, the *in situ* small artery VSM is significantly less polarized than *in vitro*, even after sympathetic denervation. In contrast, this was not observed in the small veins, where after denervation the mean *in situ* E_m in the SHR and WKY groups became equal to their respective *in vitro* counterparts. These data suggest that an elevated sympathetic neural input can account for all of the venous depolarization that exists in these vessels *in situ* (and hence all of the increased venous tone, assuming tight electromechanical coupling).

The reason for a smaller *in situ* magnitude of E_m in VSM of the denervated small mesenteric arteries from both SHR and WKY compared to respective *in vitro* magnitudes is not clear, especially if removal of the small artery from its normal environment does not significantly alter its ionic gradients, its membrane pump activity, or its membrane permeability properties. One cause could be the presence of one or more as-yet unidentified circulating agonists that exert a selective and equal depolarizing effect on the small artery, but not small vein, VSM in both SHR and WKY. Another possible cause could be a myogenically induced reduction in E_m resulting from the *in situ* intraluminal pressure not present *in vitro*. However, no difference was evident between the SHR and WKY mean E_m *in situ* following denervation despite the significant difference in mean arterial pressure.[100] Further, to date we have been able to detect a maximum depolarization of only 4 ± 1.3 mV (SHR) and 3 ± 2.0 mV (WKY) depolarization in the small mesenteric arteries when mounted isometrically on wires in the Mulvany-Halpern-type myograph[117] and passively stretched to a pressure equivalent to 200 mmHg).[244] However, Harder et al.[213] have observed an approximately 30 mV depolarization in VSM of SHR and 20 mV depolarization in VSM of WKY measured *in vitro* in the middle cerebral artery mounted as a blind pouch on a small pipette and pressurized to 150 mmHg. These depolarizations were accompanied by a myogenically mediated attenuation of the diameter increase with increasing intraluminal pressure. The attenuation was significantly greater in the SHR cerebral vessels and was Ca^{2+}-mediated as demonstrated by verapamil blockade. Thus, the SHR cerebral vessels exhibit a greater Ca^{2+}-dependent, pressure regulated, myogenic tone that is correlated with a greater VSM depolarization.

These data suggest that the myogenically active VSM in SHR cerebral vessels exhibits a greater stretch-induced increase in P_{Ca} than VSM in WKY control vessels.[213] Such a suggestion is of great current interest for several reasons. First, it addresses the general question concerning mechanisms underlying an altered P_{Ca} across VSM and possibly endothelial cells in hypertensive animals and man. Support for an elevated P_{Ca} in hypertension, particularly in response to stimuli, can also be derived from a variety of other studies including:

1. Increased peripheral vascular resistance upon intravenous infusion of Ca^{2+} into hypertensive but not normotensive patients[214]
2. Increased rate of force development of isolated femoral artery strips from DOCA-salt hypertensive rats upon restoration of Ca^{2+} to the bath PSS[215]
3. Increased NE-dependent Ca^{2+} sensitivity in small mesenteric arteries of SHR[7,163-165]
4. Increased Ca^{2+} influx into VSM of SHR caudal artery in response to NE, but not K^+, stimulation[216]
5. Increased tension response upon restoration of normal Ca^{2+} concentration in PSS bathing isolated strips of aorta from SHR but not WKY[217]

Evidence is conflicting for an elevated P_{Ca} under basal conditions in VSM from hypertensive animals (i.e., with the nonstimulated *in vitro* vessel preparations maintained in normal PSS). Noon et al[218] observed relaxation of aortic strips from SHR, but not WKY, following removal of Ca^{2+} from the bath PSS. From this observation they concluded that cell membranes of VSM in SHR aorta are inherently more leaky to Ca^{2+} than those in WKY aorta. If so, this is not a common defect for all SHR VSM since equal Ca^{2+} influx was measured in nonstimulated VSM of isolated caudal artery rings from SHR and WKY.[216] Thus, it appears that P_{Ca} of Ca^{2+} leak channels in VSM plasma membranes is not altered under basal conditions, at least in caudal arteries of SHR. Another reason for current interest in the inverse relation between pressure-induced decreases in VSM E_m, P_{Ca}, and contractile force is the potential for such measurements to establish the relative contribution made by myogenically induced tone in specific vascular beds to the elevated TPR in hypertensive animal models. A third reason is the potential to further clarify the mechanisms by which abnormal endothelial cell function can contribute to VSM tone in hypertension.

As summarized by Kulberg,[219] numerous recent studies indicate widespread occurrence and functionally diverse stretch-activated ion channels in both animal and bacterial cell membranes. By applying different amounts of suction via patch clamp pipettes sealed to whole cell membrane preparations, these channels have been shown to be gated by membrane expansion or distortion rather than by membrane voltage changes or ligand activation.[219] Of particular interest are the stretch-activated membrane channels in aortic endothelial cells that have been shown to be approximately six times more permeable to Ca^{2+} than to Na^+.[220] Their opening frequency is directly proportional to the membrane stretch supplied by suction. From their results, Lansman et al.[220] suggest that the endothelial cells may act as mechanotransducers. In this capacity they could mediate the arterial contraction demonstrated in response to stretch or pressure[185-188] and the vasodilation demonstrated in response to blood flow mediated shear stress.[221,222] Lansman et al.[220] further propose that the stretch-activated Ca^{2+} influx through channels in endothelial cell membranes may serve as a second messenger to mediate synthesis and release of prostaglandin and EDRF. Possible aberrations in the function of such stretch-activated Ca^{2+} channels in VSM of hypertensive subjects remains to be demonstrated.

As described in Section II (Equations 1 to 3), the passive diffusion component of the E_m in VSM is a function of the concentration gradients and membrane conductances (and permeabilities) for specific ions (e.g., Na^+, K^+, Cl^- and Ca^{2+}). The electrogenic component of this E_m is a function of active transport of these specific ions across the VSM cell membrane. By far, the most intensively studied electrogenic active transport system in VSM of isolated blood vessels from hypertensive subjects is the Na/K pump.[7,12,70,80-86,93,95,96,98,100] This interest stems from the fact that altered Na/K pump activity may play both a causal[95] and compensatory[12,83] role in hypertension.

However, relatively few of the many studies of the role of altered Na/K pump activity in hypertension have incorporated measurements of E_m changes. One of the earliest was that of Hermsmeyer[70] in which he utilized microelectrode measurements of E_m in VSM of *in vitro* caudal artery preparations to demonstrate a compensatory role for the Na/K pump in SHR with established hypertension. In this electrophysiological study, Hermsmeyer indirectly demonstrated a lower K^+_i activity in the VSM cell of SHR caudal artery by linear extrapolation of the E_m vs. log K^+_o relationship to $0\ E_m$. Hence K^+_i activity (not concentration) in VSM of caudal artery was 153 mM in SHR and 171 mM in WKY. This method of assessing K^+_i assumes that it does not change with increasing concentrations of K^+_o in the PSS suffusate. This assumption remains to be verified. According to Hermsmeyer,[70,83] the smaller K^+_i and the associated smaller K^+ transmembrane electrochemical gradient, when coupled with an elevated Na_i activity, would cause the resting E_m to be less negative in VSM of the SHR caudal artery relative to that of the WKY. However, the lack of a difference in E_m upon direct measurement was taken as evidence for an increased activity of electrogenic ion transport in the SHR VSM (i.e., an increased electrogenesis). This increase would at least partially compensate for the increased Na^+_i and decreased K^+_i. Additional evidence for enhanced activity of an electrogenic Na/K pump in VSM of SHR caudal artery was obtained from comparison of the 12 mV (SHR) vs. 5 mV (WKY) ouabain-sensitive hyperpolarization upon elevating K^+_o of the suffusate to 30 mM after a 10 min suffusion with 0 mM K^+_o (see Section II.C).

Fundamental to this interpretation of the E_m data is the hypothesis that the smaller electrochemical gradient for K^+ is the result of an increased P_K (and possibly P_{Na}) across the VSM membrane in the SHR caudal artery. Such increased VSM membrane permeability for Na^+ and

K^+ is considered to be an inherent property present in VSM of SHR, even in the prehypertensive state. As summarized by Jones[71,85] and by Friedman,[223,224] much evidence, based on ion flux and intracellular ionic concentration measurements, is available in support of a prehypertensive elevation in VSM membrane permeability for Na^+, K^+ and Cl^-. This has been demonstrated in several salt-sensitive animal models of hypertension (e.g., SHR, DOCA-salt, and aldosterone hypertensive rats) and in blood cells of humans with essential hypertension. Concomitant with these elevated ion permeabilities is an enhanced compensatory activity of the Na/K pump.[85,224]

Hermsmeyer[70] observed an increased electrical and mechanical sensitivity of denervated, *in vitro,* SHR caudal artery preparations over a range of NE concentrations (i.e., 10^{-7} to 10^{-5} M). In order to explain this increased sensitivity and its possible endogenous contribution to the elevated TPR in the SHR, he postulated that NE can virtually eliminate the electrogenic component of E_m by "short circuiting" it (i.e., by reducing r_m of the VSM membrane due to elevation of g_{Na}, g_K, and g_{Cl}) (see Section II.C). In the absence of the electrogenic component, the remaining diffusion potential component of E_m is smaller in the VSM of SHR tail artery due to the smaller ionic gradient for K^+ (and possibly elevated gradient for Na^+). Consequently, the E_m for the SHR tail artery VSM (but not that for the WKY) would fall in the range for effective electromechanical coupling (i.e., between approximately -47 and -30 mV).[225] Though this interesting and unique hypothesis can explain at least one of the mechanisms that may contribute to an elevated VSM sensitivity in a specific SHR vessel, its supporting data is not universally accepted. First, as described above, the evidence for an increased intrinsic mechanical sensitivity of isolated and denervated SHR caudal artery to exogenous NE is conflicting.[70,155-158] Second, in a more recent study, Cheung[226] showed that the mean E_m of VSM in *in vitro* caudal artery segments from SHR at 8 to 10 weeks of age was 8 mV less negative than that of WKY controls. Third, in his study Cheung also reported that 10^{-3} M ouabain depolarized the *in vitro* caudal artery from both SHR and WKY at 8 to 10 weeks of age but that the magnitude of depolarization was significantly less (approximately 7 mV) in the VSM of SHR vessels. From these data he concluded that the smaller baseline E_m and smaller response to ouabain in SHR with established hypertension is due to a decrease in ouabain-sensitive electrogenic pumping.

However, Cheung's conclusion does not agree with evidence based on measurements of transmembrane flux and intracellular concentration for Na^+, K^+, and Cl^-. As discussed earlier, the latter evidence supports the conclusion that activity of the Na/K pump is enhanced to compensate for elevated ion permeabilities across the VSM membrane in SHR with established hypertension.[85,224] In addition, our own *in vitro* E_m data obtained from VSM of small mesenteric arteries and veins of 12- to 15-week old SHR and WKY also indicate that the SHR VSM membrane Na/K pump activity is increased.[100] Thus first, we found no significant difference in *in vitro* mean E_m between SHR and WKY small arteries (approximately -56 mV) and small veins (approximately -52 mV). Denervation with 6-OHDA had no effect on these mean E_m. Second, the magnitude of the ouabain-sensitive hyperpolarization in response to 15 mM K^+_o (after a 30-min suffusion with 0 mM K^+_o) was 8-fold larger in the SHR small artery and 3-fold larger in the SHR small vein relative to respective WKY controls.[100] These increases could be eliminated completely by 10^{-3} M ouabain. Third, the lack of a difference in mean E_m of denervated VSM in SHR vs. WKY small mesenteric arteries or veins measured *in situ* also does not support a reduction of Na/K pump activity in the SHR VSM. Thus, our *in situ* and *in vitro* E_m measurements support the data of Hermsmeyer and favor an elevated rather than a reduced Na/K pump activity in the mesenteric vessels from SHR with established hypertension. Furthermore, initial results from our current studies indicate that Na/K pump function is not elevated in small mesenteric vessel preparations from young (4- to 5-week-old) SHR before TPR is significantly elevated. Thus baseline mean E_m in VSM of small mesenteric artery or vein of young SHR do not differ from respective mean E_m in young WKY (e.g., approximately -52 mV for small artery and -51 mV for small vein). Mean E_m in each vessel type from the young rats also do not differ from respective values in the older SHR and WKY. In addition, for each vessel type in the young rats, the hyperpolarizing responses to 15 mM K^+_o did not differ between SHR and WKY (approximately 26 mV for small artery and 29 mV for small vein). It is important to note that the hyperpolarizing responses to 15 mM K^+_o in both vessel types from the young WKY were approximately 15-fold greater than responses of respective vessels in the 12- to 15-week-old WKY. The response to 15 mM K^+_o in the young SHR was 2-fold greater for each vessel type compared to the response in the 12- to 15-week-old SHR. Taken together, these data suggest the following hypotheses: (1) the ionic permeabilities (e.g., P$_{Na}$, P$_K$, and possibly P$_{Cl}$) of the VSM membrane in both small mesenteric arteries and veins and in both SHR and WKY decrease with increasing age and (2) this decrease with age is attenuated in the SHR small mesenteric vessels.

Possible mechanisms underlying such attenuation of age-related decreases in VSM membrane permeability to ions are not clear. However, it is tempting to speculate that a gradually increasing sympathetic efferent neural input to both the small resistance and capacitance vessels that develops with age may contribute significantly to this attenuation. Thus, there are several E$_m$ changes that correlate with a greater age-related sympathetic efferent modulation of ion permeabilities in VSM of SHR vessels. These include:[100] (1) a relatively greater depolarization of VSM in SHR vessels upon suffusion with 0 mM K^+_o for a fixed time interval and (2) a relatively greater hyperpolarizing response by the Na/K pump in SHR VSM membrane upon changing from 0 to 15 mM K^+_o; (3) a relatively greater depolarization of VSM in SHR vessels after a fixed time interval at 16°C. These observations are in accord with the reported elevation in calculated P$_{Na}$ and P$_K$ of VSM membranes in aorta and caudal artery of SHR with established hypertension.[85,224] Hence, the greater E$_m$ responses in SHR suggest that the increasing sympathetic neural input significantly attenuates an age-related decrease in P$_{Na}$ and P$_K$ of VSM membranes in SHR vessels. This would induce an increase in electrogenic transport of these ions in order to maintain normal ion concentration gradients across the VSM membrane. Such an hypothesis is in agreement with the results of Campbell et al.[227] who developed a caudal artery transplantation and cross-innervation technique in which vessel segments from SHR or WKY could be placed either into an innervated or denervated anterior chamber of the eye in host SHR or WKY. These investigators demonstrated that cross-transplantation of donor vessel segments into host animals caused crossover conversion of ion transport and NE sensitivity in these vessels to those of the host animal only when the donor vessel was from 2-week-old animals. There was no alteration in VSM membrane properties of the donor vessels when they were taken from 12-week-old SHR.[227] In a further study[228] they found that sympathetic denervation of the eye prevented the crossover of membrane properties. This suggested that it was the sympathetic neural input that accounted for the changes in membrane properties produced by cross transplantation. Thus, on the basis of these data, they postulated that an alteration in VSM membrane ion transport caused by a neural trophic factor precedes, and most likely causes, the increased contractile strength in SHR with established hypertension.[83]

The studies of Pamnani et al.[229] also support an elevated Na/K pump activity in the VSM membrane of SHR with established hypertension. These investigators measured an increase in both ouabain-sensitive and -insensitive ^{86}Rb uptakes in *in vitro* SHR tail artery segments. Their data, coupled with a large number of ^{86}Rb uptake studies in isolated caudal artery from a variety of other animal models of hypertension, form the basis for a dual hypothesis proposed by Haddy and co-workers[95,230,231] to explain the relationship between blood volume, VSM P$_{Na}$, Na/K pump activity, and the elevated TPR. One part of this hypothesis states that VSM membrane Na/K pump activity is elevated in the SHR and Dahl S genetic models of hypertension secondarily in response to an elevated P$_{Na}$ in the VSM cell membrane. These postulated elevations are based on an observed increase in both ouabain-sensitive and -insensitive uptake of ^{86}Rb by the VSM in isolated caudal artery. Na/K pump activity is also assumed to be elevated in the one kidney dexamethasone-treated rat as a result of an observed increase in the ouabain-sensitive fraction of ^{86}Rb uptake. However, the elevation in the Na/K pump activity is attributed to an elevation of membrane-bound Na$^+$-K$^+$ ATPase activity rather than an elevation of VSM P$_{Na}$.[231] Thus, this part of the dual hypothesis agrees with results obtained from ion flux measurements and VSM E_m responses to changes in K^+_o, indicating an elevated Na/K pump activity in genetic hypertension.

As briefly outlined in Section II.C, the second part of Haddy's dual hypothesis invokes an increased plasma concentration of a circulating Na/K pump inhibitor to explain the elevated natriuresis, VSM tone, and TPR observed in low renin, presumably volume-expanded, animal models of hypertension. Such models include one kidney, one wrap dog; one kidney, one clip (1K,1C) rat; one kidney DOCA-salt rat; reduced renal mass rat (RRM). An elevated circulating Na/K pump inhibitor is also postulated in low renin, human essential hypertension.[95,230,231] Current evidence characterizes this inhibitor as a heat- and acid-stable, low molecular weight molecule with ouabain-like action, but with different VSM membrane receptor sites.[232] Its site of storage and/or release is probably in the hypothalamus.[232] The primary evidence supporting the second part of the dual hypothesis is an observed reduction in ouabain-sensitive ^{86}Rb uptake measured *in vitro* in caudal artery segments from each of the above-listed low renin hypertensive models.[95,230,231] Additional evidence includes observation of a reduced ouabain-sensitive ^{86}Rb uptake by caudal artery segments from a normal rat acutely volume expanded (2 h) with iso-osmotic solutions of NaCl or mannitol. Furthermore, supernatants of boiled plasma from saline-expanded rats (and dogs) reduced steady-state ^{86}Rb uptake when applied to caudal arteries from normotensive rats.[233]

Thus, there is much functional evidence to suggest that a natriuretic factor, which inhibits renal tubular Na^+ reabsorption and Na/K pump activity of both the VSM membrane and adrenergic neural terminal membrane,[231] may play a causal role in low renin, volume-expanded hypertension in animals and man.[95,230-232] However, this second part of the Haddy hypothesis is much more controversial than the first for several reasons. One is that the postulated circulating Na/K pump inhibitor still remains to be identified and biochemically characterized.[231,232] A second reason stems from a methodological question concerning the effect of in vitro incubation time on activity of VSM membrane-bound Na/K inhibitor when measured in isolated vessel preparations. According to Haddy,[231] prolonged *in vitro* incubation periods of vessel preparations before measurements are made (example, 4 h) can wash away the inhibitor. He suggests this explanation as a possible reason why his co-workers observed a decrease in Na/K pump activity in isolated tail artery from the one-kidney, DOCA-saline model of hypertension,[234] whereas Friedman[224] and Jones[85] observed an increase. It is important to note that in the absence of an Na/K inhibitor, data from all three of these investigators support an increase in Na/K pump activity in this model because DOCA (and aldosterone) increase P_{Na} of the VSM membrane.

A third source of controversy concerning the role of an Na/K pump inhibitor in elevating TPR in volume-expanded forms of hypertension is the evidence provided by the current studies of Overbeck and co-workers[235-237] refuting the hypothesis that pump suppression in VSM characterizes volume-expanded forms of hypertension. For example, these investigators measured an increase in plasma volume in the hypertensive Dahl S rat on a high salt diet, relative to normotensive Dahl R on a high salt diet and to Dahl S and R rats on a low salt diet. However, despite such plasma volume expansion, they could find no evidence for a decrease in VSM Na/K pump activity in the hypertensive Dahl S rat relative to the normotensive controls (based on measurements of ouabain-sensitive ^{86}Rb uptakes in caudal artery). In fact, ouabain-sensitive uptakes in all Dahl S rats exceeded those of all Dahl R rats. Also, because experimental elevation of Na_i in control rats to levels 60 to 80% above normal did not increase pump activity, the increased pump activity in the high salt Dahl S rats was not attributed to an elevated Na_i. Rather, suggested possibilities included increased pump site density in the VSM membrane, increased surface area of plasma membrane per unit tissue weight, and faster turnover rate per pump site.[235] Similar results were obtained in studies in which ^{86}Rb uptakes were measured to assess Na/K pump activity in caudal artery and aorta in chronic one and two kidney-one clip Goldblatt models of hypertension.[236] As in the Dahl S rat on high salt diet, increases in the activity of the VSM membrane Na/K pump were also observed in the renal models of hypertension. However, unlike the Dahl S rat on a high salt diet, these models (on normal salt intake) were not volume expanded. Again, in this study ^{86}Rb uptake in normotensive aortic control vessels was shown to be independent of Na$_i$ produced by experimental Na$^+$ loading. From the ^{86}Rb uptake measurements with these Goldblatt rat models of hypertension, it was concluded that Na/K pump activity in isolated caudal artery and aorta is not decreased, but increased. Further, these increases did not appear to be related to altered activity of the renin-angiotensin system; to changes in body fluid volumes; or to increases in VSM Na^+_i. As in the Dahl S rat on a high salt diet, the increase in Na/K pump activity in these hypertensive models was attributed to increases in density of VSM membrane pump molecules and/or their turnover rates.[236] To explain the discrepancy between their results and those of Haddy and co-workers[95,230,231] using the same animal models and vessel preparations, Overbeck and Grisette[236] have suggested that a greater severity of hypertension may have been present in the rat models used in the Haddy studies. This may have caused deterioration of renal function and depression of Na/K pump activity due to uremia;[238] however, data for comparison of renal function in these two studies are not available. In a third study by Overbeck,[237] small vessel resistance responses to NE were compared to controls in initially relaxed, blood perfused hind limbs of rats with chronic, benign 1K,1C hypertension (and on high NaCl intake for volume expansion). As in their other studies with *in vitro* conduit vessel preparations from Dahl S and renal hypertensive rat models, this study also did not provide any evidence for a circulating Na/K pump inhibitor which would produce a physiologically significant inotropic enhancement of the vascular resistance response to NE.

The lack of agreement concerning the role of altered Na/K pump activity as a causal agent in genetic, volume-expanded, and nonvolume-expanded renal forms of hypertension stresses the need for other parameters to assess Na/K pump function at the VSM cell level. Thus, in addition to ^{86}Rb uptake measurements, more recent studies of this problem have included E$_m$ measurements in VSM. As proposed in the early studies of the mechanism of K$^+$ vasodilation by Haddy[101,239] and by Overbeck,[102] reduction in the electrogenic Na/K pump activity in VSM also should be accompanied by partial depolarization (i.e., reduction in magnitude of E$_m$) with a consequent increase in VSM tone and/or increase in sensitivity to neural and humoral stimuli.

In one of the first studies of E$_m$ changes in the *in vitro* caudal artery preparation taken from 1K,1C hypertensive rats, Pamnani et al.[240] observed that VSM from hypertensive rats was approximately 7 mV less polarized than VSM from one-kidney sham-clipped normotensive controls. Additionally, plasma supernatants from hypertensive animals significantly depolarized VSM from normotensives but had no effect on E$_m$ from hypertensives. Ouabain depolarized the VSM of caudal artery from normotensives but not from hypertensives. From these results Pamnani et al.[240] concluded that the plasma from the 1K,1C hypertensive rat contains a humoral pump inhibitor which can increase VSM sensitivity through voltage-dependent vasoconstriction and in this manner can contribute to the genesis and maintenance of this type of hypertension. Similar results were obtained in the 1K,1C hypertensive rat in a later follow-up study.[241] In addition, E$_m$ measurements were made in VSM of *in vitro* caudal arteries from a 70 to 80% reduced renal mass (RRM) rat model maintained on 1% NaCl drinking solution (RRM-S). The magnitude of E$_m$ in VSM of caudal artery from the RRM-S vessels did not differ significantly from RRM controls maintained on a 0.02% NaCl drinking solution (RRM-DW). However, when plasma supernatant from an RRM-S rat was applied to one-half of a caudal artery from a normal (i.e., non-RRM) rat, the VSM depolarized by 6 mV. Plasma supernatants from an RRM-DW rat had no effect on the other half of the caudal artery. Thus, once again it was concluded that a circulating agent from the hypertensive rats of both models causes depolarization of VSM from normotensive rats and most likely is the agent which inhibits Na/K pump activity *in situ* in VSM of peripheral vessels in these volume-expanded rat models of hypertension. The lack of difference between mean E$_m$ of RRM-S and RRM-DW rats was suggested to result from loss of inhibitor due to weak binding on VSM membrane Na/K pump sites during the 90 to 120 min of superfusion with PSS.[241]

In a more recent study, Shoemaker and Overbeck[242] observed that the mean E_m level in VSM of *in vitro* caudal artery in 1K,1C hypertensive rats was approximately 4 mV less negative than that of one kidney sham controls. However, this difference was observed only in chronic hypertensives (i.e., greater than 4 weeks). It was not observed in early (2 to 7 d) hypertensives. Also, the depolarizing effect of ouabain was attenuated in the chronic but not early hypertensives when compared to respective controls. In a concomitant study Magargal and Overbeck[243] obtained indirect evidence that fresh, unprocessed plasma from early (<7 d) 1K,1C hypertensive rats contain factors that inhibit the VSM membrane Na/K pump. On the basis of the results of these two studies,[242,243] Shoemaker and Overbeck[242] suggested that a temporal dissociation exists between levels of humoral inhibitors and depolarization and between depolarization and hypertension. They concluded further that their results do not support the hypothesis that there are causal relationships between depolarization and hypertension in volume-dependent, low renin hypertension. However, it is not clear in the studies of early 1K,1C hypertensives[242,243] what fraction of the smaller elevation in systolic blood pressure (compared to that measured in the chronic 1K,1C hypertensives) is the result of an elevated TPR. This is especially important to establish since the fresh, unprocessed plasma from the 1K,1C hypertensive rats applied to the cultured VSM cells only attenuated this increase in cellular ouabain-sensitive ^{86}Rb uptake and Na$^+$ content observed in normotensive controls. It did not produce a decrease in such uptake.[242] It is also not clear whether the plasma factor responsible for such attenuation in early 1K,1C hypertensives is the same as that attenuating ^{86}Rb uptake with VSM depolarization in the chronic 1K,1C hypertensives.

The results of these *in vitro* electrophysiological studies[241,242] emphasize the need for correlated *in situ* measurements of E_m and active VSM tension in resistance and capacitance vessels in all forms of hypertension. Such *in situ* measurements, when properly controlled, should clarify the mechanism and importance of electromechanical coupling in the enhancement of VSM tone, and hence TPR, during the etiology of various forms of hypertension.

IV. SUMMARY

The major purpose of this chapter is to establish the importance of correlative electrical and mechanical measurements in studies designed to clarify extrinsic and intrinsic mechanisms involved in regulation of VSM structure and function in hypertension. It is clear that the extrinsic neural, humoral, and ionic mechanisms controlling VSM tone *in vivo* act through intrinsic structural channels in the VSM membrane to regulate specific ion permeabilities. This regulation is reflected in both the electrical and mechanical responses of the VSM cell. Thus, both electrical and mechanical responses of VSM to intrinsic and extrinsic stimuli in both *in vitro* and *in situ* blood vessel preparations are the most informative parameters available to clarify the mechanisms generating increased active VSM tone in both resistance and capacitance vessels in hypertension. Though less appreciated than the well-established elevation in TPR, a decrease in venous compliance is an equally important hemodynamic change necessary to sustain many forms of hypertension. Thus, a clear need exists for correlative measurement of changes in electrical and mechanical properties of VSM on the venous as well as arterial side of the circulation during the development and maintenance of hypertension.

One of the key electrical properties that can provide useful information about the etiology of hypertension is the transmembrane potential in VSM. As in other electrically excitable cells, the E_m of VSM, though variable in magnitude in different vessels as a function of their VSM membrane properties, is a steady-state variable dependent upon a constant supply of metabolic energy for its maintenance. This is true both for its diffusion potential and electrogenic potential component.

The magnitude of the diffusion potential is a function of both the VSM transmembrane gradients for K$^+$, Na$^+$, Cl$^-$, and the relative membrane permeabilities (or electrical conductances) of these ions. These conductances, in turn, are a function of the surface density and selectivity properties of gated membrane channels for specific ions. Under resting conditions, the diffusion potential component is determined primarily by the gradient for K^+ due to its relatively high resting permeability. Electrical, neural, humoral, and ionic stimulation causes opening of channels specific for each of the above ions and Ca^{2+}. This leads to a concurrent reduction in E_m magnitude and an increase in active contractile force.

The magnitude of the electrogenic component of E_m is primarily a function of the permeability of Na^+ relative to K^+ which, in turn, regulates the rate of the VSM membrane Na/K pump, the coupling ratio for efflux of Na^+ and influx of K^+ (approximately 1.5) and the electrogenic current across the membrane resistance. In VSM the magnitude of the electrogenic component of E_m ranges between approximately 5 and 15 mV. Thus, when this E_m component is "short-circuited" by agonists which increase membrane conductances for K^+, Na^+, and Cl^- (e.g., NE), the VSM E_m is significantly reduced. If the reduction is sufficient, excitation-contraction coupling is initiated and VSM membrane sensitivity to neurohumoral stimuli is increased. In addition to neurohumoral agonists, electrogenic Na/K pump activity is also modulated by changes in VSM membrane permeability for the same ions involved in the maintenance of the diffusion potential component and hence VSM tone. Thus, intense interest has been focused on the relation between changes in VSM tone and the electrogenic Na/K pump in studies designed to explain the elevated TPR in hypertension.

Since changes in electrical properties of VSM are as important to understand as changes in their mechanical properties in order to explain the elevated VSM tone on both the arterial and venous side of the circulation in hypertension, special effort has been expended in this review to establish the importance of electromechanical coupling in VSM. Considerable evidence has been presented in support of the key hypothesis stating that E_m changes in VSM are tightly coupled to changes in VSM active tone over the range of E_m values that exist *in vivo*. Such electromechanical coupling also has been firmly linked to regulation of the VSM intracellular Ca^{2+} activity that, in turn, regulates VSM tone. Though pharmacomechanical coupling has been demonstrated *in vitro* primarily in large diameter vessels, its physiological importance *in vivo* has not been well established. The key question, namely whether endogenous vasoconstrictors and vasodilators, acting via VSM membrane phosphoinositides and endothelial cells, respectively, can exert their effects by pure nonelectrical mechanisms in normally polarized cells *in vivo*, remains to be answered. New methods for measuring electrical currents in single specific ion channels (e.g., patch clamp technique) should provide new data critical for the determination of the relative importance of electromechanical, pharmacomechanical, and "mechano-mechanical" (i.e., stretch-activated) coupling in regulating VSM tone in normo- and hypertensive subjects. Similarly, these methods should also help determine the relative contribution of receptor-operated channels vs. potential-operated channels in regulating VSM tone both in normo- and hypertensive subjects. Current pharmacological evidence for the existence of separate ROCs and POCs in the VSM membrane is indirect and open to criticism. However, recent evidence derived from patch clamp studies lends support to the concept of ROCs for Ca^{2+} when activated by ATP. It is clear that more studies with newer techniques are needed to resolve this question.

It has been well established that both structural changes in the vascular wall as well as functional changes in the VSM cells situated in its media contribute to the elevated TPR (and possible reduction of venous capacitance) in the generation and maintenance of hypertension. The pioneering studies by Folkow and co-workers have conclusively established the importance of a pressure-mediated increase in blood vessel wall to lumen ratio for maintenance of an elevated TPR in virtually all forms of hypertension. Elevations in this ratio have been demonstrated even on the low pressure venous side of the circulation. Consequently, in genetic forms of hypertension an inherent predisposition has been suggested as a cause for the hypertrophy of the vascular wall. There is general agreement that the elevated wall to lumen ratio increases the geometric gain of resistance vessels such that they undergo a greater reduction in their lumen diameters upon neural or humoral stimulation. Thus, it is proposed that this mechanism makes a significant contribution to the elevated TPR in established hypertension. The morphological evidence supporting the concept that the increased wall to lumen ratio also includes a reduction in lumen diameter even under relaxed basal conditions is controversial primarily because of differences in fixation techniques.

Though a great number of studies designed to demonstrate an increased neurohumoral sensitivity of the VSM cell in vessels from both genetic and investigator-generated models of hypertension have been reported, this question still remains to be answered. To date, conflicting affirmative and negative evidence abounds in the literature. Such conflict can be attributed to a variety of factors stemming from the type of hypertension, vessel heterogeneity, mechanical conditions of measurement, extent of local innervation, and condition of the VSM endothelium. Clear evidence from the studies of Mulvany and co-workers with small resistance vessels from SHR supports an elevated NE-dependent Ca^{2+} sensitivity of VSM in resistance vessels. However, the physiological significance of such increased sensitivity as a contributing factor *in situ* to the elevated TPR in hypertension remains to be established since no differences were observed in SHR vessel sensitivity to Ca^{2+} at concentrations normally present *in vivo*.

Thus, most evidence for an increased VSM sensitivity to agonists in hypertension is conflicting. However, fairly clear evidence is available supporting a lesser active outward transport of activator Ca^{2+} by VSM membrane vesicles prepared from small and large arteries of both SHR and DOCA-salt hypertensive rats, even when their pressures are minimally elevated. Thus, reduced Ca^{2+} extrusion from the VSM cell may be a predisposing factor for hypertension. With the discovery of the modulating role played by the vascular endothelium in regulating VSM tone, much interest is being focused currently on its possible role in regulating VSM sensitivity in hypertension. To date, initial evidence from studies performed on both conduit and resistance arteries and arterioles suggests that the maximal response to endothelium-dependent vasodilators is compromised in genetic, Dahl S, renal, and coarctation models of hypertension. However, other evidence indicates that the loss of endothelium-dependent vasodilation is a result, rather than a cause of the hypertension.

An increasing number of studies have been performed that demonstrate the value of VSM E_m measurements in clarifying the mechanisms responsible for elevated active VSM tone in hypertension. *In situ* E_m measurements from our own laboratory support an elevated sympathetic efferent neural input to both resistance and capacitance vessels in the intestinal mesenteric and skeletal muscle beds of the SHR with established hypertension. However, such sympathetic input is not elevated to these beds in young SHR when blood pressure is minimally elevated. These data suggest that sympathetic neural input gradually increases to both resistance and capacitance vessels in SHR. Hemodynamically this would contribute to both the elevated TPR and decreased venous compliance observed in this hypertensive model. Much additional evidence in support of an elevated sympathetic input in SHR is available from direct measurements of sympathetic neural activity, vascular tissue content of NE, and NE turnover at adrenergic neural terminals.

The question concerning the level of activity of the Na/K pump in VSM of various models of hypertension and the existence of a circulating inhibitor for this pump also remains to be settled. On the basis of both ^{86}Rb uptake measurements and *in vitro* E_m measurements in caudal arteries, Haddy and co-workers have obtained considerable evidence for a circulating ouabain-like Na/K pump inhibitor in low renin, volume-expanded models of hypertension. In genetic models of hypertension their evidence indicates that Na/K pump activity in VSM is elevated most likely as a result of an increased P_{Na} across the VSM cell membrane. Their results for the SHR artery are in agreement with the electrophysiological measurements of Hermsmeyer and the ion flux measurements of Jones and Friedman. However, there is disagreement about the level of activity of the Na/K pump in the other rat models of hypertension that are presumably volume expanded. Thus, in the Dahl S and 1K,1C models, Overbeck and co-workers measured an increase in Na/K pump activity in caudal artery on the basis of an increased ^{86}Rb uptake. Hence, these investigators find no evidence for a circulating Na/K pump inhibitor in these rat models of hypertension.

The opposite results of both the ^{86}Rb and electrophysiological studies concerning levels of Na/K pump activity and ion permeability in VSM of these hypertensive rat models emphasize the need for correlated *in situ* measurements of E_m and active tension in resistance and capacitance blood vessels in all forms of hypertension. Properly controlled *in situ* measurements of these two variables should clarify the mechanisms and importance of electromechanical coupling in the enhancement of VSM tone on both the arterial and venous side of the circulation during the etiology of various forms of hypertension.

ACKNOWLEDGMENTS

This work was supported by a grant from the National Institutes of Health (HL 29587).

LIST OF ABBREVIATIONS

E_{diff}: Diffusion potential component of E_m (function of concentration gradients of diffusible ions not in electrochemical equilibrium and their conductances (chord equation) or permeabilities (G.H.K. equation))

E_m: Total electrical potential difference across VSM cell membrane (sum of E_{diff} + E_p)

E_p: Electrogenic potential component of E_m (product of I_p and r_m)

G.H.K. Eq.: Goldman, Hodgkin, Katz equation for E_{diff}

g_{ion}: VSM membrane electrical conductance of designated ion (e.g., g_{Na}, g_K, g_{Ca}, g_{Cl})

Σ_g: Total ionic conductance across VSM cell membrane

Ion_o: Extracellular "ion activity" of designated ion (e.g., Na^+_o, K^+_o, Ca^{2+}_o, Cl^-_o)

Ion_i: Intracellular "ion activity" of designated ion (e.g., Na^+_i, K^+_i, $Ca^{2+}i$, Cl^-_i

I_p: Net ionic current across VSM membrane (due to active transport by Na/K pump with Na-K coupling ratio greater than unity)

Na/K pump: VSM membrane electrogenic sodium-potassium ion pump (reflecting activity of VSM membrane Na-K ATPase)

P_{ion}: VSM membrane permeability for designated ion (e.g., P_{Na}, P_K, P_{Ca}, P_{Cl})

r_m: VSM transmembrane electrical resistance (equal to $1/\Sigma_g$)

r_{in}: Total resistance of amplifier input circuit (including microelectrode and VSM membrane)

*: The "ion activity" is equal to the product of f_{ion} x (concentration)$_{ion}$ where f_{ion}, defined as the activity coefficient, is a function of ion binding with solute and solvent particles in solution.

REFERENCES

1. **Lund-Johansen, P.,** Hemodynamics in essential hypertension, *Clin. Sci.,* 59 (Suppl. 6), 343s, 1980.
2. **Folkow, B.,** Physiological aspects of primary hypertension, *Physiol. Rev.,* 62, 347, 1982.
3. **Tarazi, R. C.,** The hemodynamics of hypertension, in *Hypertension, Physiopathology and Treatment,* 2nd ed., Genest, J., Kuchel, O., Hamet, P., and Cantin, M., Eds., McGraw-Hill, New York, 1983, chap. 2.
4. **Mulvany, M. J.,** Pathophysiology of vascular smooth muscle in hypertension, *J. Hypertension,* 2 (Suppl. 3), 413, 1984.
5. **Frohlich, E. D.,** Is the spontaneously hypertensive rat a model for human hypertension?, *J. Hypertension,* 4 (Suppl. 3), S15, 1986.
6. **Bohr, D.,** What makes the pressure go up? A hypothesis, *Hypertension,* 3 (Suppl. II), 160, 1981.
7. **Mulvany, M. J.,** Do resistance vessel abnormalities contribute to the elevated blood pressure of spontaneously hypertensive rats?, *Blood Vessels,* 20, 1, 1983.
8. **Haeusler, G.,** Contraction, membrane potential, and calcium fluxes in rabbit pulmonary arterial muscles, *Fed. Proc.,* 42, 263, 1983.
9. **Hermsmeyer, K., Trapani, A., and Abel, P. W.,** Membrane potential-dependent tension in vascular muscle, in *Vasodilation,* Vanhoutte, P. M. and Leusen, I., Eds., Raven Press, New York, 1981, 273.
10. **Trapani, A., Matsuki, N., Abel, P. W., and Hermsmeyer, K.,** Norepinephrine produces tension through electromechanical coupling in rabbit ear artery, *Eur. J. Pharmacol.,* 72, 87, 1981.
11. **Harder, D. R., Abel, P. W., and Hermsmeyer, K.,** Membrane electrical mechanism of basilar artery constriction and pial artery dilation by norepinephrine, *Circ. Res.,* 49, 1237, 1981.
12. **Hermsmeyer, K.,** Electrogenic ion pumps and other determinants of membrane potential in vascular muscle, *The Physiologist,* 25, 454, 1982.
13. **Harder, D. R.,** Membrane electrical activation of arterial smooth muscle, in *Vascular Smooth Muscle: Metabolic, Ionic and Contractile Mechanisms,* Crass, J. F. and Barnes, C. D., Eds., Academic Press, New York, 1982, 71.
14. **Harder, D. R. and Waters, A.,** Electrical activation of arterial muscle, *Int. Rev. Cytol.,* 89, 137, 1984.
15. **Okamoto, K. and Aoki, K.,** Development of a strain of spontaneously hypertensive rats, *Jpn. Circ. J.,* 27, 282, 1963.
16. **Yamori, Y.,** Pathogenetic similarities and differences among various strains of spontaneously hypertensive rats, in *Hypertensive Mechanisms,* Rascher, W., Clough, D., and Ganten, D., Eds., F. K. Shattauer, Stuttgart, 1982, 66.
17. **McGiff, J. C. and Quilley, C. P.,** The rat with spontaneous genetic hypertension is not a suitable model of human essential hypertension, *Circ. Res.,* 48, 455, 1981.
18. **Rushmer, R. F.,** *Cardiovascular Dynamics,* 4th ed., W. B. Saunders, Philadelphia, 1976, 206.
19. **Genest, J., Kuchel, O., Hamet, P., and Cantin, M., Eds.,** *Hypertension, Physiopathology and Treatment,* 2nd ed., McGraw-Hill, New York, 1983.
20. **Guyton, A. C.,** *Circulatory Physiology III: Arterial Pressure and Hypertension,* W.B. Saunders, Philadelphia, 1980.
21. **Guyton, A. C.,** Mean circulatory pressure, mean systemic pressure and mean pulmonary pressure and their effect on venous return, in *Circulatory Physiology: Cardiac Output and its Regulation,* W. B. Saunders, Philadelphia, 1973, 193.
22. **Richardson, T. Q., Stallings, J. O., and Guyton, A. C.,** Pressure-volume curves in live, intact dogs, *Am. J. Physiol.,* 201, 471, 1961.
23. **Smith, T. L. and Hutchins, P. M.,** Central hemodynamics in the developmental stage of spontaneous hypertension in the unanesthetized rat, *Hypertension,* 1, 508, 1979.
24. **Pfeffer, M. A. and Frohlich, E. D.,** Hemodynamic and myocardial function in young and old normotensive and spontaneously hypertensive rats, *Circ. Res.,* 32/33 (Suppl. I), 28, 1973.
25. **Ferrone, R. A., Walsh, G. M., Tsuchiya, M., and Frohlich, E. D.,** Comparison of hemodynamics in conscious spontaneous and renal hypertensive rats, *Am. J. Physiol.,* 236, H403, 1979.
26. **Coleman, T. G. and Guyton, A. C.,** Hypertension caused by salt loading in the dog. III. Onset transients of cardiac output and other circulatory variables, *Circ. Res.,* 25, 153, 1969.
27. **Manning, R. D., Jr., Coleman, T. G., Guyton, A. C., Norman, R. A., Jr., and McCaa, R. E.,** Essential role of mean circulatory filling pressure in salt-induced hypertension, *Am. J. Physiol.,* 236, R40, 1979.
28. **Ledingham, J. M.,** Blood pressure regulation in renal failure, *J. R. Coll. Physicians London,* 5, 103, 1971.
29. **Ferrario, C. M. and Page, I. H.,** Current views concerning cardiac output in the genesis of experimental hypertension, *Circ. Res.,* 43, 821, 1978.
30. **Frohlich, E. D.,** Hemodynamics of hypertension, in *Hypertension, Physiopathology and Treatment,* Genest, J., Koiw, E., and Kuchel, O., Eds., McGraw-Hill, New York, 1977, chap. 3.
31. **Safar, M. E., Weiss, Y. A,. London, G. M., Simon, A. C., and Chau, N. P.,** Hemodynamic changes in mild early hypertension, in *Hypertension in the Young and the Old,* Onesti, G., and Kim, K. E., Eds., Grune & Stratton, New York, 1981, chap. 3.

32. **Ricksten, S. E., Yao, T., and Thorén, P.,** Peripheral and central vascular compliances in conscious, normotensive and spontaneously hypertensive rats, *Acta Physiol. Scand.,* 112, 169, 1981.

33. **Safar, M. E. and London, G. M.,** Arterial and venous compliance in sustained essential hypertension, *Hypertension,* 10, 133, 1987.

34. **Julius, S. and Esler, M.,** Autonomic nervous cardiovascular regulation in borderline hypertension, *Am. J. Cardiol.,* 36, 685, 1975.

35. **Messerli, F. H., deCarvalho, J. G. R., Christie, B., and Frohlich, E. D.,** Systemic and regional hemodynamics in low, normal and high cardiac output in borderline hypertension, *Circulation,* 58, 441, 1978.

36. **Yamori, Y.,** Pathophysiology of the various strains of spontaneously hypertensive rats, in *Hypertension, Physiopathology and Treatment,* 2nd ed., Genest, J., Kuchel, O., Hamet, D., and Cantin, M., Eds., McGraw-Hill, New York, 1983, chap. 36.

37. **Herron, E., Green, A., and Cowley A. W., Jr.,** Early hemodynamic changes in reduced renal mass high sodium water hypertension in conscious rats, *Fed. Proc.,* 45 (Abstr.), 301, 1986.

38. **Prosser, C. L., Burnstock, G., and Kahn, J.,** Conduction in smooth muscle. Comparative structural properties, *Am. J. Physiol.,* 199, 545, 1960.

39. **Rhodin, J. A. G.,** Fine structure of vascular walls in mammals with special reference to smooth muscle component, *Physiol. Rev.,* 42 (Suppl. 5), 48, 1962.

40. **Funaki, S.,** Studies on membrane potentials of vascular smooth muscle with intracellular microelectrodes, *Proc. Jpn. Acad.,* 34, 534, 1958.

41. **Ling, G. and Gerard, R. W.,** The normal membrane potential of frog sartorius fibers, *J. Cell. Comp. Physiol.,* 34, 383, 1949.

42. **Graham, J. and Gerard, R. W.,** Membrane potentials and excitation of impaled single muscle fibers, *J. Cell. Comp. Physiol.,* 28, 99, 1946.

43. **Johansson, B. and Somlyo, A. P.,** Electrophysiology and excitation-contraction coupling, in *Handbook of Physiology,* Section II, Vol. 2, Bohr, D. F., Somlyo, A. P., and Sparks, H. V. Jr., Eds. American Physiol. Society, Bethesda, MD, 1980, 301.

44. **Horn, L.,** Electrophysiology of vascular smooth muscle, in *Microcirculation,* Vol. 2, Kaley, G. and Altura, B. M., Eds., University Park Press, Baltimore, 1978, 119.

45. **Hermsmeyer, K.,** Integration of mechanisms in single vascular muscle cells, *Fed. Proc.,* 42, 269, 1983.

46. **Harder, D. R., Contney, S. J., Willems, W. J., and Stekiel, W. J.,** Norepinephrine effect on *in situ* venous membrane potential in spontaneously hypertensive rats, *Am. J. Physiol.,* 240, H837, 1981.

47. **Stekiel, W. J., Contney, S. J., Lombard, J. H., and Willems, W. J.,** Effect of adrenergic denervation on small mesenteric vessel membrane potential response to noradrenaline in spontaneously hypertensive and Wistar-Kyoto rats, in *Hypertensive Mechanisms, The SHR as a Model to Study Human Hypertension,* Rascher, W., Clough, D., and Ganten, D., Eds., F. K. Schattauer, Stuttgart, 1982, 252.

48. **Burke, M. J., Stekiel, W. J., and Lombard, J. H.,** Electromechanical coupling in mesenteric arteries of spontaneously hypertensive and Wistar-Kyoto rats, *Fed. Proc.,* 43(Abstr.), 507, 1984.

49. **Bolton, T. B.,** Mechanisms of action of transmitters and other substances on smooth muscle, *Physiol. Rev.,* 59, 606, 1979.

50. **Bean, B. P., Sturek, M., Puga, A., and Hermsmeyer, K.,** Calcium channels in smooth muscle cells from mesenteric arteries, *J. Gen. Physiol.,* 86, 23a, 1985.

51. **Benham, C. D. and Tsien, R. W.,** Calcium-permeable channels in vascular smooth muscle: voltage-activated, receptor operated, and leak channels, in *Cell Calcium and Control of Membrane Transport,* Mandel, L. J. and Eaton, D. C., Eds., Rockefeller University Press, New York, 1987, 46.

52. **Bean, B. P., Sturek, M., Puga, A., and Hermsmeyer, K.,** Calcium channels in muscle cells isolated from rat mesenteric arteries: modulation by dihydropyridine drugs, *Circ. Res.,* 59, 229, 1986.

53. **Vanhoutte, P. M.,** Heterogeneity in vascular smooth muscle, in *Microcirculation,* Vol. 2, Kaley, G. and Altura, B. M., Eds., University Park Press, Baltimore, 1978, 181.

54. **Hendrickx, H. and Casteels, R.,** Electrogenic sodium pump in arterial smooth muscle cells, *Pfluegers Arch.,* 346, 299, 1974.

55. **Hermsmeyer, K.,** Sodium pump hyperpolarization-relaxation in rat caudal artery, *Fed. Proc.,* 42, 246, 1983.

56. **Hille, B.,** *Ionic Channels of Excitable Membranes,* Sinauer Associates, Sunderland, MA, 1984, 13.

57. **Goldman, D. E.,** Potential, impedance, and rectification in membrane, *J. Gen. Physiol.,* 27, 37, 1943.

58. **Harder, D. R. and Sperelakis, N.,** Membrane electrical properties of vascular smooth muscle from the guinea pig superior mesenteric artery, *Pfluegers Arch.,* 378, 111, 1978.

59. **Sperelakis, N. and Lehmkuhl, D.,** Effect of current or transmembrane potentials in cultured chick heart cells, *J. Gen. Physiol.,* 47, 895, 1964.

60. **Eisenberg, R. S. and Engel, E.,** The spatial variation of membrane potential near a small source of current in a spherical cell, *J. Gen. Physiol.,* 55, 536, 1970.

61. **Hirst, G. D. S. and Nield, T. O.,** An analysis of excitatory junction potentials recorded from arterioles, *J. Physiol.,* 280, 87, 1978.

62. **Harder, D. R. and Sperelakis, N.,** Action potentials induced in guinea-pig arterial smooth muscle by tetraethylammonium, *Am. J. Physiol.,* 237, C75, 1979.

63. **Benos, D. J.,** Amiloride: a molecular probe of sodium transport in tissues and cells, *Am. J. Physiol.,* 242 (*Cell Physiol.,* 11), C131, 1982.

64. **Marty, A. and Neher, E.,** Tight seal whole cell recording, in *Single Channel Recording,* Sakmann, B. and Neher, E., Eds., Plenum Press, New York, 1983, 107.

65. **Lecar, H. and Smith, T. G., Jr.,** Voltage clamping small cells, in *Voltage and Patch Clamping with Microelectrodes,* Smith, T. G., Jr., Lecar, H., Redman, S. J., and Gage, P. W., Eds., American Physiol. Society, Bethesda, MD, 1985, 231.

66. **Lux, H. D.,** Observations in single calcium channels, in *Single Channel Recording,* Sakmann, B. and Neher, E., Eds., Plenum Press, New York, 1983, 437.

67. **Reuter, H., Stevens, C. F., Tsien, R. W., and Yellen, G.,** Properties of single calcium channels in cardiac cell culture, *Nature (London),* 297, 501, 1982.

68. **Hodgkin, A. L. and Horowicz, P.,** Potassium contractures in single muscle fibers, *J. Physiol. (London),* 153, 386, 1960.

69. **Harder, D. R.,** Comparison of electrical properties of middle cerebral and mesenteric artery in cat, *Am. J. Physiol.,* 239, (*Cell Physiol.,* 8), C23, 1980.

70. **Hermsmeyer, K.,** Electrogenesis of increased norepinephrine sensitivity of arterial vascular muscle in hypertension, *Circ. Res.,* 38, 362, 1976.

71. **Jones, A. W.,** Content and fluxes of electrolytes, in *Handbook of Physiology,* Section II, Vol. 2, Bohr, D. F., Somlyo, A. P., and Sparks, H. V., Jr., Eds., American Physiol. Society, Bethesda, MD, 1980, 253.

72. **Kreye, V. A. W., Bauer, P. K., and Vilhauer, I.,** Evidence for furosemide-sensitive active chloride transport in vascular smooth muscle, *Eur. J. Pharmacol.,* 73, 91, 1981.

73. **Kreye V. A. W. and Ziegler, F. W.,** Anions and vascular smooth muscle function, *Adv. Microcirc.,* 11, 144, 1982.

74. **Mekata, F. and Niu, H.,** Biophysical effects of adrenaline on the smooth muscle of the rabbit common carotid artery, *J. Gen. Physiol.,* 59, 92, 1972.

75. **Wahlstrom, B.A.,** A study on the action of noradrenaline on ionic content and sodium, potassium and chloride effluxes in the rat portal vein, *Acta Physiol. Scand.,* 89, 522, 1973.

76. **Droogmans, G., Raeymaekers, L., and Casteels, R.,** Electro- and pharmacomechanical coupling in the smooth muscle cells of the rabbit ear artery, *J. Gen. Physiol.,* 70, 129, 1977.

77. **Toda, N.,** Mechanical responses of isolated dog cerebral arteries to reduction of external K, Na, and Cl, *Am. J. Physiol.,* 234, H404, 1978.

78. **Betz, E. and Heuser, D.,** Actions and interactions of cations and anions on pial arteries, in *Advances in Neurology,* Vol. 20, Cervos-Navarro, J., Betz, E., Ebhardt, G., Ferzt, R., and Wullenweber, R., Eds., Raven Press, New York, 1978, 71.

79. **Hilton, S. M., Hudlicka, O., and Marshall, J. M.,** Possible mediators of functional hyperemia in skeletal muscle, *J. Physiol. (London),* 282, 131, 1978.

80. **Thomas, R. C.,** Electrogenic sodium pump in nerve and muscle cells, *Physiol. Rev.,* 52, 563, 1972.

81. **Fleming, W. W.,** The electrogenic Na^+, K^+-pump in smooth muscle: physiologic and pharmacologic significance, *Annu. Rev. Pharmacol. Toxicol.,* 20, 129, 1980.

82. **Mulvany, M. J.,** Change in sodium pump activity and vascular contraction, *J. Hypertension,* 3, 429, 1985.

83. **Hermsmeyer, K.,** Altered arterial muscle ion transport mechanism in the spontaneously hypertensive rat, *J. Cardiovasc. Pharmacol.,* 6, S10, 1984.

84. **Daniel, E. E.,** Role of altered vascular smooth muscle function in hypertension, in *Vasodilation,* Vanhoutte, P. M. and Leusen, I., Eds., Raven Press, New York, 1981, 381.

85. **Jones, A. W.,** Ionic dysfunction and hypertension, *Adv. Microcirc.,* 11, 134, 1982.

86. **Schwartz, A. and Collins, J. H.,** Na^+/K^+ ATPase. Structure of the enzyme and mechanism of action of digitalis, in *Membranes and Transport,* Vol. 1, Martonosi, A., Ed., Plenum Press, New York, 1982, 521.

87. **Heidlage, J. F. and Jones, A. W.,** The kinetics of ouabain-sensitive ionic transport in the rabbit carotid artery, *J. Physiol.,* 317, 243, 1981.

88. **Mullins, L. J. and Noda, K.,** The influence of sodium-free solutions on the membrane potential of frog muscle fibers, *J. Gen. Physiol.,* 47, 117, 1963.

89. **Sjodin, R. A. and Ortiz, O.,** Resolution of the potassium ion pump in muscle fibers using barium ions, *J. Gen. Physiol.,* 66, 269, 1975.

90. **Hermsmeyer, K.,** Membrane potential mechanisms in hypertension, in *New Trends in Arterial Hypertension,* Worcel, M., Bonvalet, J. P., Langer, S. Z., Menard, J., and Sassard, J., Eds., Elsevier/North Holland, Amsterdam, 1981, 175.

91. **Kuffler, S. W., Nicholls, J. G., and Martin, A. R.,** *From Neuron to Brain,* 2nd ed., Sinauer Associates, Sunderland, MA, 1984, 196.

92. **Taylor, G. S., Paton, D. M., and Daniel, E. E.,** Effect of rubidium and cesium on electrogenic sodium pumping in rat myometrium, *Comp. Biochem. Physiol.,* A38, 251, 1971.

93. **Overbeck, H. W., Pamnani, M. B., Akera, T., Brody, T. M., and Haddy, F. J.,** Depressed function of a ouabain-sensitive sodium-potassium pump in blood vessels from renal hypertensive dogs, *Circ. Res.,* 38 (Suppl. II), 48, 1976.

94. **Akera, T., Choi, Y. R., and Yamamoto, S.,** Potassium-induced changes in Na,K-ATPase: influences on the interaction between cardiac glycosides and enzymes, in *Na,K-ATPase Structure and Kinetics,* Skou, J. C. and Nordby, J. C., Eds., Academic Press, New York, 1979, 405.

95. **Haddy, F.J. and Pamnani, M.B.,** The vascular Na$^+$K$^+$ pump in low renin hypertension, *J. Cardiovasc. Pharmacol.,* 6, S61, 1984.

96. **Wong, S.W., Westfall, D.P., Menear, D., and Fleming, W.W.,** Sodium-potassium pump sites, as assessed by ^{3}H-ouabain binding in aorta and caudal artery of normotensive and spontaneously hypertensive rats, *Blood Vessels,* 21, 211, 1984.

97. **Khalil, F., Hopp, L., Searle, B.M., Tokushige, A., Tamura, H., Kino, M., and Aviv, A.,** [^{3}H] binding to cultured rat vascular smooth muscle cells, *Am. J. Physiol.,* 246 (*Cell Physiol.,* 15), C551, 1984.

98. **Deray, G., Pernollot, M.-G., Devynck, M.-A., Zingraff, J., Touam, A., Rosenfeld, J., and Meyer, P.,** Plasma digitalislike activity in essential hypertension or end-stage renal disease, *Hypertension,* 8, 632, 1986.

99. **Widdicombe, J. H.,** The ionic properties of the sodium pump in smooth muscle, in *Smooth Muscle,* Bulbring, E., Brading, A. F., Jones, A. W., and Tomita, T., Eds., University of Texas Press, Austin, 1981, 93.

100. **Stekiel, W. J., Contney, S. J., and Lombard, J. H.,** Small vessel membrane potential sympathetic input, and electrogenic pump rate in SHR, *Am. J. Physiol.,* 250 (*Cell Physiol.,* 19), C547, 1986.

101. **Chen, W. T., Brace, R. A., Scott, J. B., Anderson, D. K., and Haddy, F. J.,** The mechanism of the vasodilator action of potassium, *Proc. Soc. Exp. Biol. Med.,* 140, 820, 1972.

102. **Overbeck, H. W.,** Vascular responses to cations, osmolality and angiotensin in renal hypertensive dogs, *Am. J. Physiol.,* 223, 1358, 1972.

103. **Murphy, R. A., Gerthoffer, W. T., Trevethick, M. A., and Singer, H. A.,** Ca^{2+}-dependent regulatory mechanisms in smooth muscle, in *Vasodilator Mechanisms,* Vanhoutte, P. M. and Vatner, S. F., Eds. S. Karger, Basel, 1984, 99.

104. **Casteels, R. and Droogmans, G.,** Cell membrane responsiveness and excitation-contraction coupling in smooth muscle, *J. Cardiovasc. Pharmacol.,* 6, (Suppl. 2), S-304, 1984.

105. **van Breemen, C.,** Calcium requirement for activation of intact aortic smooth muscle, *J. Physiol.,* 272, 317, 1977.

106. **Hartshorne, D. J. and Gorecka, A.,** Biochemistry of the contractile proteins of smooth muscles, in *Handbook of Physiology,* Section II, Vol. 2, Bohr, D. F., Somlyo, A. P., and Sparks H. V., Jr., Eds., American Physiol. Society, Bethesda, MD, 1980, 93.

107. **Su, C., Bevan, J. A., and Ursillo, R. C.,** Electrical quiescence of pulmonary artery smooth muscle during sympathomimetic stimulation, *Circ. Res.,* 15, 20, 1964.

108. **Somlyo, A. V. and Somlyo, A. P.,** Electromechanical and pharmacomechanical coupling in vascular smooth muscle, *J. Pharmacol. Exp. Ther.,* 159, 129, 1968.

109. **Somlyo, A. P. and Somlyo, A. V.,** Vascular smooth muscle. I. Normal structure, pathology, biochemistry and biophysics, *Pharmacol. Rev.,* 20, 197, 1968.

110. **Somlyo, A. P. and Somlyo, A. V.,** Vascular smooth muscle. II. Pharmacology of normal and hypertensive vessels, *Pharmacol. Rev.,* 22, 249, 1970.

111. **Hermsmeyer, K.,** Calcium antagonist effects on vascular muscle membrane potentials and intracellular Ca^{2+}, in *Calcium in Biological Systems,* Rubin, R. P., Weiss, G. B., and Putney, J. W., Jr., Eds., Plenum Press, New York, 1985, 423.

112. **Bohr, D. F.,** Vascular smooth muscle updated, *Circ. Res.,* 32, 665, 193, 1973.

113. **Bohr, D. F.,** Vascular smooth muscle, in *Peripheral Circulation,* Johnson, P. C., Ed., John Wiley & Sons, New York, 1978, 13.

114. **Cauvin, C., Lukeman, S., Cameron, J., Hwang, O., Meisheri, K., Yamamoto, H., and van Breemen, C.,** Theoretical basis for vascular selectivity of Ca^{2+} antagonists, *J. Cardiovasc. Surg.,* 6, S638, 1984.

115. **Casteels, R., Kitamura, K., Kuriyama, H., and Suzuki, H.,** Excitation-contraction coupling in the smooth muscle cells of the rabbit main pulmonary artery, *J. Physiol.,* 271, 63, 1977.

116. **Kitamura, K. and Kuriyama, H.,** Effects of acetylcholine on the smooth muscle cell of isolated main coronary artery of the guinea-pig, *J. Physiol.,* 293, 119, 1979.

117. **Mulvany, M. J. and Halpern, W.,** Contractile properties of small arterial resistance vessels in spontaneously hypertensive and normotensive rats, *Circ. Res.,* 41, 19, 1977.

118. **Mulvany, M. J., Nilsson, H., and Flatman, J. A.,** Role of membrane potential in the response of rat small mesenteric arteries to exogenous noradrenaline stimulation, *J. Physiol.,* 332, 363, 1982.

119. **Bolton, T. B., Lang, R. J., Takewaki, T., and Clapp, L. H.,** Autonomic receptors and cell membrane potential, in *Vasodilator Mechanisms,* Vanhoutte, P. M. and Vatner, S. F., Eds., S. Karger, Basel, 1984, 109.

120. **Casteels, R., Kitamura, K., Kuriyama, H., and Suzuki, H.,** The membrane properties of the smooth muscle cells of the rabbit main pulmonary artery, *J. Physiol.,* 271, 41, 1977.

121. **Jones, A. W. and Miller, L. A.,** Ion transport in tonic and phasic vascular smooth muscle and changes during desoxycorticosterone hypertension, *Blood Vessels,* 15, 83, 1978.

122. **Haeusler, G.,** Contraction of vascular muscle as related to membrane potential and calcium fluxes, *J. Cardiovasc. Pharmacol.,* 7 (Suppl. 6), S3, 1985.

123. **Haeusler, G.,** Relationship between noradrenaline-induced depolarization and contraction in vascular smooth muscle, *Blood Vessels,* 15, 46, 1978.

124. **Haeusler, G.,** α-Adrenoceptor mediated contractile and electrical responses of vascular smooth muscles, *J. Cardiovasc. Pharmacol.,* 4, S97, 1982.

125. **van Breemen, C., Aaronson, P., and Loutzenhizer, R.,** Sodium-calcium interactions in mammalian smooth muscle, *Pharmacol. Rev.,* 30, 167, 1979.

126. **Cauvin, C., Loutzenhizer, R., and van Breemen, C.,** Mechanisms of calcium antagonist-induced vasodilation, *Annu. Rev. Pharmacol. Toxicol.,* 23, 373, 1983.

127. **Cauvin, C. and van Breemen, C.,** Different Ca^{2+} channels along the arterial tree, *J. Cardiovasc. Pharmacol.,* 7, S4, 1985.

128. **Meech, R. W.,** The sensitivity of Helix aspersa neurones to injected calcium ions, *J. Physiol.,* 237, 259, 1974.

129. **Bassingthwaighte, J. B., Fry, C. H., and McGuigan, J. A. S.,** Relationship between internal calcium and outward current in mammalian ventricular muscle: a mechanism for the control of the action potential duration?, *J. Physiol.,* 262, 15, 1976.

130. **Walsh, J. V. and Singer, J. J.,** Penetration-induced hyperpolarization as evidence for Ca^{2+} activation of K^+ conductance in isolated smooth muscle cells, *Am. J. Physiol.,* 239, (*Cell Physiol.,* 8), C182, 1980.

131. **Somlyo, A. V., Vinall, P., and Somlyo, A. P.,** Excitation-contraction coupling and electrical events in two types of vascular smooth muscle. *Microvasc. Res.,* 1, 354, 1969.

132. **Kuriyama, H. and Suzuki, H.,** The effects of acetylcholine on the membrane and contractile properties of smooth muscle cells of the rabbit superior mesenteric artery, *Br. J. Pharmacol.,* 64, 493, 1978.

133. **Keatinge, W. R.,** Electrical and mechanical response of arteries to stimulation of sympathetic nerves, *J. Physiol.,* 185, 701, 1966.

134. **Su, C. and Bevan, J. A.,** The electrical response of pulmonary artery muscle to acetylcholine, histamine and serotonin, *Life Sci.,* 4, 1025, 1965.

135. **Vanhoutte, P. M. and Miller, V. M.,** Heterogeneity of endothelium-dependent responses in mammalian blood vessels, *J. Cardiovasc. Pharmacol.,* 7 (Suppl. 3), S12, 1985.

136. **Furchgott, R. F., Jothianadan, D., and Cherry, P. O.,** Endothelium-dependent responses. The last three years, in *Vasodilator Mechanisms,* Vanhoutte, P. M. and Vatner, S. F., Eds., S. Karger, New York, 1984.

137. **Meisheri, K. D., Hwang, O., van Breemen, C.,** Evidence for two separate Ca^{2+} pathways in smooth muscle plasmalemma, *J. Membr. Biol.,* 59, 19, 1981.

138. **Tobian, L. and Binion, J. T.,** Tissue cations and water in arterial hypertension, *Circulation,* 5, 754, 1952.

139. **Jones, A. W.,** Reactivity of ion fluxes in rat aorta during hypertension and circulatory control, *Fed. Proc.,* 33, 133, 1974.

140. **Jones, A. W.,** Vascular smooth muscle and alterations during hypertension, in *Smooth Muscle,* Bülbring, E., Brading, A. F., Jones, A. W., and Tomita, T., Eds., University of Texas Press, Austin, 1981, chap. 19.

141. **Tobian, L.,** Interrelationships of electrolytes, juxtaglomerular cells and hypertension, *Physiol. Rev.,* 40, 280, 1960.

142. **Folkow, B.,** The Fourth Volhard Lecture. Cardiovascular structural adaptation: its role in the initiation and maintenance of primary hypertension, *Clin. Sci. Mol. Med.,* 55, 3s, 1978.

143. **Yamori, Y., Nakada, T., and Lovenberg, W.,** Effect of antihypertensive therapy on lysine incorporation into vascular protein of the spontaneously hypertensive rat, *Eur. J. Pharmacol.,* 38, 349, 1976.

144. **Lee, R. M. K. W.,** Vascular changes at the prehypertensive phase in the mesenteric arteries from spontaneously hypertensive rats, *Blood Vessels,* 22, 105, 1986.

145. **Lee, R. M. K. W., Triggle, C. R., Cheung, D. W. T., and Coughlin, M. D.,** Structural and functional consequences of neonatal sympathectomy in blood vessels of spontaneously hypertensive rats, *Hypertension,* 10, 328, 1987.

146. **Lee, R. M. K. W., Garfield, R. E., Forrest, J. B., and Daniel, E. E.,** Morphometric study of structural changes in the mesenteric blood vessels of spontaneously hypertensive rats, *Blood Vessels,* 20, 57, 1983.

147. **Mulvany, M. J., Hansen, P. K., and Aalkjaer, C.,** Direct evidence that the greater contractility of resistance vessels in spontaneously hypertensive rats is associated with a narrower lumen, a thicker media and a greater number of smooth muscle cell layers, *Circ. Res.,* 43, 854, 1978.

148. **Mulvany, M. J.,** Role of vascular structure in blood pressure development of the spontaneously hypertensive rat, *J. Hypertension,* 4 (Suppl. 3), S61, 1986.

149. **Lee, R. M. K. W., Forrest, J. B., Garfield, R. E., and Daniel, E. E.,** Ultrastructural changes in mesenteric arteries from spontaneously hypertensive rats, *Blood Vessels,* 20, 72, 1983.

150. **Warshaw, D. M., Mulvany, M. J., and Halpern, W.,** Mechanical and morphological properties of arterial resistance vessels in young and old spontaneously hypertensive rats., *Circ. Res.,* 45, 250, 1979.

151. **Brayden, J. E., Halpern, W., and Brann, L. R.,** Biochemical and mechanical properties of resistance arteries from normotensive and hypertensive rats, *Hypertension,* 5, 17, 1983.

152. **Folkow, B.,** The structural cardiovascular factor in primary hypertension — pressure dependence and genetic reinforcement, *J. Hypertension,* 4 (Suppl. 3), S51, 1986.

153. **Webb, R. C.,** Vascular changes in hypertension, in *Cardiovascular Pharmacology,* 2nd ed., Antonaccio, M., Ed., Raven Press, New York, 1984, 215.

154. **Bohr, D. F. and Webb, R. C.,** Vascular smooth muscle function and its changes in hypertension, *Am. J. Med.,* 77(4A), 3, 1984.

155. **Webb, R. C. and Vanhoutte, P. M.,** Sensitivity to noradrenaline in isolated tail arteries from spontaneously hypertensive rats, *Clin. Sci.,* 57, 31s, 1979.

156. **Triggle, C. R. and Laher, I.,** A review of changes in vascular smooth muscle functions in hypertension: isolated tissue versus *in vivo* studies, *Can. J. Physiol.,* 63, 355, 1985.

157. **Fouda, A. -K., Marazzi, A., Boillat, N., Sonnay, M., Guillan, H., and Atkinson, J.,** Changes in the vascular reactivity of the isolated tail arteries of spontaneous and renovascular hypertensive rats to endogenous and exogenous noradrenaline, *Blood Vessels,* 24, 63, 1987.

158. **Mulvany, M. J., Nilsson, H., Nyborg, N., and Mikkelsen, E.,** Are isolated femoral resistance vessels or tail arteries good models for the hindquarter vasculature of spontaneously hypertensive rats?, *Acta Physiol. Scand.,* 116, 275, 1982.

159. **Whall, C. W., Myers, M. M., and Halpern, W.,** Norepinepherine sensitivity, tension development and neuronal uptake in resistance arteries from spontaneously hypertensive and normotensive rats, *Blood Vessels,* 17, 1, 1980.

160. **Mulvany, M. J., Aalkjaer, C., and Christensen, J.,** Changes in noradrenaline sensitivity and morphology of arterial resistance vessels during development of high blood pressure in spontaneously hypertensive rats, *Hypertension,* 2, 664, 1980.

161. **Coskinas, E. and Price, J. M.,** Length-dependent sensitivity of vascular smooth muscle in normotensive and hypertensive animals, *Am. J. Physiol.,* 253 (*Heart Circ. Physiol.,* 22), H402, 1987.

162. **Bevan, J. A. and Nyborg, N.,** Increased sensitivity of mesenteric resistance arteries of spontaneously hypertensive rats to norepinepherine is associated with increased α_1-adrenoreceptor affinity, *Hypertension,* 10(3)(Abstr.), 361, 1987.

163. **Mulvany, M. J. and Nyborg, N.,** An increased calcium sensitivity of mesenteric resistance vessels in young and adult spontaneously hypertensive rats, *Br. J. Pharmacol.,* 71, 585, 1980.

164. **Mulvany, M. J., Korsgaard, N., and Nyborg, N.,** Evidence that the increased calcium sensitivity of resistance vessels in spontaneously hypertensive rats is an intrinsic defect of their vascular smooth muscle, *Clin. Exp. Hypertension,* 3, 749, 1981.

165. **Nilsson, H. and Mulvany, M. J.,** Prolonged exposure to ouabain eliminates the greater noradrenaline-dependent calcium sensitivity of resistance vessels in spontaneously hypertensive rats, *Hypertension,* 3, 691, 1981.

166. **Pegram, B. L. and Ljung, B.,** Neuroeffector function of isolated portal vein from spontaneously hypertensive and Wistar-Kyoto rats: dependence on external calcium concentration, *Blood Vessels,* 18, 89, 1981.

167. **Mulvany, M. J.,** Resistance vessel abnormalities in spontaneously hypertensive rats, *J. Cardiovasc. Pharmacol.,* 6, S656, 1984.

168. **Aoki, K. and Asano, M.,** Effects of dihydropyridine calcium agonist and antagonist on femoral arteries isolated from spontaneously hypertensive rats, *J. Hypertension,* 4 (Suppl. 5), S138, 1986.

169. **MacKay, M. J. and Cheung, D. W.,** Increased reactivity in the mesenteric artery of spontaneously hypertensive rats to phorbol esters, *Biochem. Biophys. Res. Commun.,* 145, 1105, 1987.

170. **Gleason, M. M. and Flaim, S. F.,** Phorbol ester contracts rabbit thoracic aorta by increasing intracellular calcium and by activating calcium influx, *Biochem. Biophys. Res. Commun.,* 138, 1362, 1986.

171. **Aoki, K., Yamashita, K., Tomita, N., Tazumi, K., and Hotta, K.,** ATPase activity and Ca^{2+} binding activity of subcellular membrane of arterial smooth muscle in spontaneously hypertensive rat, *Jpn. Heart J.,* 15, 180, 1974.

172. **Webb, R. C. and Bhalla, R.,** Altered calcium sequestration by subcellular fractions of vascular smooth muscle from spontaneously hypertensive rats, *J. Mol. Cell. Cardiol.,* 8, 651, 1976.

173. **Kwan, C. -Y., Belbeck, L., and Daniel, E. E.,** Abnormal biochemistry of vascular smooth muscle plasma membrane as an important factor in the initiation and maintenance of hypertension in rats, *Blood Vessels,* 16, 259, 1979.

174. **Kwan, C. -Y., Belbeck, L., and Daniel, E. E.,** Abnormal biochemistry of vascular smooth muscle plasma membrane isolated from hypertensive rats, *Mol. Pharmacol.,* 17, 137, 1980.

175. **Kwan, C. -Y. and Daniel, E. E.,** Calcium transport by plasma membrane vesicles isolated from vascular smooth muscle of normal and hypertensive rats, in *Vasodilation,* Vanhoutte, P. M. and Leusen, I., Eds., Raven Press, New York, 1981, 405.

176. **Furchgott, R. F. and Zawadzki, J. V.,** The obligatory role of endothelial cells in the relaxation of arterial smooth muscle by acetylcholine, *Nature (London),* 288, 373, 1980.

177. **Furchgott, R.,** Role of endothelium in responses of vascular smooth muscle, *Circ. Res.,* 53, 557, 1983.
178. **Peach, M. J., Loeb, A. L., Singer, H. A., and Saye, J.,** Endothelium-derived vascular relaxing factor, *Hypertension,* 7 (Suppl. I), 94, 1985.
179. **Rapoport, R. M. and Murad, F.,** Endothelium-dependent and nitrovasodilator-induced relaxation of vascular smooth muscle: role of cyclic GMP, *J. Cyclic Nucleotide Protein Phosphor. Res.,* 9, 281, 1983.
180. **Vanhoutte, P. M., Rubanyi, G., Miller, V. M., and Houston, D. S.,** Modulation of vascular smooth muscle contraction by the endothelium, *Annu. Rev. Physiol.,* 48, 307, 1986.
181. **Fridovitch, I., Hagen, P. -O., and Murray, J. J.,** Endothelium derived relaxing factor: in search of the endogenous nitroglycerin, *News Physiol. Sci.,* 2, 61, 1987.
182. **De Mey, J. G. and Gray, S. D.,** Endothelium-dependent reactivity in resistance vessels, *Prog. Appl. Microcirc.,* 8, 181, 1985.
183. **Owen, M. P. and Bevan, J. A.,** Acetylcholine induced endothelial-dependent vasodilation increases as artery diameter decreases in the rabbit ear, *Experientia,* 41, 1057, 1985.
184. **Cocks, T. M. and Angus, J. A.,** Endothelium-dependent relaxation of coronary arteries by noradrenaline and serotonin, *Nature (London),* 305, 627, 1983.
185. **Hickey, K. A., Rubanyi, G. M., Paul, R. J., and Highsmith, R. F.,** Characterization of a coronary vasoconstrictor produced by cultured endothelial cells, *Am. J. Physiol.,* 248, C550, 1985.
186. **Vanhoutte, P. M.,** Endothelium and control of vascular tissue, *News Physiol. Sci.,* 2, 18, 1987.
187. **Katusic, Z., Shepherd, J. T., and Vanhoutte, P. M.,** Endothelium-dependent contraction to stretch in canine basilar arteries, *Am. J. Physiol.,* 252 (*Heart Circ. Physiol.,* 21), H671, 1987.
188. **Harder, D. R.,** Pressure-induced myogenic activation of cat cerebral arteries is dependent on intact endothelium, *Circ. Res.,* 60, 102, 1987.
189. **Lüscher, T. F. and Vanhoutte, P. M.,** Endothelium-dependent contractions to acetylcholine in the aorta of the spontaneously hypertensive rat, *Hypertension,* 8, 344, 1986.
190. **Cauvin, C. and Pegram, B.,** Decreased relaxation of isolated mesenteric resistance vessels from two-kidney, one-clip Goldblatt hypertensive rats, *Clin. Exp. Hypertension,* A5, 383, 1983.
191. **Konishi, M. and Su, C.,** Role of endothelium in dilator responses of spontaneously hypertensive rat arteries, *Hypertension,* 5, 881, 1983.
192. **Winquist, R. J., Bunting, P. B., Baskin, E. P., and Wallace, A. A.,** Decreased endothelium-dependent relaxation in New Zealand genetic hypertensive rats, *J. Hypertension,* 2, 541, 1984.
193. **Lockette, W., Otsuka, Y., and Carretero, O.,** The loss of endothelium-dependent vascular relaxation in hypertension, *Hypertension,* 8 (Suppl. II), 61, 1986.
194. **Van de Voorde, J. and Leusen, I.,** Endothelium-dependent and independent relaxation of aortic rings from hypertensive rats, *Am. J. Physiol.,* 250 (*Heart Circ. Physiol.,* 19), H711, 1986.
195. **Lüscher, T. F., Rau, L., and Vanhoutte, P. M.,** Endothelium-dependent vascular responses in normotensive and hypertensive Dahl rats, *Hypertension,* 9, 157, 1987.
196. **Carvalho, M. H. C., Scivoletto, R., Fortes, Z. B., Nigro, D., and Cordellini, S.,** Reactivity of aorta and mesenteric microvessels to drugs in spontaneously hypertensive rats: role of the endothelium, *J. Hypertension,* 5, 377, 1987.
197. **Lüscher, T. F., Vanhoutte, P. M., and Rau, L.,** Antihypertensive treatment normalizes decreased endothelium-dependent relaxations in rats with salt-induced hypertension, *Hypertension,* 9 (Suppl. III), 193, 1987.
198. **Winquist, R. J.,** Altered vasodilator and endothelium-dependent responses in hypertension, *Drug Dev. Res.,* 7, 311, 1986.
199. **De Chastonay, C., Gabbiani, G., Elemer, G.M., and Huttner, I.,** Remodeling of the rat aortic endothelial layer during experimental hypertension, *Lab. Invest.,* 48, 45, 1983.
200. **Contney, S. J., Stekiel, W. J., Roman, R. J., Greene, A. S., and Lombard, J. H.,** Neural contribution to vascular smooth muscle membrane potentials of small arteries and veins in SHR, Dahl S and DOCA salt hypertensive rats, *Fed. Proc.,* 46 (Abstr.), 523, 1987.
201. **Thorén, P. and Ricksten, S. E.,** Recordings of renal and splanchnic sympathetic nervous activity in normotensive and spontaneously hypertensive rats, *Clin. Sci.,* 57, 1972, 1979.
202. **Nilsson, H. and Folkow, B.,** Range of transmitter release modulation in small arteries of spontaneously hypertensive and normotensive rats, *Prog. Appl. Microcirc.,* 8, 188, 1982.
203. **Lee, T. J. and Saito, A.,** Altered cerebral vessel innervation in the spontaneously hypertensive rat, *Circ. Res.,* 55, 392, 1984.
204. **Burnstock, G., Folkow, B., Karlström, G., Nilsson, H., and Sjöblom, N.,** How do changes in diameter at the precapillary level affect cardiovascular function?, *J. Cardiovasc. Pharmacol.,* 6, 280, 1984.
205. **Head, R. J., Cassis, L. A., Robinson, R. L., Westfall, D. P., and Stitzel, R. T.,** Altered catecholamine contents in vascular and nonvascular tissues in genetically hypertensive rats, *Blood Vessels,* 22, 196, 1985.
206. **Touda, K., Kuchii, M., Kusuyama, Y., Hano, T., Nishio, I., and Masuyama, Y.,** Neurotransmitter release and vascular reactivity in spontaneously hypertensive rats, *Jpn. Circ. J.,* 48, 1263, 1984.

207. **Cassis, L. A., Stitzel, A. E., and Head, R. J.,** Hypernoradrenergic innervation of the caudal artery of the spontaneously hypertensive rat: an influence upon neuroeffector mechanisms, *J. Pharmacol. Exp. Ther.,* 234, 792, 1985.

208. **Galloway, M. P. and Westfall, T. C.,** The release of endogenous norepinephrine from the coccygeal artery of spontaneously hypertensive and Wistar-Kyoto rats, *Circ. Res.,* 51, 225, 1982.

209. **Nagatsu, T., Ikuta, K., Numata, Y., Kato, T., Sano, M., Nagatsu, I., Umezawa, H., Matsuzaki, M., and Takeuchi, Z.,** Vascular and brain dopamine B-hydroxylase activity in young spontaneously hypertensive rats, *Science,* 191, 290, 1976.

210. **Shimamura, K., Shimada, T., Yamamoto, K., Sunano, S., and Okamoto, K.,** Noradrenaline content and release in the mesenteric artery of stroke-prone spontaneously hypertensive rats (SHRSP) and a new strain of SHRSP (M-SHRSP), *Blood Vessels,* 24, 334, 1987.

211. **De Champlain, J., Farley, L., Cousineau, D., and Van Amerigen, M. R.,** Circulating catecholamine levels in human and experimental hypertension, *Circ. Res.,* 38, 109, 1976.

212. **Crabb, G. A., Head, R. J., Hempstead, J., and Berkowitz, B. A.,** Altered disposition of vascular catecholamines in hypertensive (DOCA-salt) rats, *Clin. Exp. Hypertension,* 2, 129, 1980.

213. **Harder, D. R., Smeda, J., and Lombard, J.,** Enhanced myogenic depolarization in hypertensive cerebral arterial muscle, *Circ. Res.,* 57, 319, 1985.

214. **Vlachakis, N. D., Frederics, R., Velasquez, M., Alexander, N., Singer, F., and Maronde, R. F.,** Sympathetic system function and vascular reactivity in hypercalcemic patients, *Hypertension,* 4, 452, 1982.

215. **Holloway, E. T., Sitrin, M .D., and Bohr, D. F.,** Calcium dependence of vascular smooth muscle from normotensive and hypertensive rats, in *Hypertension, 1972,* Genest, J. and Kouiw, E., Eds., Springer-Verlag, Berlin, 1972.

216. **Aqel, M. B., Sharma, R. V., and Bhalla, R. C.,** Increased ^{45}Ca influx in response to α_1-adrenoceptor stimulation in spontaneously hypertensive rat caudal artery, *J. Cardiovasc. Pharmacol.,* 10, 205, 1987.

217. **Fitzpatrick, D. F. and Szentivanyi, A.,** The relationship between increased myogenic tone and hyporesponsiveness in vascular smooth muscle of spontaneously hypertensive rats, *Clin. Exp. Hypertension,* 2, 1023, 1980.

218. **Noon, J. P., Rice, P. J., and Baldessarini, P. J.,** Calcium leakage as a cause of the high resting tension in vascular smooth muscle from the spontaneously hypertensive rat, *Proc. Natl. Acad. Sci. U. S. A.,* 75, 1605, 1978.

219. **Kulberg, R.,** Stretch-activated ion channels in bacteria and animal cell membranes, *Trend. Neurosci.,* 10, 387, 1987.

220. **Lansman, J. B., Hallam, T. J., and Rink, T. J.,** Single stretch-activated ion channels in vascular endothelial cells as mechanotransducers?, *Nature (London),* 325, 811, 1987.

221. **Pohl, U., Holtz, J., Busse, R., and Bassenge, E.,** Crucial role of endothelium in the vasodilator response to increased flow *in vivo, Hypertension,* 8, 37, 1986.

222. **Kaiser, L. and Sparks, H. V.,** Mediation of flow-dependent arterial dilation by endothelial cells, *Circ. Shock,* 18, 109, 1986.

223. **Friedman, S. M.,** Sodium ions and regulation of vascular tone, *Adv. Microcirc.,* 11, 20, 1982.

224. **Friedman, S. M.,** Cellular ionic perturbations in hypertension, *J. Hypertension,* 1, 109, 1983.

225. **Hermsmeyer, K.,** Cellular basis for increased sensitivity of vascular smooth muscle in spontaneously hypertensive rats, *Circ. Res.,* 38 (Suppl. II), 53, 1976.

226. **Cheung, D. W.,** Membrane potential of vascular smooth muscle and hypertension in spontaneously hypertensive rats, *Can. J. Physiol. Pharmacol.,* 62, 957, 1984.

227. **Campbell, G. R., Chamley-Campbell, J., Short, N., Robinson, R., and Hermsmeyer, K.,** Effect of cross-transplantation in normotensive and spontaneously hypertensive rat arterial muscle membrane, *Hypertension,* 3, 534, 1981.

228. **Abel, P. W. and Hermsmeyer, K.,** Sympathetic cross-innervation of SHR and genetic controls suggests a trophic influence on vascular muscle membranes, *Circ. Res.,* 49, 1311, 1981.

229. **Pamnani, M. B., Clough, D. L., Huot, S. J., and Haddy, F. J.,** Na+-K+ pump activity in tail arteries of spontaneously hypertensive rats, *Jpn. Heart J.,* 20 (Suppl. 1), 228, 1979.

230. **Haddy, F. J.,** Abnormalities of membrane transport in hypertension, *Hypertension,* 5 (Suppl. V), 66, 1983.

231. **Haddy, F. J.,** The role of a humoral Na+, K+-ATPase inhibitor in regulating precapillary vessel tone, *J. Cardiovasc. Pharmacol.,* 6, S 439, 1984.

232. **De Wardener, H. E. and Clarkson, E. M.,** Concept of natriuretic hormone, *Physiol. Rev.,* 65, 658, 1985.

233. **Pamnani, M. B., Clough, D. L., Huot, S. J., and Haddy, F. J.,** Sodium-potassium pump activity in experimental hypertension, in *Vasodilation,* Vanhoutte, P. M. and Leusen, I., Eds., Raven Press, New York, 1981, 391.

234. **Pamnani, M. B., Clough, D. L., and Haddy, F. J.,** Altered activity of the sodium-potassium pump in arteries of rats with steroid hypertension, *Clin. Sci. Mol. Med.,* 55, 41s, 1978.

235. **Overbeck, H. W., Ku, D. D., and Rapp, J. P.,** Sodium pump activity in arteries of Dahl salt sensitive rats, *Hypertension,* 3, 306, 1981.

236. **Overbeck, H. W. and Grisette, D. E.,** Sodium pump activity in arteries of rats with Goldblatt hypertension, *Hypertension,* 4, 132, 1982.

237. **Overbeck, H. W.,** Effect of ouabain in arteriolar responses to norepinephrine in chronic, benign, volume-expanded hypertension, *Hypertension,* 6 (Suppl. I), 82, 1984.

238. **Haddy, F. J. and Overbeck, H. W.,** The role of humoral agents in volume-expanded hypertension, *Life Sci.,* 19, 935, 1976.

239. **Haddy, F. J.,** Local control of vascular resistance as related to hypertension, *Arch. Intern. Med.,* 133, 916, 1974.

240. **Pamnani, M. B., Harder, D. R., Huot, S. J., Bryant, H. J., Kutyna, F. A., and Haddy, F. J.,** Vascular smooth muscle membrane potential and a ouabain-like humoral factor in one-kidney, one-clip hypertension in rats, *Clin. Sci.,* 63, 31s, 1982.

241. **Pamnani, M. B., Bryant, H. J., Harder, D. R., and Haddy, F. J.,** Vascular smooth muscle membrane potentials in rats with one-kidney, one-clip and reduced renal mass saline hypertension: the influence of humoral pump inhibitor, *J. Hypertension,* 3 (Suppl. 3), S29, 1985.

242. **Shoemaker, R. L. and Overbeck, H. W.,** Vascular smooth muscle membrane potential in rats with early and chronic one-kidney, one-clip hypertension (42288), *Proc. Soc. Exp. Biol. Med.,* 181, 529, 1986.

243. **Magargal, W. W. and Overbeck, H. W.,** Effect of hypertensive rat plasma on ion transport of cultured vascular smooth muscle, *Am. J. Physiol.,* 251 (*Heart Circ. Physiol.,* 20), H984, 1986.

244. **Stekiel, W. J.,** unpublished observations.

245. **Rusch, N.,** personal communication.

INDEX

A

B

C

in DOCA-salt hypertension, 81
functional, 76, 99
functional implications of, 84—85
future trends and, 85—86
in humans, 77—78
mechanisms leading to, 82—84
microcirculation and, 93—94
in pulmonary hypertension, 81—82
in renovascular hypertension, 80—81
in SHR, 78—80
structural, 76
transcapillary exchange and, 85
Receptor-operated calcium channels (ROC), 141,
142
Red blood cells, see Erythrocytes
Relaxation, 103
Relaxation factors, 51—52, 58—60, see also specific
types
Renal disease, 137, see also specific types
Renal function, 97, 100
Renal hypertension, 93, 99, 100, 102, 143, 156
Renal hypertensive rat (RHR), 5, 6, 9
Renin, 96
Renovascular hypertension, 80—81
RHR, see Renal hypertensive rat
ROC, see Receptor-operated calcium channels
Rubidium, 136, 155

S

Sarcoplasmic reticulum, 140
Sausage (bead-string) phenomenon, 27
Scavengers of free radicals, 27, 57, see also specific
types
Serotonin, 45, 137
Shear stress, 153
SHR, see Spontaneously hypertensive rat
SHRSP, see Spontaneously hypertensive stroke-
prone rat
Skeletal muscle, 92, 95, 98
Slow depolarization, 114, 116, 118—120
Small arterioles, 72—76
Smooth muscle
depolarization of, 101
endothelium interactions with, 44
inhibitory actions of endothelium on growth of,
50—51
membrane properties of, 104
protection of from vasoactive agents, 44—45
transmembrane potential of, 98
vascular, see Vascular smooth muscle
Smooth muscle growth modulators, 50—51, see also
specific types
Sodium, 96, 104, 114, 131
Sodium channels, 133
Sodium-potassium electrogenic membrane pump,
134
Sodium-potassium exchange coupling ratio, 135
Sodium-potassium exchange pump, 131, 134
Sodium-potassium pump inhibitor, 137, 156
SP, see Substance P

Spinotrapezius muscle, 92, 95
Spontaneously hypertensive rate, 129, 130
Spontaneously hypertensive rat (SHR), 5, 97, 151
arteriole constriction in, 92
blood-brain barrier and, 30
catecholamine fluorescence in, 5—6
chronic hypertension in, 22
innervation in, 113
neuromuscular transmission in, 118—120
norepinephrine in, 7—9
presynamptic mechanisms in, 113, 114
rarefaction of microvessels in, 78—80
sympathetic innervation in, 150
synaptic cleft distance in, 9
Spontaneously hypertensive stroke-prone rat
(SHRSP), 22, 25, 30, 151
Steady state, 131
Stress, 153, see also specific types
Stretch-activated ion channels, 153
Stroke, 20, 22
Structural rarefaction of microvessels, 76
Substance P (SP), 13, 47, 54, 147
Superoxide anion radicals, 28
Superoxide dismutase, 27, 57
Sympathectomy, 112, 145
Sympathetic innervation, 150
Sympathetic nerves, 13, see also specific types
activities of, 13, 92, 96, 100
in acute hypertension, 31
in cerebral blood flow, 30—32
in chronic hypertension, 31
origins of, 9—13
peripheral, 112
trophic effects of, 97
Sympathetic tone, 94
Synaptic cleft distance, 9

T

Tachykinins, 54, see also specific types
TEA, see Tetraethylammonium
Tension, 128
Tetraethylammonium (TEA), 36, 133
Tetrodotoxin, 97—99, 103
Thrombin, 54, 147
Thromboxane, 48
Thromboxane A (TXA), 59
Tissue blood flow, 99
Tissue metabolism, 99
Tissue perfusion, 94, 97, 104, 105
TNS, see Transmural nerve stimulation
Total peripheral resistance (TPR), 128—131
TPR, see Total peripheral resistance
Transcapillary exchange, 85
Transmembrane potential, 128, 131—142
diffusion potential and, 131—134
electromechanical coupling and, 137—142
pharmacomechanical coupling and, 137—142
Transmural nerve stimulation (TNS), 5, 13
Transmural pressure, 101, 104
Transplantations, 155, see also specific types

Printed and bound by CPI Group (UK) Ltd, Croydon, CR0 4YY

17/10/2024

01775700-0020